Nutrition for the Culinary Arts

Nutrition for the Culinary Arts

Nancy Berkoff
RD, EdD, CCE, AAC

PEARSON
Prentice Hall
Upper Saddle River, New Jersey 07458

Library of Congress Cataloging-in-Publication Data
Berkoff, Nancy.
Nutrition for the culinary arts / Nancy Berkoff.—1st ed.
p. cm.
Includes index.
ISBN 0-13-094628-1
1. Nutrition. 2. Cookery. 3. Table setting and decoration. I. Title.
RA776.B496 2004
613.2—dc22
2003020977

Editor-in-Chief: Stephen Helba
Executive Editor: Vernon R. Anthony
Executive Assistant: Nancy Kesterson
Editorial Assistant: Beth Dyke
Director of Manufacturing and Production: Bruce Johnson
Managing Editor: Mary Carnis
Production Liaison: Adele M. Kupchik
Manufacturing Manager: Ilene Sanford
Manufacturing Buyer: Cathleen Petersen
Interior Design & Formatting: Pine Tree Composition, Inc.
Production Editor: John Shannon, Pine Tree Composition, Inc.
Cover Designer: Miguel Ortiz
Cover Image: Leigh Beisch, Food Pix/Getty Images
Senior Marketing Manager: Ryan DeGrote
Marketing Assistant: Elizabeth Farrell
Senior Marketing Coordinator: Adam Kloza
Printer/Binder: Phoenix Book Tech
Cover Printer: Phoenix Book Tech

Pearson Education, Ltd., London
Pearson Education Australia Pty. Limited, Sydney
Pearson Education Singapore, Pte. Ltd.
Pearson Education North Asia Ltd., Hong Kong
Pearson Education Canada, Ltd., Toronto
Pearson Educaçion de Mexico, S.A. de C.V.
Pearson Education—Japan, Tokyo
Pearson Education Malaysia, Pte. Ltd.

10 9 8 7 6 5 4 3 2 1
ISBN 0-13-094628-1

This book is dedicated to Bob, a man of ethics, science, passion, adventure and patience—a gourmand, not only of cuisine, but of life and to Ezra, who knew that food was the way to go!

Contents

Preface

Culinary Nutrition

Occam's Razor: If many explanations are possible, choose the simplest
Leonardo Di Vinci: Simplicity is the ultimate sophistication
Brooklyn Cab Driver: KISS (keep it simple, stupid)

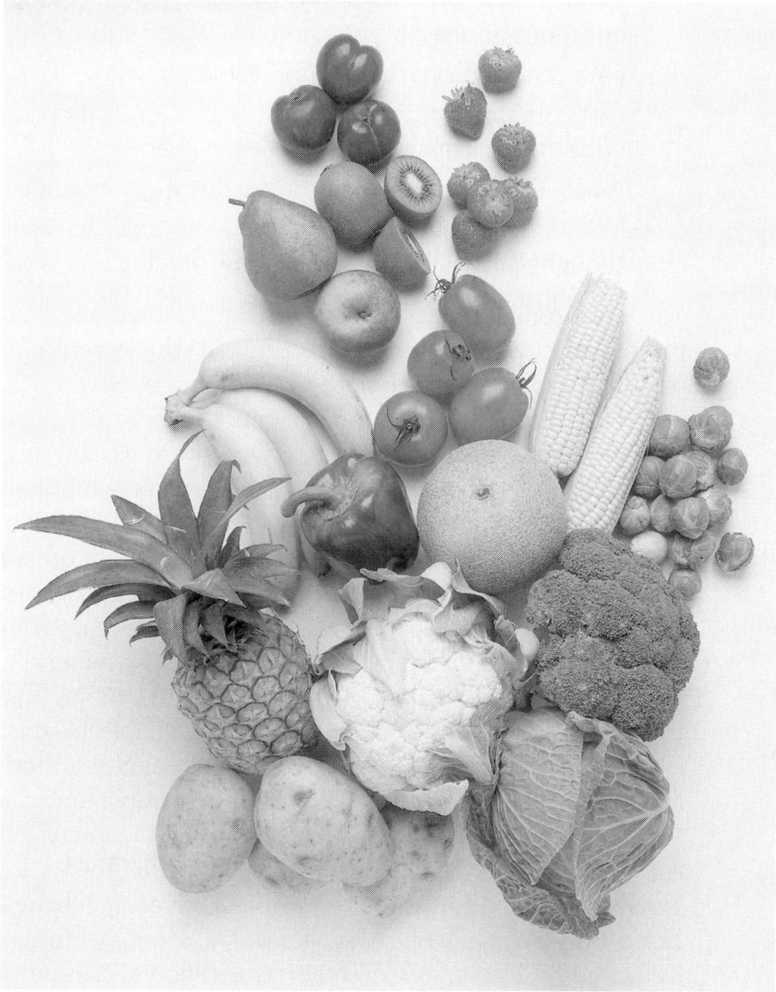

Why do hospitality, food service management, and culinary students need to study nutrition? The answer is simple. People need to eat. People like to eat. People would like to eat foods that taste good and that are good for them (or at least, not bad for them).

Another part of this simple explanation is that nutrition sells. You will have a difficult time finding a menu that does not have a bit of "nutrition" on it. Steak houses are adding grilled fish items, seafood restaurants are adding vegetarian entrees and bakeries are adding sugar-free and low-fat items to their traditional product lines. If you want to do nutrition, then you have to understand it.

This book was written to given an overview of culinary nutrition. It will provide the background you need to design healthy menus, write healthy recipes, market healthy food programs, and train food-service staff in healthy preparation and service techniques.

In each chapter you will find:

1. Chapter Overview: a guide to covered topics
2. Objectives: as you read through the chapter, glance back at the objective questions and see if you can understand them
3. FYI: topical culinary nutrition subjects
4. Critical Application Exercises: real-life nutrition problems to be solved with the information found in each chapter
5. Nutri-Words: to help build your nutrition vocabulary
6. Whaddaya Think?: you should be able to answer these nutrition thought-provoking questions after reading and reviewing the chapter.

You will also find margin notes, side bars, tables, and charts to enhance chapter information. The appendices provide supplementary information that will be useful to you in the class room and on the job.

Nutrition is a very broad science, touching aspects of biology, chemistry, physiology and psychology. To convey the message of good nutrition to the public, the culinarian needs to have a handle on a bit of all these sciences. This text will guide you through the right balance of nutrition and food service.

This text is the culmination of twenty years of teaching culinary nutrition at community colleges and universities, health care facilities, corporate hotels, correctional facilities and cruise ships in the United States, above the Arctic Circle and at the Equator to culinary olympians, executive chefs, food service executives, culinary and nutrition students, homeless shelter volunteers, and firefighters. Their input was invaluable in including information that is timely and useful in the world of culinary arts and food service. I would also like to thank the following reviewers for their invaluable suggestions and comments: Mary Tabacchi, Cornell School of Hospitality Management; Debra May Louis, DTR, Long Beach City College; Teresa L. Boehr, George Fox University; Joan Aronson, New York University; James Mbugua, California State Polytechnic University, Pomona; Connie Holt, Widener University; Kelly Kohls, University of Nebraska–Lincoln; Lesley Johnson, Ph.D., RD, University of Nevada Las Vegas; and Robert M. Zeit, M.D.

Nutrition for the Culinary Arts

Chapter 1

Introducing Nutrition

Chapter Overview

Objectives

After reading this chapter, the student should be able to:

1. *Identify customer populations that are receptive to nutrition-based menus.*
2. *Define the concept of nutritional health.*
3. *Explain the government's interests and interventions to ensure good nutritional health.*
4. *Determine which nutrition professionals are qualified to perform particular nutritional tasks.*
5. *List the nutritional qualifications of certified chefs, registered dietitians, food technologists, and other allied professionals.*
6. *Develop menu concepts based on the USDA and ethnic food guide pyramids.*

7. *Develop several menu courses based on the Exchange Lists for Meal Planning.*
8. *Analyze the information contained on a nutrition label.*
9. *Explain how nutritional foods need not be boring or plain.*

Introduction

What's all the noise about the need for nutrition knowledge? Why would food-service professionals give a Twinkie about good nutrition? Don't customers want to have a good time when they dine out? Do customers really care about nutrition? Of course, the important part of any business is the bottom line—making a profit. In truth, the bottom line is always about coinage. And the culinary truth is that nutrition sells.

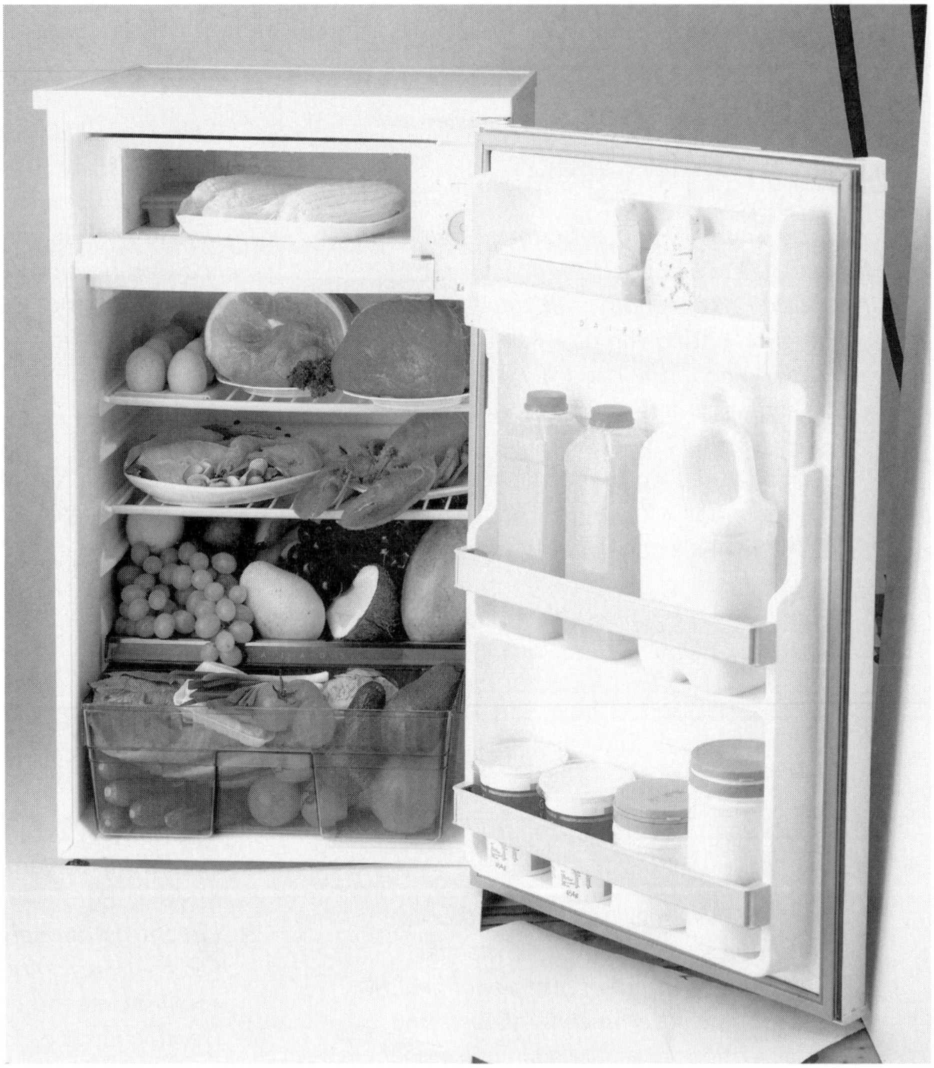

Rate this refrigerator in terms of nutritional and culinary ingredients.

WHAT DOES EVERYBODY WANT?

Food-service operators are in a unique position. At no time in history have more people been eating out, been more knowledgeable about food, and been more concerned about their health. When McDonald's starts putting **radicchio** in its green salads and using low-fat milk for its milkshakes, you know that something is up. That something is nutrition when eating out.

Baby Boomers don't want to cook, **Generation-Xers** don't have the time to cook and Generation-Yers think the microwave is an advanced form of cookery. In the year 2000, the same amount of food dollars were spent in the grocery store as were spent in restaurants. When you add in that Baby Boomers are fast becoming seniors concerned about maintaining their health and more Generation-Xers are vegetarians than ever before, you better get the clue that offering nutrition on the menu is pretty important for attracting and keeping customers. Take a clue from your customers. Good nutrition equals good health. Good health means a better and longer life. Offering healthy menus means a longer, more profitable life for your business (*Healthy People,* p. 3).

We will discuss what individual chefs and corporate food-service operators are doing about adding nutrition to their menus. You may want to check

Meal decisions need to be based on many things, including activity level.

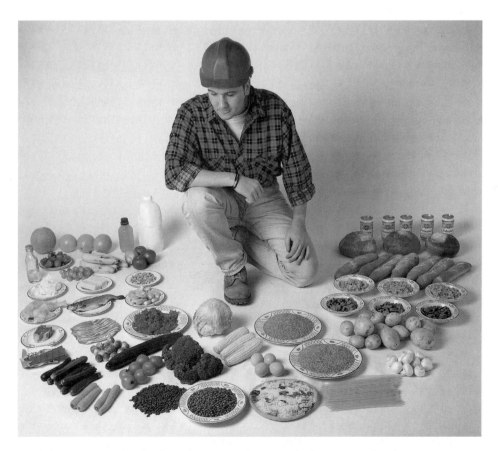

out nutrition accents you see on restaurant and food-service menus. For example, fast-food chains offer printed and web nutritional information about their burgers, shakes, and fried fish. Cruise lines are offering lower-salt, lower-fat "spa" menus. Fitness clubs offer gourmet menus analyzed by consultant nutritionists. Hotel chefs are expected to offer macrobiotic menu items prepared with organic ingredients. Airlines offer an array of calorie-, sodium-, and fat-modified meals along with vegetarian selections. School and university food services are adding soy milk, tofu, and veggie burgers to their traditional offerings. Nutrition has entered every aspect of food service. Culinarians are expected to know enough about nutrition to write recipes and menus, purchase ingredients, design promotions, train staff, and interact with customers.

Does this mean you need a degree in nutrition? No, but you should be able to do some or all of the following:

1. Create low-fat menus or recipes for healthy menu promotions.
2. Present consumer classes or demos linked to healthy menu promotions.
3. Determine ingredients necessary for producing healthy menus. For example, can nonfat yogurt be used in recipes to replace some or all of the sour cream? What are some low-fat ingredients you can offer to top baked potatoes?
4. Write press releases or media copy promoting healthy menus. Nutrition information has to be accurate and truthful.
5. Train front-of-the-house staff about healthy promotions. Staff will need to be versed in the details of the healthy menu, how to answer customers' questions, know how foods can and cannot be modified (yes, we can broil/poach the salmon; yes, we can serve the sauce on the side; no, we cannot omit the sodium from the gazpacho).
6. Analyze recipes and menus for calories, fat, and sodium content.
7. Design special menus for customer requests, such as low-salt, low-cholesterol, 1,200-calorie, high-protein, or macrobiotic.
8. Read and interpret labels to determine if products are appropriate for healthy recipes and menus.
9. Create healthy food items, such as salad dressing, desserts, and sauces, rather than purchasing ready-to-use products.
10. Participate in the creation of processed healthy food items, such as frozen entrees, canned soups, or dessert mixes.
11. Explain healthy food preparation techniques to food service staff.

WHAT DO YOU WANT?

But we speak so much about other people. What about you? Wouldn't you like to feel physically healthy and mentally alert? Wouldn't you like to be able to enjoy your educational and professional career, rather than just dragging through it? Before you save the world, you've got to rescue yourself. Good personal nutrition can help you think more clearly, have lots of energy, and avoid some illnesses. But it sounds so boring.

Yes, we know. Who would want to give up the excitement of bubbly diet cola or a frothy cappuccino for a glass of water? No one says you have to give it up (although it is a thought!), but you can broaden your horizons. The more caffeine you drink, the more calcium you leech from your body. Caffeine makes your kidneys work overtime, filtering excess chemicals. Not a pretty picture. So be good to yourself. If you must, reach for that morning jolt of Joe. Then, make yourself an icy fruit smoothie or order one at a local juice bar. How about orange-banana-cranberry with a swirl of honey? Or a blueberry-banana yogurt with a heat-flash of ginger? Not too hard to take.

If you eat good, you feel good. If you offer menus that make your customers feel good and improve or maintain their health, you make money and do good things. Read on.

WHO SAYS SO?

Over half a century ago the **World Health Organization (WHO)** defined the term "health" as a state of complete physical, mental, and social well-being and not merely the absence of disease or infirmity. In other words, people should be in good shape, not just avoiding the doctor. One of the WHO's key items for maintaining the health of the world was to provide adequate amounts of safe and healthy food.

Governments have a reason for wanting their citizens to be healthy. Healthy citizens can work, which means they earn money. Some of that money goes to taxes, and some of it is put back into the economy when citizens spend their hard-earned dough. Healthy citizens can work, produce, invent, and build. Unhealthy citizens cost the government money in health-care dollars and lost time and cannot contribute, monetarily or otherwise, to the fiscal and physical improvement of the country.

Since nutrition is a very important component of health, the government takes a strong interest in it. Many governmental nutrition interventions have benefited the consumer, such as enrichment and fortification of food. Food labeling and nutrition education programs came about because of government concern about the health of the citizens (Johnson & Kennedy, p. 1). And you thought your sugar crunchies had all those extra, added vitamins and minerals because the manufacturers were so concerned about your health!

Uncle Sam Wants You (to Have Your Iodine)

In the early 1900s, it was found that a large amount of the population was suffering from **goiter,** a symptom of a poorly functioning thyroid. The **thyroid** is the "alternator" for the body, controlling metabolism rates and other important functions. Interestingly, thyroid disease was widespread in communities located inland, such as in the Midwest or in the southern mountain areas. It was rarely, if ever, seen on either coast or in the Gulf of Mexico area. Research revealed that the thyroid needed trace amounts of **iodine** for proper functioning. Iodine is found in the ocean. Breathing the air along the coast supplied

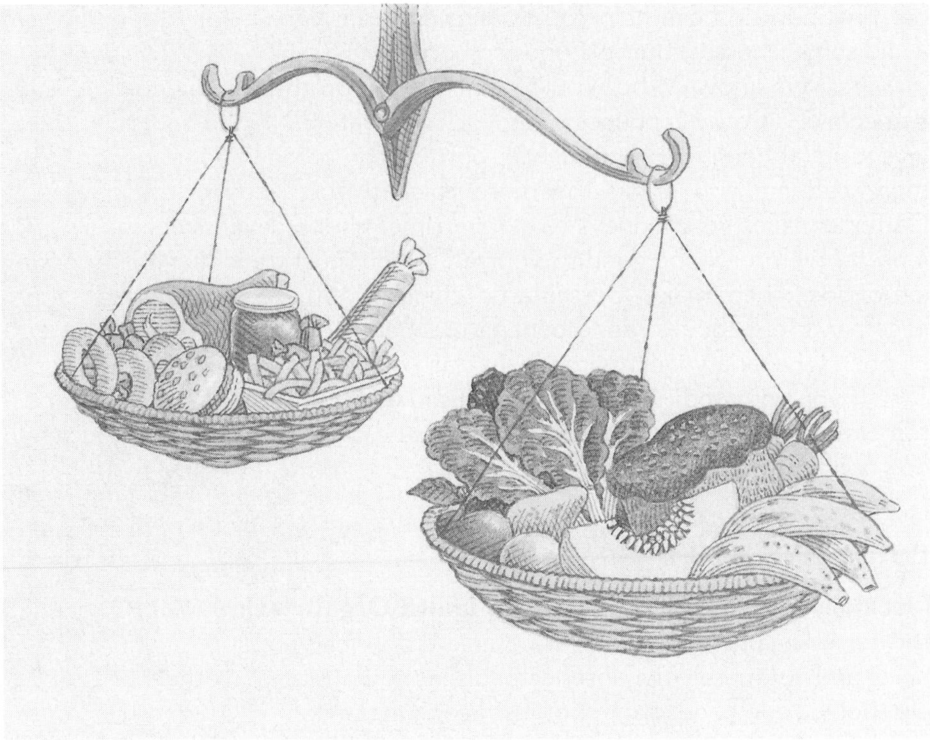

Culinarians need to "weigh" the nutrients in all foods.

dissolved iodine, and eating food products grown along the coast supplied sufficient amounts of iodine. Eating fish or vegetables, such as nori or seaweed, supplied lots of iodine as well. People living in coastal areas had lots of access to iodine, but those living inland did not.

Inland communities just accepted goiter as a condition that could not be avoided. The government became concerned because having a large number of people with poorly functioning thyroid glands meant having a large number of citizens who were not able to work well, serve in the armed forces, or make a decent contribution to the economy. The government had to figure out a way to get iodine to people that would be effective and affordable. The solution was to mandate that salt companies add iodine to their product. In those days, every household kept a good supply of salt. The relationship between salt and high blood pressure was yet to be discovered and most people felt that salt was an important part of their daily intake. Iodized salt was born out of a concern by the federal government to keep the population well-nourished.

The enrichment and fortification of dairy milk with vitamins A and D and wheat-based products, such as flour and cereals, with B vitamins and iron are additional examples of government-mandated "good nutrition." Look at the labels of some of your less "nutritional" foods. You'll be surprised to see some vitamins and minerals in cheese puffs, sugary cold cereal, canned chili, and frozen pizza. We're not suggesting this is the way to go to obtain optimal nutrition. We just want you to be aware that it's hard to escape nutrition, even in the strangest places.

HOW DO YOU DEFINE IT?

What does good nutrition mean? It means different things to different people. For an infant, good nutrition results in adequate growth and physical and mental development. For a college athlete, good nutrition may mean the ability to give maximum performances on the playing field and in the classroom. For a senior citizen, good nutrition may mean strong bones and physical and mental acuity.

Some nutritional needs are the same over a lifetime, and some are specific for certain points of the life cycle. In the following chapters, we will take each nutrient and discuss it in some detail. Right now, let's talk about the people and the tools that can help you work with nutrition.

NUTRITION PROFESSIONALS

Food-service professionals and nutrition professionals occupy similar but parallel universes. Sometime these universes meet, depending on the needs and desires of the clientele or employees. Figure 1–1 lists some professional food organizations and councils concerned with various aspects of nutrition.

Consciously or not, people eat to supply their bodies with necessary nutrients. We're not saying that everyone succeeds or cares, but all the food that is taken in has to be broken down and processed one way or another by the body. Some foods, such as fresh oranges, may help the body. Other foods, such as beer or diet soda, may make the body work hard to filter out unnecessary chemicals.

Food professionals go at nutrition in different ways. A dietitian may suggest that fresh seasonal vegetables be lightly sautéed or quickly steamed, to ensure that the maximum amount of nutrients are preserved. A chef will want to prepare fresh veggies the same way, not necessarily because nutrition is utmost on his or her mind, but because vegetables prepared in this way can be presented at the peak of their flavor and color. A college food-service director might direct kitchen staff to prepare vegetables by the batch method (cooking only what you need at the time you need it), to reduce the shrinkage that comes with overcooking. Not only will the vegetables look good, the food-service director is making sure to get the most profit out of every pound of carrots. A caterer preparing vegetables for a day-care account would lightly cook vegetables, knowing that young children prefer vegetables that are still crisp and crunchy.

Each method described above protected the nutrients naturally contained in the food. Only one of the food professionals mentioned above consciously thought about nutrition, but all presented a nutritious menu item.

Nutrition with a Moral

What's the moral to this story? One moral could be that high food quality and maximum nutrition are not mutually exclusive. If you present nicely textured, crisp, firm, herbed, steamed vegetables, they are both a culinary and a nutri-

1. American Dietetic Association
216 West Jackson Blvd.
Chicago, IL 60606-6995
(312) 899-0040
www.eatright.org
2. American Culinary Federation
10 San Bartola Drive
Saint Augustine, FL 32086
(800) 624-9458
www.acfchefs.org
3. Foodservice Educators Network International
959 Melvin Road
Annapolis, MD 21403
(410) 268-5542
www.feni.org
4. Institute of Food Technologists
211 North LaSalle Street, Suite 300
Chicago, IL 60601-1291
(312) 782-8424
www.ift.org
5. International Association of Culinary Professionals
304 W. Liberty, Suite 201
Louisville, KY 40202
(800) 928-4227
www.iacp-online.org
6. Oldways Preservation & Exchange Trust
266 Beacon Street
Boston, MA 02116
(617) 421-5500
www.oldwayspt.org
7. Research Chefs Association
304 W. Liberty, Suite 201
Louisville, KY 40202
(502) 992-0438
www.researchchef.com
8. Council for Responsible Nutrition
1875 Eye Street NW, Suite 400
Washington, DC 20006
(202) 872-1588
www.crnusa.org
9. Nutrition Information Center Rockefeller University
1230 York Avenue, Box 246
New York, NY 10021
(212) 327-7707
10. Second Harvest Network
116 South Michigan Avenue, Suite 4
Chicago, IL 60603
(312) 263-2303
www.secondharvest.org
11. United Soybean Board
16640 Chesterfield Grove Road, Suite 130
Chesterfield, MO 63005
(314) 530-1777
www.unitedsoybean.org
12. American Wine Society
3006 Latta Road
Rochester, NY 14612
(716) 225-7613
www.vicon.net
13. International Dairy Association
1250 H Street, NW Suite 900
Washington, DC 20005
(202) 737-4332
www.idfa.org
14. National Yogurt Association
2000 Corporate Ridge, Suite 1000
McLean, VA 22102
(703) 821-0770
www.affi.com
15. United Fresh Fruit and Vegetable Assn
727 N. Washington Street
Alexandria, VA 22314
(703) 836-3410
www.uffva.org
16. Rare Fruit Council International
12255 SW 73rd Avenue
Miami, FL 33256
(305) 378-4457
17. USA Rice Federation
6699 Rookin Road
Houston, TX 77074
(713) 270-6699
www.usarice.com
18. National Pasta Association
2101 Wilson Boulevard, Suite 920
Arlington, VA 22201
(703) 841-0818
www.ilovepasta.org
19. International Olive Oil Council
515 East 71st Street, Suite 904
New York, NY 10021
(800) 232-6548
20. Organic Trade Association
PO Box 547
Greenfield, MA 01301
(413) 774-7511
www.ota.com
21. National Seafood Educators
PO Box 60006
Richmond Beach, WA 98160
(206) 546-6410
22. American Spice Trade Association
560 Sylvan Avenue
Englewood Cliffs, NJ 07632
(201) 568-2163
www.astaspice.org
23. The Vinegar Institute
5775 Peachtree-Dunwoody Road, Suite 500-G
Atlanta, GA 30342
(404) 252-3663
www.versatilevinegar.org
24. Vegetarian Resource Group
PO Box 1463
Baltimore, MD 21203
(410) 366-8343
www.vrg.org

Figure 1–1 Professional Info to Get You Started

A. Institute of Food Technologists
www.ift.org
Certification: Member, Professional Member, Fellow

B. Research Chefs Association
www.rca.org
Certifications: CRC (Certified Research Chef); pending is CCS (Certified Culinary Scientist)

C. International Food Service Executives Association
www.ifsea.org
Certifications: Certified Food Service Executive

D. International Association of Culinary Professionals
304 West Liberty Street, Suite 201, Louisville, KY 40202
(502) 581-9786
iacp@hqtrs.com
Certification: CCP (Certified Culinary Professional)

E. National Restaurant Association
1-800-352-6700
www.nraef.org
Certification: ServSafe Certified Food Handling Instructor. Several courses lead to an NRA certificate of completion in nutrition, supervision, sanitation, bar management and professional service. These certificates can be used as continuing education credits for other professional organizations and are recognized by many employers.

Figure 1–2 Various Professional Food Organizations and Their Certifications

tion masterpiece. Soggy, overcooked green beans lose both their culinary and nutritional appeal. The other moral could be that you can't always leave nutrition to chance. Most food professionals have some interest or training (or both) in nutrition. We've included some designations awarded by several professional food organizations in Figure 1–2. Most of these organizations have Web sites or toll-free numbers if you are interested in finding out the qualifications necessary for the designations.

Who's Who in the Food-Service World

Certified Chefs

The **American Culinary Federation (ACF)** is the certifying board for chefs in the United States. The ACF belongs to the World Association of Cooks' Society (WACS). WACS offers international certifications. The ACF credentials post-secondary culinary arts programs in community colleges, four-year colleges or universities, private culinary academies, and organized apprenticeship programs. Every student or professional chef who seeks ACF certification must complete a thirty-hour course in nutrition, with a refresher course every five years. The ACF realizes how important nutrition is to the culinary world and wants to ensure its certified members are knowledgeable about providing both interesting and healthy menus.

Certified Culinarian (CC)
Certified Sous Chef (CSC)
Certified Chef de Cuisine (CCC)
Certified Executive Chef (CEC)
Certified Master Chef (CMC)
Certified Culinary Educator (CCE)
Certified Pastry Chef (CPC)
Certified Executive Pastry Chef (CEPC)
Certified Master Pastry Chef (CMPC)

Figure 1–3 Certification Levels for the American Culinary Federation

Certified chef-members of the ACF must take thirty-hour courses in nutrition, sanitation, and supervision. Certification is valid for five years, at which time refresher courses must be taken. This means that ACF-certified chefs should be current in basic nutrition.

Food Technologists

The **Institute of Food Technologists (IFT)** is a professional organization of food scientists, research and development scientists, packaging engineers, cereal and meat chemists, flavor experts and food microbiologists, to name a few. Most members of the IFT have at least a bachelor's degree, with most having advanced degrees. Food science degrees are a mixture of organic chemistry, nutrition, biology and physiology, biochemistry, microbiology, and specific courses in food science that pertain to ingredient preparation, food preservation, food packaging, and food production. For example, one undergraduate food-science course might take a student from milk pasteurization, enrichment and fortification, to cheese and ice cream production, in both theory and application. Many university food-science departments have pilot plant equipment that allows the student to experience commercial food production up close and personal. At the University of Washington at Pullman and at Rutgers University in New Jersey, food-science students pasteurize milk obtained from agricultural colleges' dairy herds. The milk is processed by the students into cheeses, ice cream, and butter, which is sold locally and on-line.

Food technologists may not be chefs or dietitians, but they know everything there is to know about food interactions. Frozen entrees, canned soups, shelf-stable bakery items, and bottled beverages were perfected and packaged by food technologists. A food technologist can show you how to fortify orange juice with calcium, ice cream with extra vitamin A and D, or pack twenty essential nutrients into a breakfast bar.

The **Research Chefs Association (RCA)** has a lot in common with the IFT. Chefs can work in a million different areas of the food world. Some enjoy the challenge of working with food scientists, and some seek to perfect the art of vinegar production. You will find research chefs working with food technologists and business people to perfect the art and science of all aspects of food. Research chefs have developed allied courses with the food-technology departments at several universities, marrying the arts and sciences of culinary technique with nutrition and technology.

Registered Dietitians and Dietetic Technicians

The **American Dietetic Association (ADA)** is the certifying board for dietitians (**registered dietitian,** or **RD**) and dietetic technicians (**registered dietetic technicians,** or **DTR**) in the United States. Someone wanting to become an RD must complete an ADA-approved undergraduate program. Course work resembles a pre-med course, with lots of chemistry, biology, nutrition, psychology, economics, and administration courses. After attaining a BS in nutrition, a student must complete a supervised internship, usually health-care affiliated and about twelve to eighteen months long, or obtain a masters degree.

DTRs can complete their course work at an ADA-approved program at a two-year or four-year school, completing about 1,000 hours of clinical internship. DTRs cannot assume all the medical responsibilities that an RD can, but they are quite knowledgeable in many areas of nutrition. Chefs wanting to increase their nutrition knowledge and credibility sometimes pursue a DTR license.

So, if you find the need for a nutrition professional, you have an idea where to look. Among other things, RDs and DTRs can nutritionally analyze recipes and menus, present seminars on how to get more nutrition into

RD (Registered Dietitian)
RDs may add additional certifications to their general RD status that deal with advanced training in specialized areas such as pediatric nutrition or diabetes education. The ADA also has a "fellow" status for RDs who have distinguished themselves in the nutrition field.

RDs must complete an American Dietetic Association–approved undergraduate program plus advanced training that is a combination of graduate-level courses and directed professional experience. After completing advanced training, a graduate may take a national licensing examination.

To maintain an RD license, the RD must complete approved continuing-education hours.

DTR (Registered Dietetic Technician)
DTRs complete a two- or four-year undergraduate AS or BS from an American Dietetic Association–approved program. After completing directed professional experience, the DTR can take a national or state licensing examination.

The DTR must maintain licensure by completing continuing-education hours.

Figure 1–4 American Dietetic Association Registration Levels menus, and can help to design food-service plans for various menu modifications, such as lower salt or higher fiber. ACF-certified chefs can identify nutritious ingredients and set up a menu plan for healthy cuisine, can plan menus for vegetarians or athletes, and advise on nutritious ingredient selection. Members of the IFT or RCA can take your award-winning pizza and convert it into a frozen product.

Walk the Walk and Talk the Talk

Many people call themselves "nutritionists" or "nutrition advisors." There is no such thing as a licensed "nutritionist." Many people may have extensive nutrition backgrounds and some may not. If you require accurate nutrition information, it is your responsibility to check out the backgrounds of the people you hire.

Say your customers have asked you to add some low-fat or sugar-free items to your menu. Or say you want to advertise a portion of your menu as meeting the USDA Guidelines for Healthy Americans (discussed below). Many restaurants and food-service establishments are doing this. You'll need a nutrition professional to look at your ideas and make sure that they do what they say they do. You don't want to poison your customers, nor do you want to get into a false-advertising lawsuit.

An RD or DTR can do the type of job you need. They should provide you with a written report that details how your menu meets the criteria you're claiming. A food scientist, certified chef, or member of the RCA may be able to provide you with this information. More importantly, the people listed above would be acknowledged and accepted by government agencies.

A local nutrition professor, with a doctorate in nutrition, is not necessarily certified by any organization. Membership in the ACF, ADA, IFT, or RCA is voluntary, not mandatory, so you can't always look for initials after people's names. You can, however, check out their background to ensure that they have the necessary qualifications to act as a nutrition expert. Just because someone has worked in food service for many years does not make him or her a nutrition maven. If it's your money and your reputation, ask some questions before you hire a nutrition person of your very own.

Now that we've discussed the people, let's discuss the equipment you'll need to enhance your nutrition knowledge. There are many nutrition tools with which you'll want to become familiar so you can devise nutritional recipes and menus of your own.

NUTRITION TOOLS

Nutrition tools come in all shapes and colors, depending on your needs and your nutrition background. The **food guide pyramids** were designed to be simple, effective, and accessible to everyone. Initially, there was one food guide pyramid, designed very generally to meet the needs of lots of people. As time went by, food guide pyramids were developed for different ethnic groups' diets. Where the food guide pyramids deal with whole foods, like dairy products or nuts, the **RDAs (the Recommended Dietary**

Allowances) deal with individual nutrients. It takes a bit more nutrition expertise to plug an individual's specific need for calcium into a recipe. **The USDA Guideline for Healthy Americans** is a very general guide for nutritional health, offering advice on daily levels of saturated fat or sodium. The ADA's **Exchange Lists for Meal Planning** provides a fast way to analyze recipes and menus for calories, carbohydrates, proteins, and fats. Let's discuss each one of these nutrition tools.

Walk Like An Egyptian: Food Guide Pyramids

The Food Guide Pyramids are discussed in this chapter's FYI. The Food Guide Pyramids are helpful for figuring out if you are eating a reasonably healthy diet or if you've designed a reasonably healthy menu. If you want to really scare yourself, do this fast Pyramid exercise:

Go over the principles of the Pyramid; compare an ethnic Pyramid with the American Pyramid. Think about your shopping and meal planning, with a particular Pyramid in mind. Hold a small picture or poster of the Pyramid in your hand. Do you fit the Pyramid plan this way? If not, then invert the Pyramid. How would you like to live in a building with such a shaky foundation (the narrow top of the Pyramid)? Is your diet or menu as shaky as the inverted Pyramid? Think about it!

RDA Every Day

The Recommended Dietary Allowances are listed in Appendix 1. The main RDA table gives recommendations for protein, eleven vitamins, and seven minerals. Other RDA tables give energy needs for various ages and tentative recommendations for two more vitamins and eight minerals. Before you use the RDAs, understand the following:

1. RDA are not minimum requirements, but *recommended* amounts. The RDA are not mandatory or required, but an allowance based on the most recent scientific evidence. The RDA are reviewed and revised periodically by scientists selected by the National Academy of Science.
2. The RDA are estimates of needs for healthy people. The allowances are generous (except for energy, or calorie, needs) but still may not cover every person for every nutrient. For example, if you are anemic, the RDA for iron may not be enough for you. If you are overweight, then the RDA for energy (meaning calories) may be too much for you.
3. Separate recommendations are made for different groups. Be sure to look up the RDA appropriate for you. There are different recommendations for different age groups, for example.
4. The RDA are not meant to be used as an exact guide and are not meant for people with particular health issues. For example, an anemic teenager cannot use the RDA for iron as an intake guide, nor can an obese, hypertensive fifty-year-old man use the RDA for energy needs for his daily intake.

Understand that the RDAs are a flexible approximation. The RDAs are usually used with a combination of other nutrition tools, such as a diet history and

The Food Guide Pyramid emphasizes foods from the five major food groups shown in the three lower sections of the Pyramid. Each of these food groups provides some, but not all, of the nutrients you need. Foods in one group can't replace those in another. No one food group is more important than another—for good health, you need them all.

The small tip of the Pyramid shows fats, oils, and sweets. These are foods such as salad dressings and oils, cream, butter, margarine, sugars, soft drinks, candies, and sweet desserts. These foods provide calories and little else nutritionally. Most people should use them sparingly.

On the next level of the Food Guide Pyramid are two groups of foods that come mostly from animals: milk, yogurt, cheese; and meat, poultry, fish, dry beans, eggs, and nuts. These foods are for protein, calcium, iron, and zinc. The next level includes foods that come from plants—vegetables and fruits. Most people need to eat more of these foods for the vitamins, minerals, and fiber they supply.

At the base of the Food Guide Pyramid are breads, cereals, rice, and pasta—all foods from grains. You

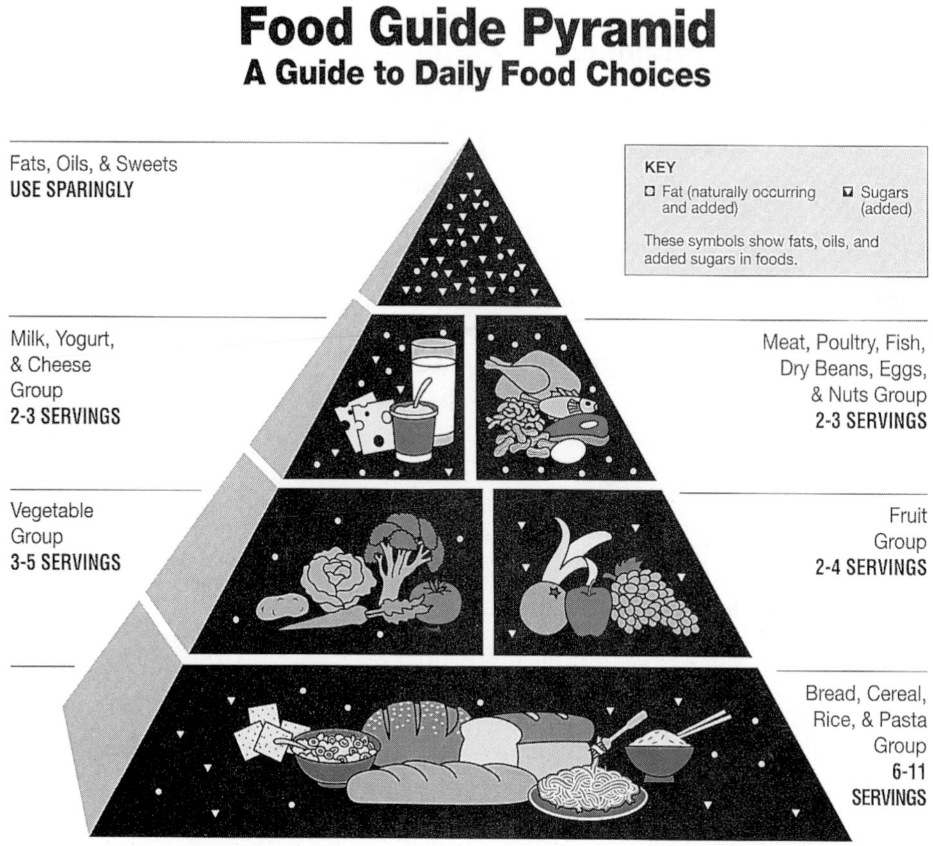

Figure 1–5 American Food Guide Pyramid (*Source:* USDA.)

the USDA Guideline for Americans. The RDA can be used to assess, in a small range, the adequacy of an individual's diet. Remember that the RDA can direct an individual to an adequate intake, but excess intake of energy or nutrients are hard to assess.

The RDAs do not address the issues of under- or overnutrition. Undernutrition may be a lack of adequate calories, or can be a lack of adequate vitamins or minerals. Undernutrition may lead to depressed immunity, anemia, decreased healing, and retardation of growth and development. Overnutrition, which is an intake of too much energy, can lead to heart disease, diabetes, cancer and liver disease, as well as circulatory and physical problems.

Another index, called the RDI, or reference dietary index, is more useful for people who may not be in the best of health or for people who are seeking to prevent certain disease states. The RDI states the highest RDA advisable for

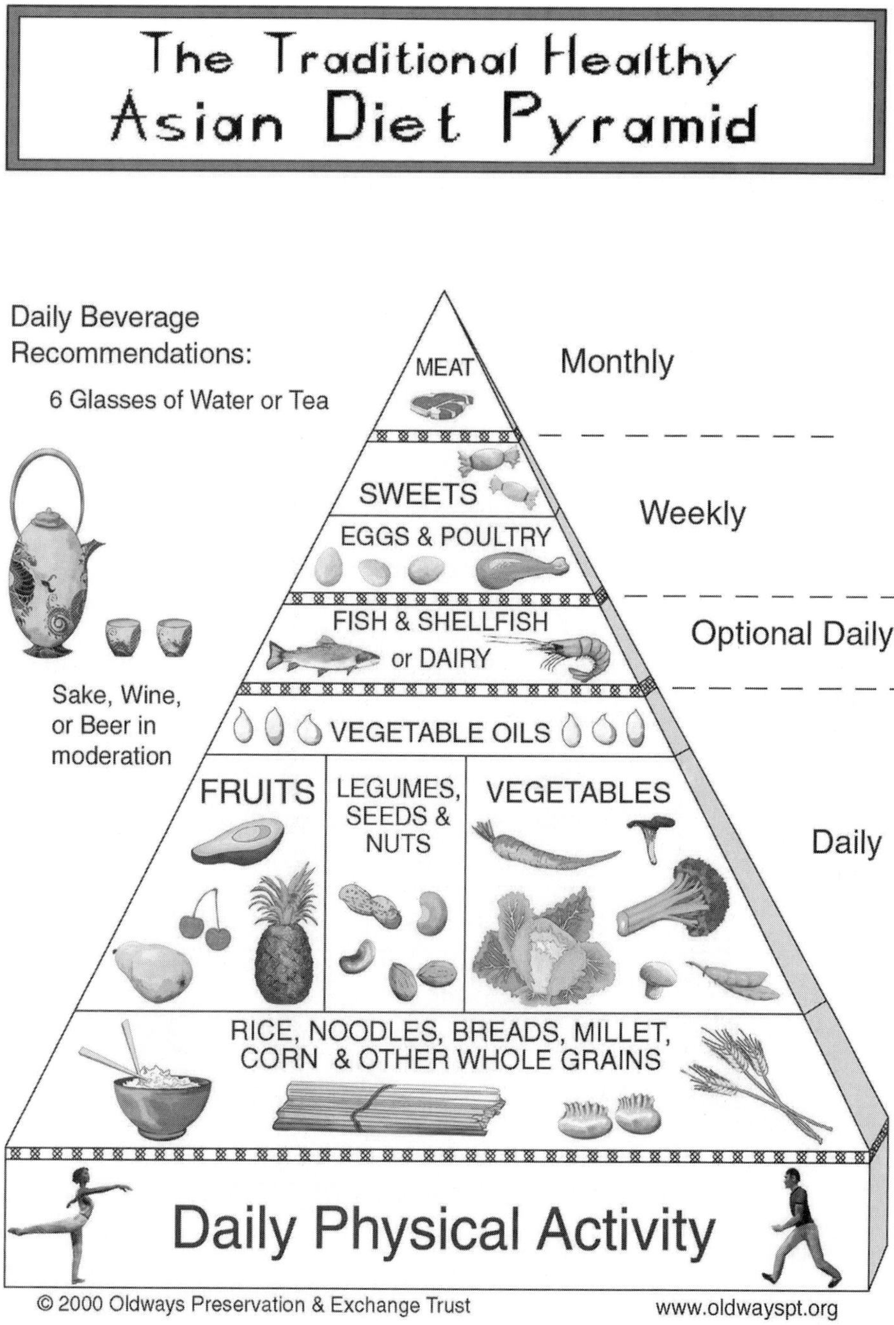

Figure 1–6 Asian Diet Pyramid *(Courtesy of Oldways Preservation and Exchange Trust)*

many nutrients. Many health-care professionals suggest following the RDIs for nutrients that have been demonstrated to help in the prevention of disease.

USDA Guidelines for Healthy Americans

Back in the good old days, there were the four food groups. Easy to remember, pretty easy with which to comply. You had your meat, your dairy, your fruit and vegetables, your bread. Period. Simple to understand. Unfortunately,

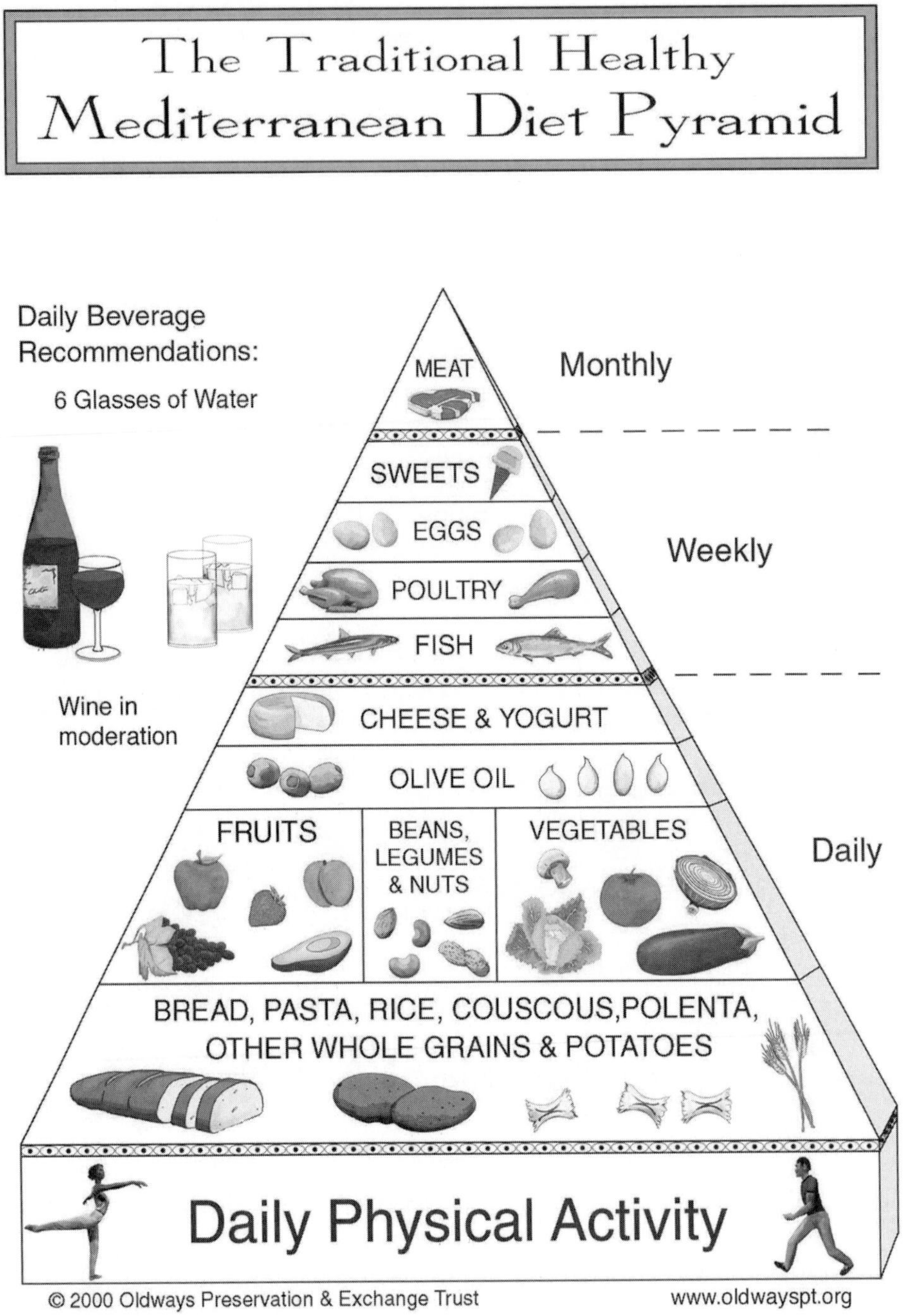

Figure 1–7 Mediterranean Diet Pyramid *(Courtesy of Oldways Preservation and Exchange Trust)*

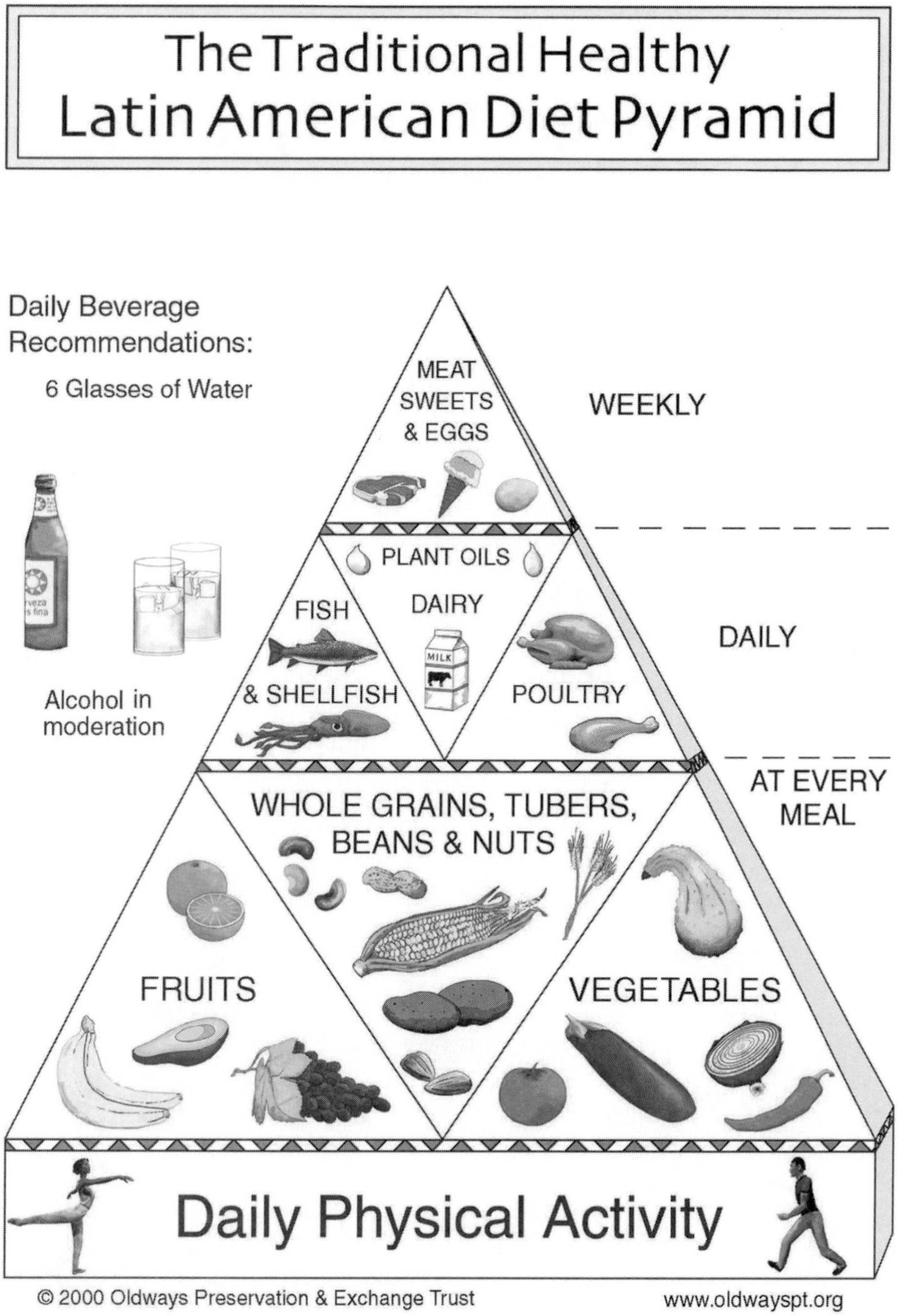

Figure 1–8 Latin American Diet Pyramid *(Courtesy of Oldways Preservation and Exchange Trust)*

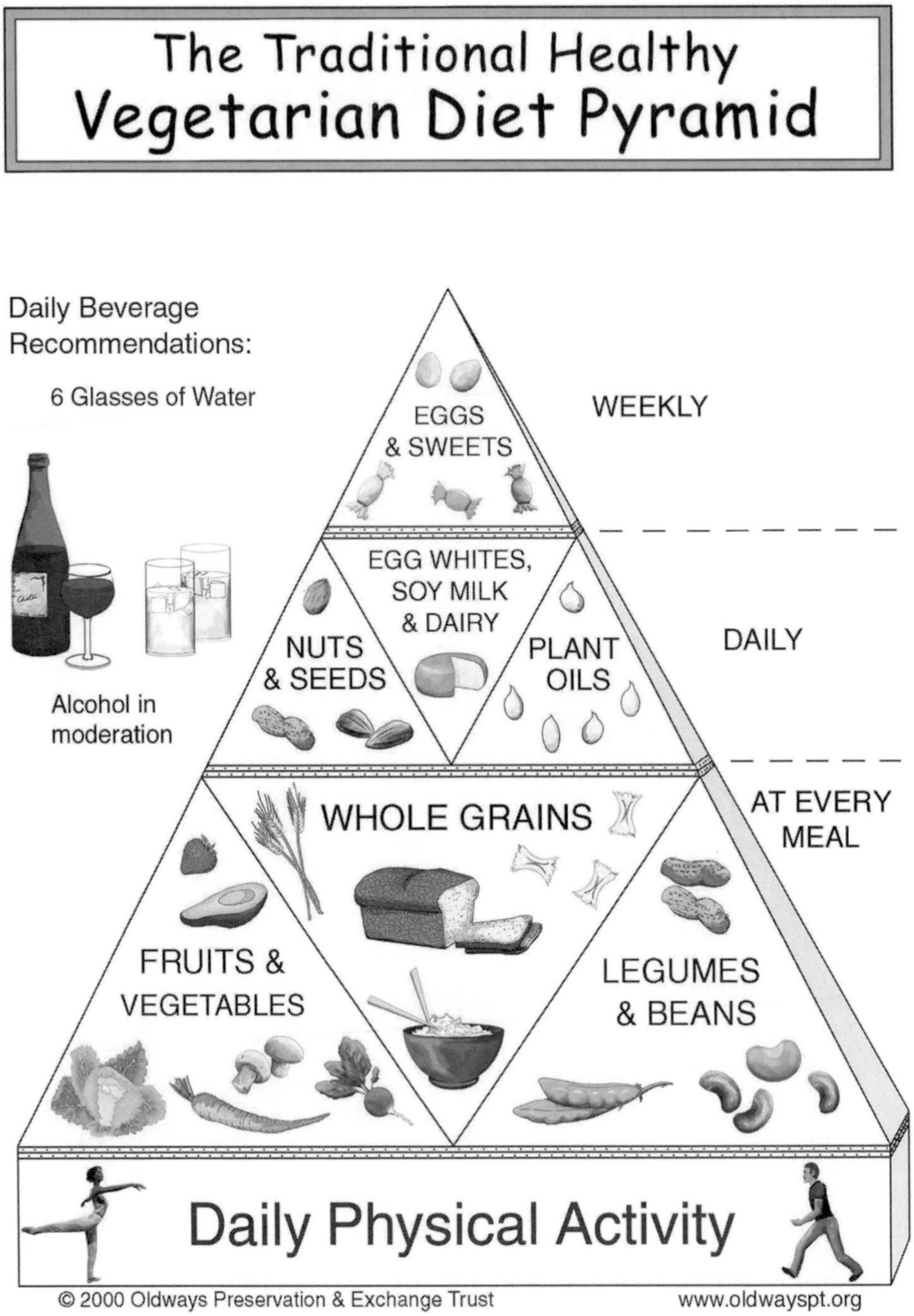

Figure 1–9 Vegetarian Diet Pyramid *(Courtesy of Oldways Preservation and Exchange Trust)*

it meant that a meal of cheese-covered nachos topped with crumbled bacon and washed down with fruit punch could constitute a healthy meal. A little fine-tuning was in order. Over the years, we have had four, six, and seven food groups; a food pyramid; and, in Canada, a food rainbow. Although they got the basics across and were adaptable to a wide audience, these tools were a bit broad.

The Feds Say

The USDA Dietary Guidelines for Americans were introduced in the 1980s and have been most recently revised in 1995 and 2000 (*Dietary Guidelines,* p. 2). The initial guidelines stressed eating a variety of foods; cutting back on fat, especially saturated fat and cholesterol; limiting salt, sodium, and sugar; including lots of fiber from fruits, vegetables, and grain products and, if using alcohol, do so in moderation.

The 1995 version included new information on the need for exercise and the tie-in between diet and exercise. "Balance the food you eat with physical activity and maintain or improve your weight," to be exact. The 2000 version organized the guidelines into the "ABCs" of healthy eating and attempted to emphasize that diet was just a part of a healthy lifestyle. The guidelines attempt to help answer the question, "What should Americans do to stay healthy?" Food-service professionals find the guidelines a useful tool for menu design.

The "eat a variety of foods" portion of the guidelines is an easy way to assure balanced nutrition. If you eat a couple of servings of different types of fruit, vegetables, grains, and low-fat dairy products every day, just by accident you'll be getting some good nutrition. Conversely, if you eat a lot of different foods, you can "stray" every once in a while and eat some things that aren't so great for you. If you do this only occasionally, then your body has time to filter out the bad stuff and recuperate.

Maintaining a diet low in fat and low in saturated fat and cholesterol is a hard one for most people. No more than 30 percent of total daily calories should come from fat, and only 10 percent of that should be from saturated fat. Lowering salt and sugar are just as difficult. We'll discuss different ways to offer foods lower in fat, salt, and sugar (that still look and taste good) in later chapters.

> FOOD FOR THE MIND
>
> Memorize the ABCs of healthy menu planning:
>
> A = adequate amounts of calories and nutrients
>
> B = balance and variety of food selections
>
> C = calorie control; not too much and not too little
>
> D = nutrient density
>
> (Adapted from "National Nutrition Month Information," American Dietetics Association, March 1998.)

Pick an Exchange, Any Exchange: Exchange Lists for Meal Planning

The Exchange Lists for Meal Planning is a quick tool for menu and diet analysis. Before there were computers or extensive data banks for menu breakdowns, there were the exchange lists. You can find an example of the exchange lists on the American Dietetic Association's Web site, *www.eatright.org* or in Appendix 3.

Exchange lists allow more fine-tuning than the Pyramids do. The exchange lists take all foods (well, not all foods, Twinkies™ and Doritos™ aren't listed) and divide them into categories, or exchanges. Each food within

1995
1. Eat a variety of foods.
2. Balance the food you eat with physical activity—maintain or improve your weight.
3. Choose a diet with plenty of grains, vegetables, and fruit.
4. Choose a diet low in fat, saturated fat, and cholesterol.
5. Choose a diet low in sugars.
6. Choose a diet low in salt and sodium.
7. If you drink alcoholic beverages, do so in moderation.

2000
1. Aim for Fitness
   a. Aim for a healthy weight.
   b. Be physically active every day.
2. Build a Healthy Base
   a. Let the food guide pyramid guide your food choices.
   b. Eat a variety of grains daily, especially whole grains.
   c. Eat a variety of fruits and vegetables daily.
   d. Keep food safe to eat.
3. Choose Sensibly
   a. Choose a diet that is low in saturated fat and cholesterol and moderate in saturated fat.
   b. Choose beverages and foods to moderate your intake of sugars.
   c. Choose and prepare foods with less fat.
   d. If you drink alcoholic beverages, do so in moderation.

Figure 1–10 USDA Dietary Guidelines for Americans

an exchange has similar characteristics in reference to protein, carbohydrates, and fat. This means that foods within each exchange can be swapped, or exchanged. Exchange lists allow people to calculate calories or grams of energy while having some food freedom.

Rather than being told that "You must have half a cup of orange juice and one medium banana," a customer can select two fruit exchanges. Portion sizes within each exchange are determined by the makeup of the food. For example, four ounces of orange juice, ten fresh grapes, and one ounce of raisins are all one fruit exchange.

Exchanges might seem like a lot to learn, but they really are easy to use and manipulate. They are an easy way to analyze recipes and menus when you can't get to a computer, and they go much faster than looking up each individual ingredient. When the Westin Hotel chain wanted to dedicate a part of their menu to healthy eating, it used the exchange lists to analyze the recipes their chefs submitted.

The exchanges are divided into the fruit, starch, vegetable, meat, dairy, and fat categories. Each have a certain number of calories. One group, the free exchanges, have little to no calories and can be eaten as desired. Make the most of the free foods exchange. A culinary nutrition class was given the challenge to design a meal almost entirely from this exchange. Here's what it came up with:

- Savory clear vegetable soup with shredded carrots, celery, green onions, and zucchini.
- Health salad with chopped cabbage, radishes, cucumbers, chilies, and spinach tossed with low-calorie salad dressing and balsamic vinegar.
- Mocha "mousse" made with espresso coffee, unsweetened cocoa powder, artificial sweetener, and unflavored gelatin.

These menu ideas add three courses to a meal without adding appreciable calories. Just think how much the customers will appreciate it! Become proficient with the exchanges so you can do the same thing.

Food Composition Tables

There are many types of food composition tables. They all list an ingredient or food item, such as bread or cheddar cheese. They then list various nutrition values for the ingredient, which can include calories, carbohydrates, protein, fats (including saturated and unsaturated fats), vitamins, minerals, and fiber, to name a few. You simply locate the food that you would like to learn about and read across the line. See Appendix I for a portion of the USDA Handbook Number 8, the grandaddy of all food composition tables. Food composition tables contain lots of information, but they can take a lot of time to use if you need to look up a lot of items.

Nutrition Labels

The **Nutrition Labeling Education Act** was passed in 1990. This bit of federal legislation changed the type and amount of information required on all packaged food. See Figure 1–6 for a run-down on label terminology. All packaged food sold in the United States must contain this information.

Just because they do not serve packaged foods, restaurateurs and other purveyors of unpackaged foods cannot breathe a sigh of relief. If you want to use any of the terms listed in Figure 1–6, such as low-fat, fresh, or healthy, then your menu items must fulfill the requirements of the definitions. When asked, by a customer or food-service inspector, you must be able to prove that your "healthy" corn chowder has only 60 milligrams or less of cholesterol. This can be proven with computerized analysis, exchange list analysis, or food composition table analysis. If you are selling a packaged clam chowder, then you can use the manufacturers' nutrition information.

Creative Writing

If you want to make healthy claims about your menu items, such as low fat, lower salt, or high fiber, you have several choices. One would be to create your own set of terms, rather then using the USDA-covered ones. How about "good for life" instead of healthy, or " fiber-packed" instead of high fiber? Another option would be not to make any nutrition claims. If you want to use the USDA terminology, you can consult one of the nutrition professionals we discussed above to help you analyze your menus, or you can learn to do it yourself! Remember, if you print it on your menu, you have to be able to prove it.

The following are USDA definitions of label terms:

a. Fresh: means that food is raw or unprocessed and has never been frozen or reheated. "Fresh" also indicates no preservatives (low-level irradiation is allowed).
b. Healthy: means that a food is low in fat and saturated fat, has no more than 60 milligrams of cholesterol per serving and has at least 10 percent of the RDA for vitamins A or C, and for protein, calcium, iron, or fiber. Healthy also means that a side dish has no more than 360 milligrams of sodium per serving and an entrée no more than 480 milligrams.
c. More: means that a food has at least 10 percent more of the RDA for a particular nutrient than a regular food. For example, calcium-fortified orange juice can make a label claim of "more calcium" than regular orange juice.
d. Light: can mean several things, as follows:
    1. "Light" can be used to describe a color or texture, as in "light wheat bread." This carries no particular nutritional meaning.
    2. Light can mean that a food contains one-third less calories or half the fat of a regular product.
    3. Light can also be used to mean that a low-fat, low-calorie food has had its sodium content reduced by half.
e. Reduced: means that a product has had its fat or sodium content lowered by 25 percent. For example, baked potato chips may be 25 percent reduced in fat and can carry a "reduced fat" label.
f. Less: means that a food contains 25 percent less calories or nutrients than a comparable product.
g. High: means that there is 20 percent or more of a particular nutrient in a serving of food.
h. Good Source: means that a food contains 10 to 19 percent of the RDA for a particular nutrient.
i. Lean and Extra Lean: lean means that there are fewer than 10 grams of fat and less than 95 milligrams of cholesterol in a meat product and extra lean means there are fewer than 5 grams of fat and 95 milligrams of cholesterol.
j. Low: can mean several different things. Low fat means less than 3 grams of fat per serving, low saturated fat means less than 1 gram of fat per serving, low sodium means no more than 140 milligrams of sodium per serving, low cholesterol means no more than 20 milligrams per serving and low calorie means no more than 40 calories per serving. The definition of "low" changes when applied to whole meals, such as frozen dinners.
k. Free: means a product contains only negligible amounts of fat, saturated fat, cholesterol, sodium, sugar, or calories.
l. Fortified: means that a manufacturer has added 10 percent or more of the RDA for a particular nutrient.

Figure 1–11 How to Read a Food Label

Many restaurants and food-service operations decide to package some of their products, such as salad dressing, barbecue sauce, or salsa. All packaged foods, nutritional claims or not, must be labeled. We are not speaking of a bakery that puts its bread in a bag so their customers can transport it or a restaurant that offers a takeaway menu. We are speaking of food that is sold as a truly packaged item, such as a bottle of salad dressing. Food technologists

At the time of this writing, the following were the allowable label health claims:

1. Calcium and osteoporesis
2. Fat and cancer
3. Soy and heart health
4. Cholesterol and heart disease
5. Cancer or heart disease and fiber
6. Sodium and hypertension
7. Folic acid and birth defects (neural tube defects)
8. Omega-3 fatty acids and heart disease

Nutrition Facts

Serving Size 1 tea bag (1g)
Servings Per Container 20

Amount Per Serving	
Calories 0	
	% Daily Value*
Total Fat 0g	**0%**
Sodium 0mg	**0%**
Total Carbohydrate less than 1g	**0%**
Sugars 0g	
Protein 0g	

Not a significant source of calories from fat, saturated fat, cholesterol, dietary fiber, vitamin A, vitamin C, calcium and iron.

*Percent Daily Values are based on a 2,000 calorie diet. Your daily values may be higher or lower depending on your calorie need.

By law, a food label must tell you the following:

1. Name of the food, the manufacturer (with contact information) and net weight or quantity.
2. Ingredients, listed in descending weight, with the heaviest ingredient first.
3. Nutrition Facts: the FDA has determined serving sizes for most foods. The manufacturer must list the amount of calories, calories from fat, total fat, saturated fat, cholesterol, sodium, total carbohydrates, dietary fiber, sugars, protein, vitamin A, vitamin C, calcium, and iron for a serving size. The only other nutrient which must be listed would be if a manufacturer makes a nutritional claim, such as "fortified with potassium."
4. The % Daily Values: these are based on a 2,000-calorie daily diet, with 30 percent of the calories coming from fat, 10 percent from protein and 60 percent from carbohydrates. Consumers have to do some division or multiplication, depending on the number of calories they eat in a day.

Figure 1–12 Dissecting a Food Label

and test kitchens offer labeling services. There are some computer programs that perform label analysis for simple foods. If you are interested in more information about creating food labeling, the Institute of Food Technologists, based in Chicago, Illinois would be a good source of information. Their Web site is *www.ift.org*.

Nutrients

We've been talking about eating "good" food, but we haven't discussed what makes food "good." The "good" parts are called **nutrients.** Nutrients are components of all foods, and help the body grow, repair, and maintain. We use the term "essential," meaning you need them and your body can't make them. Essential nutrients must be gotten from the diet. For example, the body can synthesize vitamin A from the plant source beta-carotene. So, you don't have to eat "whole" vitamin A to get it from your diet, as your body will make the vitamin A it needs from the sources you give it. On the other hand, the body cannot synthesize potassium, so you must eat potassium-rich foods to meet your potassium requirement.

Energy-giving nutrients come from carbohydrates, fats, and protein. Another group of very important nutrients that give no energy, but lots of other important stuff, are vitamins, minerals, and water. We will discuss all of these nutrients in the following chapters.

Nutrients are any of the components in food that help keep you healthy. Nutrients could be proteins, carbohydrates, certain fats, vitamins, minerals, water, and even the "good" chemicals in green tea or gingko. There are lots of ways to get adequate amounts of nutrients into your diet.

While speaking about nutrients, what about those foods that are perceived as having little nutrient value, such as coffee, chocolate, or beer? Most nutrition experts would tell you that there is no such thing as a good or bad food. It's all just a matter of proportion. We've pointed out that the USDA Guidelines for Americans suggests that you take in a variety of foods. That includes chocolate ice cream, chips and dip, and imported ale. You have to look at your degree of health, your nutritional goals and how you would like to feel, and then decide about how much of the "extra" foods you can fit into a balanced diet.

DISHING WITH JULIA

Julia Child has been influencing culinary arts for over forty years. At a time when cream of mushroom soup, prime rib, and apple pie a la mode was considered an American gourmet meal, Julia Child, the first woman with a television cooking show, dared to show America how to prepare bouillabaisse, pot au feu, and tarte tatin. Child stressed the importance of selecting high-quality ingredients and preparing them with respect and passion. Her message was not hit-you-over-the-head nutrition. She stressed enjoyment of food, including the pleasures of fresh, seasonal fruits and vegetables. She stressed fresh food that was not overcooked, drowned in gravy, or oversalted. Child attempted to get people away from canned or overprocessed foods and ingredients. Was her cuisine low-fat? Was it healthy? Yes, if taken in moderation, as all good things should be.

In a recent interview, Child was asked how she felt about the state of the American diet and people's attitudes about food. She responded that she was encouraged that the American diet is much more diverse in fresh ingredients and in fruits and vegetables than in years past. She said she liked the idea that people had more access to better eating and to many ethnic cuisines.

What bothered Child was the continuing "fear-of-food" people seemed to have. She didn't like the way people completely excluded certain ingredients, such as butter or beef from their menus. "If you can't enjoy a glass of wine, or some good cheese, if you can't enjoy your meals, how can you enjoy life?" asked Child. She continued that she didn't like to see people thinking about all the things that they couldn't eat rather than all the things they could. Child brought up the issue of moderation versus complete denial.

Child thought the best way to combat this "food as enemy" attitude is to cook good food and keep on talking about it. An example she gave is if someone didn't want to cook with butter, then they should cook Italian, and use

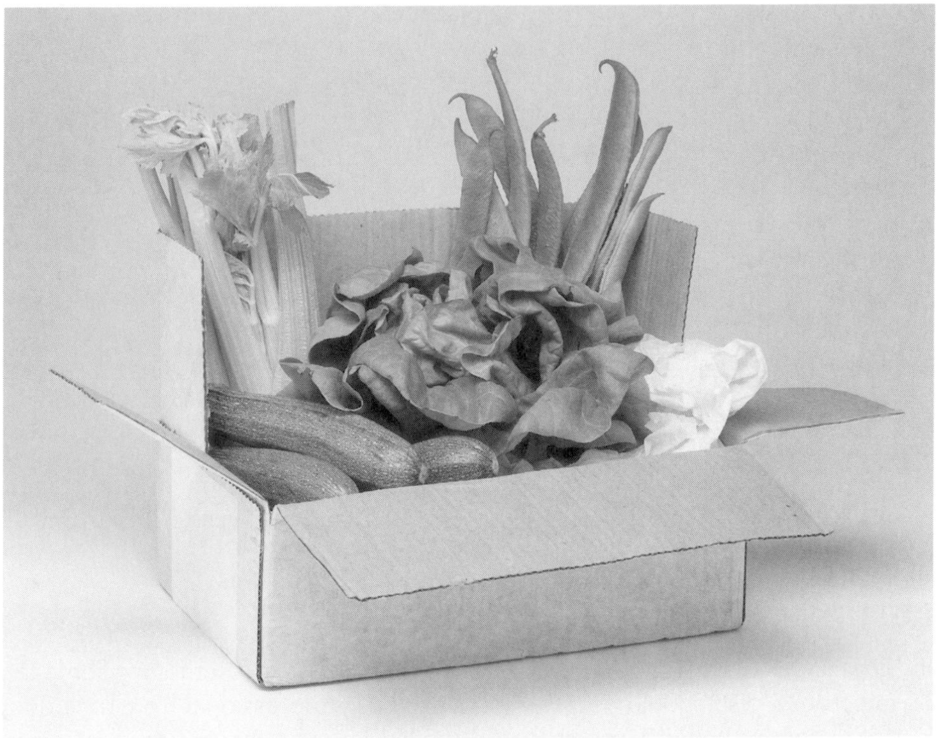

A dynamic chef can create fascinating meals with nutritious ingredients.

olive oil. But they shouldn't turn their back on the good taste of food and make a no-fat, no-flavor dish.

WHO'S ON A DIET?

Nutrition professionals like to toss around terms like "diet," "nutrients," "low-fat," and the like. What are they really trying to say? When people say they are "on a diet," it sounds like they are restricting something or eliminating certain ingredients. In reality, a diet is your normal pattern of eating. You could be on the pizza and beer diet, or on the eating lots of fruit and vegetable diet. A diet is what you typically eat. So, when someone says, "I'm on a diet, what can I order from your menu?" the first question to ask is "What kind of a diet are you on?"

For example, if someone says he or she is on a low-fat diet, you need to find out what that person means. Most people don't see in shades of gray when it comes to fat. They think they're either eating a high-fat or a low-fat diet. The general guidelines for fat intake is no more than 30 percent of your daily calories should come from fat. Any amount lower than that would be considered "low-fat." There are also clinical definitions of low-fat that calculate exactly how many grams of fat are eaten daily.

As you courageously make your way through this book, we will discuss nutrition definitions more thoroughly.

HOW DOES IT ALL RELATE?

How is drinking orange juice going to make my bones stronger? If I smoke, why should I increase the amount of vitamin C in my diet? Why should a woman who is just thinking about getting pregnant in the future maintain an adequate intake of folic acid? Why is nutrition so much like a puzzle? Because devising good nutrition plans is like fitting together the pieces of a huge jigsaw puzzle.

Nutrients do not act alone. Your body can utilize iron only if it has many supporting cast members. Vitamin C helps your body to absorb iron, as does vitamin B_{12}. Calcium blocks your body's ability to fully absorb iron. So, if you are planning a fresh spinach salad for your menu, you'd be impacting your customer's nutrition options by offering a vitamin C–containing mandarin orange vinaigrette. The citrus dressing would increase iron absorption much more than a plain vinaigrette. A buttermilk-based ranch dressing might taste good, but the calcium in the buttermilk will actually decrease the body's ability to absorb iron.

PUTTING IT ALL TOGETHER

Is "nutritious" the same thing as "boring"? It shouldn't be. Removing some fat or salt from a dish should not preclude a culinary professional from including lots of flavor. In the following chapters, we'll discuss how nutritional decisions are made, what effects certain ingredients have on health and how to put this all together for a solid understanding of culinary nutrition. With a good basis

Instead of	Think of
Potato chips or fries	Baked potato, pretzels, baked snack chips, lower-fat popcorn
Snack cakes and frosted cakes	Angel food cake with pureed raspberries or strawberries, small amount of chocolate syrup or maple syrup
Soda and no-juice fruit drinks	Sparkling water, flavored water, fruit juice–blended fruit smoothies, iced tea
Ice cream and ice cream beverages	Non-fat or low-fat frozen ice milk or yogurt sorbets or fruit ice, smoothies made with soy or rice milk or nonfat dairy milk
Cookies with cream fillings	Graham crackers with small amounts of peanut butter and fruit preserves, ginger snaps, vanilla wafers, marshmallows
Chips and dip	Veggie sticks (carrots, celery, broccoli, cauliflower, jicama, radishes, zucchini) and humus (garbanzo bean dip) or dips made with mashed beans or low-fat yogurt

Figure 1–13 Intelligent Grazing

Now that you're in the nutrition mindset, you should think about sneaking nutrition into meals. Here are some ideas to think about when you are shopping and preparing your meals:

- Add canned beans and soy beans to soups, pastas, pizzas, and stews.
- Mix edamame (fresh, cooked soy beans, available frozen) into green salads, pasta salads, eat them as a snack instead of chips or use them as hot or cold side dishes.
- Alternate peanut butter with soy butter, hazelnut butter, and almond butter.
- Flavor soups and stews with miso, pureed vegetables, and nutritional yeast to increase the soy, vitamins, and minerals in your meals.
- Check out soy "coffee cream" as a way to add soy to your menu.
- Add nuts and dried fruit to muffin and quick-bread batters, rice, couscous, and barley.
- Grate raw beets, carrots, jicama, and other root veggies into thin sticks and add to salads and soups.
- Remember lower-fat cooking techniques include steaming, poaching, barbecuing, wok-cooking, broiling, baking, and roasting; use vegetable and fruit juice, vegetable or mushroom broth and wine as a cooking liquid, rather than always using oil or margarine. Not only will this cut down on fat, it will create new taste sensations!
- All fruit is good, and some are great! A food-science professor at Rutgers University went looking for fruit that contained at least eight important vitamins and minerals per three-ounce serving. He found that kiwi, papaya, cantaloupe, strawberries, mangoes, lemons, oranges, and avocados fit the bill. Walnuts and Brazil nuts, carrots, sweet potatoes, and broccoli were pretty high up there in nutrient density, too, with lots of vitamins and minerals.
- Add nuts to sauces, salads, cooked grains, vegetable dips, pancake batter, etc. Yes, nuts are higher in calories than many foods, but their fat is unsaturated, and thought to offer many health benefits. Chop nuts and roll tofu, seitan, or tempeh in them and then bake for a crusted entrée. Puree pine nuts with basil and olive oil to make a fast pesto sauce for pasta or veggies.
- Think pasta. Pasta is low calorie (about 100 calories per half-cup serving), high in complex carbohydrates, low in fat and sodium, and generally is fortified with folic acid, niacin, riboflavin, and iron. Pasta is fast to make, stores well . . . and it tastes good! If you're really in a hurry, have fresh pasta in your refrigerator. After the water boils, it takes only about 2 to 3 minutes to cook.

When it comes to nutrition, your stomach doesn't distinguish what time of the day it is. Who of us hasn't had a bowl of corn flakes for dinner or a cold burrito for breakfast? It's not the chronology, it's the balance. Add some kiwi, tomato, and pineapple slices to that morning burrito and throw together a fruit smoothie to have with that cereal (and toss some nuts into the cereal or have half a bagel with peanut butter alongside it). Remember, you're dedicated to balance and variety on your menu.

Figure 1–14 Thinking Nutrition

in nutrition, a food-service professional can make the most particular customer happy with his or her meal while maintaining a budget and attracting lots of business.

FYI

The food guide pyramid is a colorful tool for nutrition education. You may already be familiar with it, as it appears on many food labels, is taught in many school systems and appears, in poster form, in many community health centers and medical clinics.

The food guide pyramid can be understood and used by most everyone, regardless of reading or math ability. The shape of the pyramid and the graphics make it ideal for teaching a varied audience. You'll have to look closely to achieve fine-tuning of the pyramid, because at first glance it does not seem to distinguish between high-fat meat and beans, or Captain Sugar and a bowl of oatmeal. Use the graphics already in place or develop your own to explain how to use the pyramid most effectively for good health and nutrition.

Figure 1–5 shows you the American pyramid, a familiar teaching tool. Figures 1–6 through 1–9 show the Asian, Mediterranean, Latin American, and vegetarian pyramids. Based on traditional menu selections and readily available ingredients, these pyramids attempt to reflect the melding of ethnic diets with American eating patterns.

For example, many ethnic groups tend to use whole grains and lots of vegetables and fruit in their diets and utilize meat more for flavoring than for a main course. Go with that! Remember, many dietary patterns developed in reference to the types of ingredients available, cost of ingredients, and even cost and/or availability of cooking fuel. Asian hot-pot dishes allowed the cook to prepare an entire meal in one pot, maximizing fuel use. This is a healthy outcome of limited availability. On the other hand, many ethnic groups traditionally use animal fat for cooking oil and tend to fry all the foods for an entire meal. How did this unhealthy process develop?

In many cases, animal fat was more readily available and more easily obtainable than vegetable oils. If you've slaughtered a pig or a chicken for its meat, then you'll have its remaining parts to utilize, including the rendered fat. Growing a seed crop and pressing the oil takes much more time and technology. Once you've got the fat heated, you'll want to cook all your ingredients in it, to save on fuel use.

In many countries, meat, eggs, and dairy are very expensive and considered ingredients to be used for festivities. Refrigeration may not be widely available, so a minimum amount of ingredients are purchased and are used quickly. Another unfortunate side effect of American bounty is the relative affordability and storability of ingredients. The good news is that consumers can take advantage of sale prices or the lower prices of large packages. The bad news is that many items that were formerly eaten sparingly can now be daily delights.

Get to know the ethnic eating patterns of your customers. All diets have their good news and bad news side. Think about how to continue healthy ethnic eating patterns, minimize less healthy traditions and how to moderate the "temptation" foods and cooking styles of both ethnic and American cuisines.

The food guide pyramid can be easily modified for vegetarians, those customers who do not eat animals but do eat animal products, such as eggs and yogurt, and vegans, those customers who eliminate all animals and animal products. Instead of meats and eggs, legumes, nuts, nut butters, and soy products, such as tofu, seitan, and tempeh can be chosen. "Fake" meats and meat alternatives, such as veggie burgers and soy-based "roasts" and deli slices, can be used as well. For vegetarian customers, select soy milk or rice milk fortified with vitamins A and D and calcium. Vitamin B_{12} is a nutritional concern for vegans. Some cereals and specialty products, such as some nutritional yeasts, are enriched with this important nutrient. You may want to write to manufacturers and obtain tasting samples of these products: Be sure to request recipes and consumer information as well.

Ready to scale the pyramids? Here's a rundown of each one with an accent on the healthy aspects and some hints about the unhealthy aspects:

American Pyramid:

6–11 servings of bread, cereal, rice, and pasta. You should be encouraged to select whole grains, enriched breads, corn, bagels, rice, unsweetened cereal, or tortillas.

3–5 servings of vegetables. You should be encouraged to select dark green, leafy vegetables, raw vegetables, vegetable juices, squashes, tomatoes, sweet potatoes, cruciferous vegetables, or legumes.

2–4 servings of fruit. You should be encouraged to select citrus fruit and juice, raw fruit of all types, melons, tree fruit, berries, or bananas.

2–3 servings of meat, poultry, fish, dry beans, eggs, and nuts. You should be encouraged to select lean beef, pork, lamb, veal, egg whites, fish, poultry, assorted beans, and soy foods.

2 servings of milk, yogurt, and cheese. You should be encouraged to select nonfat and 1% milk, yogurt, buttermilk, or cottage cheese and to prepare menu items with these.

Sample Dinner Menu: Baby green salad with sliced nectarines and seasonal berries (one serving fruit, one serving vegetable)

Pecan-crusted oven-roasted halibut with a ragout of white beans and tomatoes, served with tricolored rotini in a pesto sauce (the fish, nuts, and beans could be two to three servings of meat, one serving vegetables, one serving bread, one serving fat)

Caramelized apples with raisins, dried apricots and ginger, served over a cinnamon-apple sorbet (two servings fruit)

Asian Pyramid:

Add millet, rice, and rice noodles to bread group.

Add nuts and tofu to meat group. Understand that deep-frying and stir-frying are popular methods of preparation.

Understand that ginger, garlic, and rice wine and vinegar are low-sodium condiments, while soy sauce, plum sauce, oyster sauce, and hoisin sauce are high-sodium condiments. Dairy products are not frequently used; soy or rice milk may be used as a beverage rather than dairy milk.

Sample Menu:

Vegetable Hot and Sour Soup (two servings vegetables)

Wok-prepared baby bok choy with steamed tofu, fresh chilies, and rice noodles (one serving vegetables, one serving meat, one serving bread, one serving fat)

Sticky rice with sliced mango, coconut and kumquats (one serving bread, two servings fruit, one serving fat)

Mediterranean Pyramid:

Add eggplant, lentils, onions, peppers, olives, and tomatoes to vegetable group.

Add low-fat yogurt, feta cheese, and goat cheese to milk group; omit fluid milk (used infrequently).

Add dates, figs, grapes, lemons, and raisins to fruit group.

Understand that olive oil is the preparation fat of choice. Encourage nondairy calcium-rich foods, such as green leafy vegetables and seafood (with bones, such as canned salmon or sardines).

Latin American Pyramid:

Add corn and flour tortilla and rice to bread group.

Add cactus (nopales) and olives to vegetable group.

Add avocado, papaya, mango, guava, and pineapple to fruit group.

Add canned, evaporated, and condensed milk, soft white cheeses, and sour cream to milk group.

Understand that frying meat and bread are popular preparation methods, lard and butter are traditionally used for cooking, cheese and sausage are used as flavorings and garnishes. In some areas, herbal teas and beverages are popular. Encourage use of lower-fat dairy products.

Vegetarian Pyramid:

Add dark green leafy vegetables daily to vegetable group.

Omit dairy products from milk group; add soy milk, rice milk, tofu, and milk alternates to milk group.

Omit animal products, add legumes, beans, nuts, nut butters, and seeds to meat group.

If you would like to learn more about the various pyramids, especially the Mediterranean, Latin American, and Asian pyramids, than look up information about the Oldways Foundation (*www.oldwayspt.org*). Oldways is dedicated to preserving traditional healthy eating patterns and was instrumental in developing public knowledge about Mediterranean and Asian cuisines.

Nutri-Words

Words and phrases to be familiar with during your study of culinary nutrition.

American Culinary Federation (ACF): the certifying board for chefs in the United States.

American Dietetic Association (ADA): the licensing organization for dietitians and dietetic technicians in the United States.

Baby Boomer: the generation born in the years following World War II, approximately 1942 through 1960. This generation is responsible for a large growth in the population.

Exchange Lists for Meal Planning: a nutrition tool that allows the consumer to calculate the number of calories from carbohydrates, fat, and protein in a meal.

Food Guide Pyramids: nutrition tools developed by the federal government to assist the population in developing healthy eating patterns.

Generation X: the generation born in the mid 1970s.

Goiter: an enlargement of the thyroid gland due to iodine deficiency or other disease state.

Institute of Food Technologists (IFT): a professional organization whose membership includes food scientists, food chemists, food engineers, microbiologists, packaging and equipment experts, and educators.

Iodine: a micronutrient found in ocean foods and enriched food products responsible for thyroid health.

Nutrients: organic substances, such as vitamins, proteins, and water, that are required for growth and maintenance of the body.

Nutrition Labeling Education Act (NLEA): federal legislation that requires all packaged food and all menued food for which health claims are made to be labeled in accordance with federal standards.

Radicchio: a member of the chicory family with crimson and white leaves; can be eaten raw, in salads, or braised, like cabbage.

Recommended Daily Allowance (RDA) versus Reference Daily Intakes (RDI): the RDAs, first established in the late 1960s, are the recommended intakes of nutrients, including vitamins and minerals for healthy people in the United States. The RDIs are based on the highest amount of vitamins and minerals recommended by the RDAs for adults.

Registered Dietetic Technician (DTR): a licensed dietetic technician who has completed the educational and professional requirements of the ADA.

Registered Dietitian (RD): a licensed dietitian who has completed the educational and professional requirements of the ADA.

Research Chefs Association (RCA): a professional organization of chefs who are engaged in research and development, product development, food technology, and organoleptics (the science of taste).

Thyroid: an organ located near the windpipe responsible for the rate control of many bodily functions.

USDA Guidelines for Healthy Americans: nutrition information, in list form, developed by the federal government, to assist the population in adopting healthy eating habits.

World Health Association (WHO): an international organization dedicated to improving health among all the populations of the world.

Whaddaya think?

Questions to study, use as a base for further reading or research or to use for discussion.

1. Do you have some ideas how to parlay good nutrition into big bucks?
2. What would be your nutrition sales pitch to Baby Boomers? To Generation-Xers?
3. What's your definition of health?
4. Do a little salt research: Taste iodized and non-iodized salt. Ask some chefs what type of salt they prefer to use and why. Is iodizing salt still necessary today?
5. In what way can an RD help a food-service operator?
6. What types of collaborations could be formed between chefs and food technologists?
7. If someone is ACF-certified, how much nutrition background might he or she have?
8. Design a healthy, interesting, three-day menu using the Mediterranean food guide pyramid.
9. What are your RDAs for calcium and iron?
10. What do over- and undernutrition mean?
11. Explain the USDA Guidelines for Americans to a front-of-the-house staff working in a health resort.
12. Create some label terms that do not fall under the umbrella of the NLEA that impart the idea of "healthy," " low-fat," and "low-salt."
13. Give your thoughts on a holistic view of nutrition, a la Julia Child, as in have your cake (sometimes) and eat it, too.

Critical Application Exercises

1. Think of a healthy menu promotion for a midrange (cost) dinner house.
   a. Describe the promotion, giving details of menu, products, necessary training, etc.
   b. Create a tie-in product, such as a line of fat-free salad dressings.
   c. Describe how you will use various culinary and food professionals, such as American Culinary Federation certified chefs, registered dietitians, research chefs, etc.
2. Decide on an aspect of healthy eating which interests you, whether for personal health or for business.
   a. Do a Web search, finding at least ten Web sites with pertinent information.

  b. Create an information file, using Web information, that can be used as a reference by fellow students or employees.
3. Write down your favorite holiday or special occasion dinner.
  a. How does it rate on the food guide pyramid?
  b. Can you analyze it according to the Exchange Lists for Meal Planning?
  c. Does it fit into the USDA Guideline for Healthy Americans?
4. Think of a healthy menu promotion for a high-end (cost) dinner house.
  a. Describe the promotion, giving details of menu, products, necessary training, etc.
  b. Create a tie-in product, such as a line of fat-free salad dressings.
  c. Describe how you will use various culinary and food professionals, such as American Culinary Federation certified chefs, registered dietitians, research chefs, etc.

References

Johnson, R. K. & Kennedy, E. "The 2000 Dietary Guidelines for Americans: What are the Changes and Why Were They Made?" *Journal of the American Dietetic Association,* July 2000, 100:7, pp. 769–773.

Dietary Guidelines for Americans Focus Group Study. Final Report. Washington, D.C. ILSI Human Nutrition Institute, 1998.

Healthy People 2010 Objectives. Washington, D.C. US Department of Health and Human Services, Office of Public Health and Science, 1998.

Chapter 2
Thinking Nutrition

Chapter Overview

Objectives

After reading this chapter, the student should be able to:

1. *List the energy-containing nutrients and suggest healthy examples of each.*
2. *Design a nutrient-dense menu.*
3. *Evaluate the value of calories from different menu items.*
4. *Explain the benefits of good nutrition to the individual and the community.*
5. *Suggest ideas for making healthy foods interesting for the consumer.*
6. *Evaluate industry programs for healthy menus.*
7. *Decide on the purchase of organic ingredients.*
8. *Design menus for people with various food allergies.*
9. *Explain how to evaluate false or deceptive food product claims.*
10. *Design healthy menus that include a variety of ingredients.*

Introduction

The following chapter will give you a basic background in nutritional science. With this background, you will be able to decipher the latest diets, make purchasing decisions about food ingredients, design marketing plans, and keep yourself nutritionally healthy. In order to merchandise nutrition, you have to understand it and be able to explain it to staff and customers. Let's first explore some general concepts.

EXPLANATION OF ENERGY AND NON-ENERGY–CONTAINING NUTRIENTS

Nutrients, those parts of food that the body needs to grow, replenish, exercise, and feel good, are divided into two broad categories. The **energy-giving** (or calorie containing) **nutrients** are **carbohydrates, proteins,** and **fats.** The non-energy-giving (or no-calorie) nutrients are vitamins, minerals, and water. Your body can only obtain **energy,** in the form of **calories,** from carbohydrates, proteins, and fats. All carbohydrates whether popcorn, baked apples, or maple syrup, contain four calories per gram. Alcohol is considered a carbohydrate and contains seven calories per gram. However, alcohol does not have the redeeming values of vitamins, minerals, or fiber and should not be considered a nutrient. All fat, whether olive oil or bacon grease, contain nine calories per gram. All protein, whether prime rib or peanut butter, contain four calories per gram. Obviously, your body appreciates a fresh apple more than a fried-apple fritter, but when we're just talking calories, carbs are carbs, fats are fats, and proteins are proteins.

How should you divide up your nutrients? The USDA suggests that 60 percent of your calories come from carbohydrates, no more than 30 percent from fat (with the accent on unsaturated fat) and 10 percent of your daily calories should come from protein. Remember that fat contains 2.25 times more calories per gram than carbohydrates and fat, so you will consume much smaller amounts of fat than carbohydrates or protein. In other words, when you look at your plate, you should see a lot less fat ingredients than protein or carbohydrates.

FOOD FOR THE MIND

Energy = Calories

When reading a nutrient label or article on nutrition, energy and calories may be used interchangeably. Both signify the amount of work the body can do after digesting and absorbing foods.

The American Heart Association modifies this a bit, upping the calories from protein and carbohydrates and decreasing the amount coming from fat. Vitamin and mineral needs can be determined broadly by using the Food Guide Pyramids. If you follow the number of servings for each category, then you should be getting enough of all the vitamins and minerals you need. If you are healthy and don't need to change your nutritional status, you can use the RDAs as a source for determining vitamin and mineral needs. This is because the RDAs are recommendations for people who are already healthy, not for people who need to make improvements or changes in their **health.** As for water, that old stand-by rule of eight glasses (or sixty four ounces or half a gallon) of water per day is a good rule of thumb for healthy people.

You are not on your own when it comes to figuring out what you need to eat and drink to stay healthy. Although there are small variations in recommendations among the "establishment" theories, they all have the same general thrust. Be careful about following pop-culture nutrition recommendations, as they may sound easy and exciting but can have serious health consequences.

NUTRIENT DENSITY

Vending Machine Nutrition

We've said that all carbohydrates, fats, and proteins yield the same amount of calories. Does that mean if you eat a meal of potato chips (carbohydrates and fat) and chocolate ice cream (protein, fat, and carbohydrates) you're getting the same nutritive value as a meal of herb-grilled salmon (protein), potatoes au gratin (fat, protein, and carbohydrates), and honeydew sorbet (carbohydrates)?

Not exactly. Calories are calories, and your body just recognizes them as such. If you need energy right now, your body doesn't care if you give it an apple or a candy bar. It just knows you are giving it calories. However, the way your body uses the calories, and the nutrients attached to these calories is a whole other story.

Japan's Dietary Guidelines:

1. Obtain well-balanced nutrition with a variety of foods; attempt to eat thirty different ingredients per day and eat entrees, side dishes, and starches together.
2. Get exercise in proportion to the amount of energy you take in every day.
3. Eat more vegetable fats than animal fats.
4. Eat only 10 grams of sodium per day (note: that's 10,000 milligrams compared to the USDA's recommendation of no more than 2,400 milligrams per day)
5. Treasure family time and home cooking. Sit down and eat as a family.

(reference: *www.oldways.org*)

References

Squires, Sally. "When it comes to long-term weight loss, there's no magic bullet," *Los Angeles Times*, January 15, 2001, p. A24.

Figure 2–1 Comparison Shopping

Good nutrition is a long-term proposition, not a "quick, I need something to eat," putting-out-fires type of project. Although it is true that a candy bar will give you quick energy, it will not give you any nutrients and will leave you without any energy in a very short time. Your body needs a nutritional savings account of protein, vitamins, minerals, and water in order to function smoothly on a consistent basis. Living on vending machine snacks will give you fast energy, but leave you without the ability to build or repair muscles, fortify your immune system, stand up to aging or remain mentally sharp. If you live the vending machine lifestyle for too long a time, systems in your body will start breaking down, lacking the nutrients necessary for repair. Unfortunately, your body cannot tell you specifically what it wants and will go a long time before it starts to slow down. You're the controlling force and have to make the decision between beer and chips or Caesar salad and cantaloupe.

EVALUATING CALORIES

Look at the potato chip and ice cream meal. Lots of calories. Lots of calories from fat. If you are like many people, you don't require all the calories you get from this meal. That means the body will store the excess calories until needed. Fat is stored all over the body, in the fat cells. Too much stored saturated fat can lead to **heart disease** in some people (more about that in Chapter 5). Both the chips and ice cream are relatively high in sodium, another item of which most people don't need more. Does this meal have any redeeming value? Well, the potatoes may have some calcium, phosphorus, and vitamin C and the ice cream may have some calcium, vitamin A, and vitamin D, so it's not a total wash.

Now look at the salmon, potatoes, and honeydew meal. The salmon has protein and essential minerals, such as calcium and iodine. The fat, which is minimal, could be of the omega-3 fatty-acid type, the type that is supposed to help with heart health. The potatoes do have some fat and sodium with the cheese. However, if made with low-fat dairy products, the au gratin adds an acceptable amount of fat to the meal and contributes calcium, phosphorus, vitamins A and D, etc. The honeydew sorbet is made with pureed fruit that has vitamin C and potassium, so it is a source of carbohydrate with no fat or sodium.

Depending on serving size, these meals could have the same number of calories. One, however, gets its calories mostly from saturated fat with very few vitamins or minerals, while the other gets calories mostly from lean protein and carbohydrates with lots of vitamins and minerals. The second meal is what dietitians would call **nutrient dense.**

Dense Is Best

"Nutrient dense" is another way of saying "getting the most for your money with the least amount of damage." Both a fresh apple and a caramel apple have all the nutrients that apples contain. But the caramel apple has a lot of extra calories without any extra nutrients.

FOOD FOR THE MIND

Nutrient Notes

1 gram of carbohydrate = 4 calories

1 gram of protein = 4 calories

1 gram of fat = 9 calories

1 gram of alcohol = 7 calories

The concept of nutrient density is important for personal health and for designing menus. For example, a three-year-old child doesn't eat very much, yet requires enormous amounts of nutrients. Parents or caregivers need to give three-year-olds food in which every mouthful counts. A baked sweet potato would be a better choice for a three-year-old than French fries. The sweet potato is packed with vitamins A and C, potassium, and protein while the French fries are packed with fat. A customer may want to have a creamy, indulgent dessert while counting calories. A soft-serve nonfat strawberry yogurt sundae with sliced bananas, chopped dates, and figs and fresh berries is relatively low in calories but packed with calcium, vitamins A, C, and D, and iron (from the figs). Get the idea?

Baked, Not Fried

You probably already know that a candy bar is not as good a breakfast as a bowl of oatmeal. But why? They're both carbohydrates, with four calories per gram. There are different types of carbohydrates, and they are used differently by the body. A food made almost entirely of **sucrose** (white table sugar), such as a candy bar, will be broken down very quickly by the body. The resulting energy will be used very quickly as well. A more complex carbohydrate, like oatmeal, will break down slowly. This means that a slow, steady stream of energy is released for the body to use over several hours. The energy from a candy bar may last twenty minutes. The energy from a bowl of oatmeal could last three hours, depending on the type of work you are doing and the amount of energy needed to do the work.

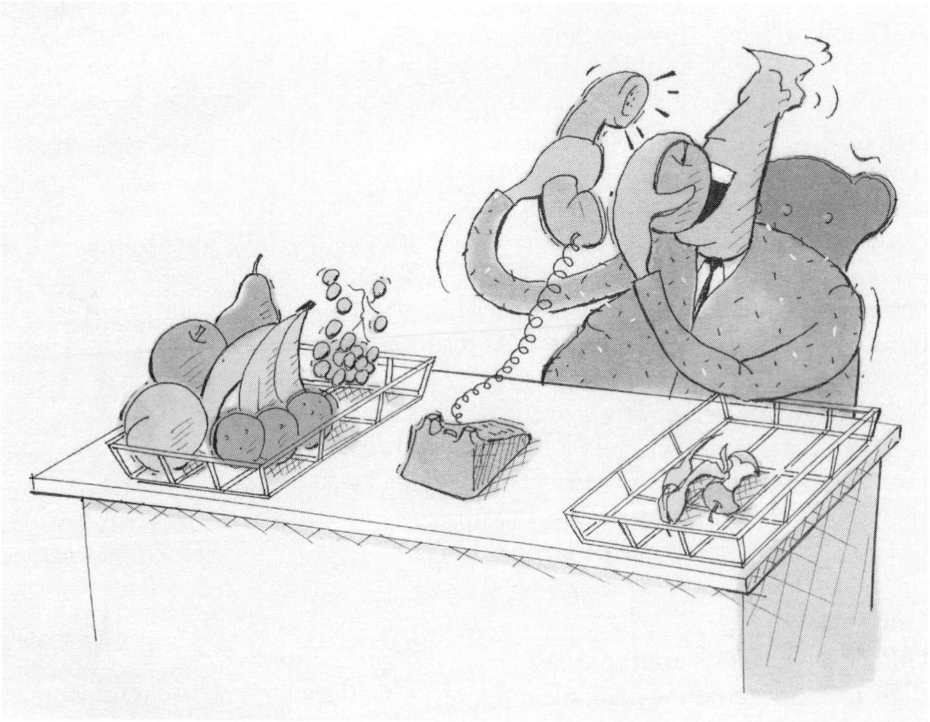

Nutrient dense snacks are best.

"Good Food," you know, that stuff your grandmother would be proud of you for choosing, can help to keep the immune system functioning at its best and can be lower in calories (and higher in nutrients).

Offer:

Fruit Instead of Cookies and Cakes for Snacks
Fresh apples, pears, oranges, grapes, bananas, peaches, apricots, melon slices and dried fruit, poached or baked apples or pears, baked bananas, apple and pear-cobblers (use low-fat granola and graham crackers for a crust)

Veggies Instead of Chips for Snacks
Carrot and celery sticks, radishes, cherry tomatoes, jicama, broccoli, cauliflower, cucumbers, bell pepper strips, roasted summer squash and eggplant, grilled carrots, baked white and sweet potatoes, baked beet, carrot and potato chips

Juice Instead of Soda
Fresh or frozen orange juice, cranberry-orange juice blends, grape juice, nectars, such as apricot, mango, peach, pears; smoothies made with fresh fruit and juice; fruit ices or sorbets made with juice, pureed fruit and sweetened with orange or apple juice concentrate.

Whole Instead of White
Whole-wheat bread and pasta, carrot and zucchini muffins, corn bread, oatmeal, graham crackers, bran and whole-grain cold cereals

Figure 2–2 Encouragement

Add nutrient density into the equation. The candy bar has calories, a little sodium, and that's about it. The oatmeal has dietary fiber, thought to reduce the amount of cholesterol in the body, some B vitamins, some minerals, and no sodium. As you can see, nutrition is just a matter of thinking about what you need and which food will be the best to supply it.

Another way to look at nutrient density is to consider which foods require the least amount of effort for your body to use with the most reward. Fat takes more energy to break down. Excess fat can force your body into unhealthy situations, taxing your liver, gallbladder and heart. The breakdown products of fat can cause some damage to the body in some people. Carbohydrates are easily broken down and absorbed by the body, with few breakdown products. So, between French fries and a baked potato, your body is voting for the baked potato. Mostly carbohydrate, the potato is easily digested and used with minimal effort. The baked potato would be considered the more nutrient-dense food.

DEFINITION OF HEALTH

Healthy Is as Healthy Does

"Health" comes from the old English word "hale," which meant having a strong mind and a strong body. What's your definition of health? Is it the absence of illness or discomfort? Is it the ability to perform normal tasks and to enjoy life? Is a healthy person the one who sleeps well, works and exercises hard, has a good appetite, and can honestly say, "I feel good?" When you think of your definition of health be sure to include mental, physical, and social aspects of "feeling good." And remember how important nutrition is for good health.

Nutrition has always been and will continue to be an important part of total health. The only problem is, nutrition is a lot like the weather. Lots of people talk about it, but not too many people do anything about it.

Whaddaya Gonna Do About It?

What can food professionals do? They can learn about good nutrition to keep themselves, their families, and their fellow workers healthy. They can realize how good nutrition can be a popular component of most menus and can increase profit and bring in more customers. You would be surprised at the popularity of "healthy" food products. Sales of "healthy" foods have soared in the past several years. With the proper merchandising and the right spin, you'll sell more whole-wheat pancakes than the buttermilk variety.

BENEFITS OF ADEQUATE NUTRITION

Good nutrition is a wonderful thing and can lead to many happy outcomes. Poor nutrition can lead to infant mortality, physical and mental developmental delays in children, illness and pain of every type for every age group, adult disability and lack of productivity, lack of independence and physical ability for seniors and increased health-care costs for everyone. Well-nourished populations are productive, successful, and have lifestyles that are the envy of their neighbors. Many business and industry companies acknowledge this and have incorporated "wellness" programs as part of their employee benefits. Many companies expect their food-service providers to offer "healthy" menus and cooking classes as part of employee perks.

That's where the food professional comes in. With good nutrition you can see:

1. More normal birth-weight babies born without birth defects.
2. Improved dental health.
3. Increased productivity in school and at work.
4. Better learning ability and success in school.
5. A reduction in the number of people with hypertension **(high blood pressure)** and heart disease.
6. A reduced incidence of childhood and adult obesity.
7. A reduced incidence of Type I (insulin dependent) and Type II (noninsulin dependent) **diabetes.**
8. A reduced incidence of prenatal, infant, childhood, and senior anemia.

9. Possible reduction of certain types of cancers.
10. A reduction in **osteoporosis** (fragile bones).

MAKING FOOD CHOICES

The Good Old Days Are Gone (Thank Goodness)

In the "good old days," people relied on family members or educated members of the community to teach them about good nutrition. This might have been as simple as which poisonous plants to avoid or as complex as what foods were important for different parts of the life cycle.

Before there was a lot of food processing, there were not a lot of food choices. Nutritional choices were easy. Eat what's available or starve. People ate foods that were in season, drying or salting some seasonal foods to be eaten in the winter. Diets were limited to what could be cultivated or caught, with a few staples, such as salt, coffee, flour and sugar, purchased on a very occasional basis. A little different from today!

In those days, the emphasis was on getting enough to eat. In other words, there was an accent on using every bit of food, preparing it in a way that was safe, so no one got sick. Menu selection was not discussed at length, as the food supply was largely seasonal.

As the food supply expanded and **food technology** offered more choices to the consumer, nutrition started entering the picture. When you have a choice, you can start thinking about nutrition. Meals were started with fresh or canned fruit or juice, entrée plates were expected to contain vegetables (even if no one ate them) and even baked goods could be made with different varieties of whole-grain wheat.

More Is Not Necessarily Better

What is interesting, as consumers had more and varied foods from which to choose, nutritional health did not greatly improve. Perhaps fewer people had obvious nutritional-deficiency disorders, like rickets or scurvy. But nutrition-related illness, such as high blood pressure, heart disease, osteoporosis, and diabetes did not decrease. They actually increased! Just because lots of healthy foods are available does not mean that people will necessarily select them.

Several interesting studies have been done with groups of people who have elevated their economic status (Squires, p. 1). When people were at the lower end of the economic scale, they tended to eat more home-cooked meals, with ingredients such as fresh vegetables, whole-grains, beans, and potatoes. As their economic situation improved, they added more meat, high-fat items, such as cheese and bacon, and ate out more often. As their income increased, they discarded the home-baked, whole-grain bread, rice-and-bean combinations, stewed vegetables and bean and vegetable soups and went for the sugar-coated cereal flakes, store-bought white bread, bacon and eggs, and restaurant meals.

High blood pressure, heart disease, gout, and diabetes used to be called "rich man's" diseases. The situation described earlier illustrates why. What can we learn from this?

Higher Prices Do Not Necessarily Mean More Nutrients

Many inexpensive foods, such as pasta, rice, and beans are low-fat and high in nutrients. Many expensive foods, such as prime rib, salad dressing, and ice cream are high in fat and salt and low in nutrients. Unfortunately, in many cases, as soon as people can afford more expensive food items, they leave the healthier, more economical items behind. In other words, when we as a nation were poor, we ate a lot of healthy foods, just not enough of them and not enough variety. Now that we've got some money, we buy the food we like and don't worry if it's good for us or not.

Food selection seems to have come full circle in the past several years. Vegetarianism is on the rise, leaner cuts of meat have become more popular, and it is not unusual to have someone order an egg white omelet. Now that the country has had years to harden its arteries and increase its blood pressure, more and more people are learning to look for foods that are "good" for their health and appealing to their palate.

Evaluating Nutritional Health or "So How Healthy Are You?"

How can you figure out if you are in good nutritional health? Nutritional health can be surmised partially by personal assessment. If the only thing you've had in the past month that resembled fruits and vegetables is a lime Lifesaver or an orange soda, than you know you've got some work to do. How you feel, how you look (as in skin, hair, and teeth) and how much energy you have are nonscientific but practical ways to assess how good your food selection is.

There are more precise ways to determine nutritional health as well. We will speak more on this in Chapter 8. Let's get a brief overview.

Height and weight charts are helpful, fast, and cheap guides. But they are not really good indicators of nutritional health. For example, someone who has been working out and eating right but doesn't lose weight has probably lost fat and built muscle. Muscle is more dense than fat. So after several months of doing the right thing, the scale can provide frustration, but not an accurate picture. As far as health goes, you are concerned about what percentage of your weight is fat, not your overall weight. Checking your weight is fine to do but doesn't give a total health picture.

Blood and urine tests look at your blood glucose (sugar) levels, cholesterol and triglyceride (another fat found in the blood that indicates heart health) levels, and they see how your kidneys and liver are working. These types of tests can help evaluate if you have enough protein in your system. They can even tell if you are a chronic alcoholic! A health-care professional can look at blood and urine work and begin to diagnose diabetes, kidney disease, heart disease, anemia, and many other nutrition-related diseases.

Healthwise Express is a two-unit quick-service, healthy food chain in Chicago that brought in over $1 million in sales in 2000. The idea for the concept came from Rosemary Deahl's film production company. The company specializes in shooting food commercials. Deahl noticed that customers seemed more and more ready for new concepts and were asking for and ordering more healthy foods.

Deahl had been a vegetarian for many years. She noticed that not only could she not grab a quick vegetarian meal on the way to or from work, but she couldn't even find quick meals that weren't loaded with fat. After a lot of research and trial and error, Deahl decided on a quick-service concept to be open from 6:30 A.M. to 5:00 P.M. (for the business crowd) with a menu that offered only 25 percent or less calories from fat. Deahl uses a combination of from-scratch and branded items, such as bottled juices or baking mixes for her mostly vegetarian menu.

HeartWise Express, a successful restaurant, has sandwiches, salads, wraps, rice bowls, smoothies, and fresh baked goods on the menu. Both units see a lot of repeat business. Breakfast and lunch hours are standing-room only. Here's a sampling of menu offerings:

HeartWise Burger: veggie burger topped with lettuce, tomato, onions, and pickles on a whole-wheat bun

Moroccan Rice Bowl: spicy pinto beans, hominy, peppers, onions, golden raisins, green onions, and cashews served on brown rice.

Killer Tofu Sandwich: A blend of tofu, celery, and onions, with a secret mix of seasonings, served on pumpernickel with lettuce and tomato

Smoothies: fresh fruit blended with bananas, non-fat or soy yogurt, sweetener, and ice.

Figure 2–3 Healthy and Quick Service Can Be Used in the Same Sentence

There are many advanced techniques for assessing nutritional status. One of the more complete, and more expensive, is a full-body CT scan. This picture of your entire insides allows health-care professionals to visualize your arteries and veins and all your internal organs. They can spot an enlarged liver or clogged arteries. Treadmill stress tests check to see how well your heart is functioning. Some stress tests include an injection of dye that allows health care professionals to see how open your arteries are. There are bone scans to detect osteoporosis, water displacement tests to measure what percentage of your body is fat, allergy tests to detect which food ingredients you are sensitive to, and glucose tolerance tests to see if you might be diabetic. There are many, many ways to measure nutritional health.

So, now you've got an overview of how a lot of your customers, employees, and peers are monitoring their health. Perhaps they have found that they need to lose weight, or get their blood pressure or cholesterol down. Or, maybe they are happy where they are and want to eat healthy meals to keep it that way. How are you going to get them to your restaurant?

Think Nutrition: Rev Up the Interest in Healthy Foods

"Diet" food has never had a popular following. Who looks forward to ordering the diet plate or eating at a restaurant called something like the "Skinny Palace"? On the other hand, **spa cuisine,** such as that served at luxury resorts, like the Golden Door in San Diego, California, has always been lusted after. Let's face it, there is no romance in the once-typical "calorie-counter" plate, composed of a broiled-to-death hamburger patty, no bun, a scoop of cottage cheese, way too many sliced tomatoes and several canned peach halves. Restaurants peddled this as a weight-loss platter for years. If you calculated the calories, you'd probably be better off with the steak and French fries.

On the other hand, think of the allure and the romance of lemon grass scented seabass served on a raft of pasta-cut summer squashes and accompanied by jasmine rice with a raspberry-pepper jus. No calories will be missed with that kind of menu!

Food professionals cannot just announce "healthy" menus to their customers. Time needs to be taken to assess what customers are interested in, and if this can be accomplished with the level of quality and budget a food establishment has.

There are lots of different types of healthy menus. Perhaps customers are just looking for a restaurant that employs low-fat, but high-flavor cooking techniques as an alternate to high-fat methods. Perhaps fat and salt are not an issue, but fresh, seasonal, and regional ingredients are what interests customers. The bicycle or running club that meets at your place every Sunday may be looking for lots of tasty carbohydrates. Other customers may not care how many calories are in the steak but want sugarless or low-calorie desserts. Do your homework before you start to order special ingredients or offer new menu items.

WHAT THE INDUSTRY IS DOING: THE RITZ CARLTON AND WESTIN HOTELS

Look at how the Ritz Carlton Hotel chain has begun to think about nutrition. Several years ago, **macrobiotic** diets were very popular among the type of clientele that frequented the Ritz. We're talking people such as Tyra Banks, the supermodel; Steve Wynn, the former owner of the Bellagio, the Mirage, and Treasure Island casinos in Las Vegas; a former Mr. Olympia; and several professional athletes. Started by Buddhist monks seeking a spiritually and physically pure life, the macrobiotic diet entails preparing foods simply, minimizing meat and dairy, maximizing fresh produce and using regional and seasonal ingredients. The idea was to give your body the type of fuel that would make it strong and healthy, able to fight off foreign invaders, like disease, and maintain structures, like the skeleton, in a strong state.

The Ritz's Marina Del Rey (California) chef saw more and more requests for "healthy" and **vegetarian** menu items and not just a few macrobiotic queries. The challenge was to add healthy menu items that could be prepared and presented with the caliber of the usual Ritz Carlton offerings.

Naked, dry chicken breast and limp steamed vegetables would not do. Here are just some of the items that appeared on the Ritz.

Carlton's healthy menu:

Heirloom tomato salad with goat cheese, basil, and tomato soup
Woked long beans and crispy garlic chip salad with citrus soy
Organic vegetable salad
Roasted eggplant, melted tomatoes, sweet peppers, and curry
Charred artichokes, fennel, Parmesan, and olive oil
Italian white beans and arugula salad
Crispy tofu braised with wild mushroom
Curry vegetable hot pot
Portobello Reuben with broccoli sprouts and brie on rye
Spicy peanut noodles with cold vegetable poached chicken breast
Vegetarian bento box with woked vegetable spaghetti
Vegetable curry udon with shrimp

To start the day, the chefs included organic fresh fruit and vegetable juice (apple, beet, carrot, wheat grass, melon, and ginger) and a Japanese bento box of miso soup, rice, nori, fruit, and sweet egg.

At their Pantheon Restaurant, the Ritz Carlton's Mediterranean-influenced operation, a duet of tomato martinis with fresh mozzarella, tomatoes, basil, and sweet onions or roasted golden beets and peppercorn-aged goat cheese, served with mustard greens and walnut, tomato and eggplant soup with toasted pine nuts and basil or olive ravioli filled with goat cheese, heirloom tomato sauce, and olive oil were offered. Check out the Mediterranean food guide pyramid; you'll find this menu offers gourmet renditions of it.

In the same vein, the Westin Hotel Chain decided several years ago to devote a certain percent of their menu to healthier items. They called the program "Smart Dining." With the help of an RD, they decided that the menu items would all be less than 20 percent fat, low in salt and calories, and, where possible, high in fiber.

Westin really pulled out all the stops with this program. They purchased healthy items from their purveyors for the mini-bars in individual guest rooms, including bagels, yogurt, sports bars, whole-grain cold cereals and bottled waters, caffeine-free sparkling waters and unsweetened teas. They offered information about healthy eating in guestroom brochures.

All the recipes for the program were developed by corporate chefs and analyzed by a consultant RD. The method of analysis was the American Dietetic Association's exchange lists. A corporate cookbook was assembled listing analyzed recipes, calorie and nutrient breakdowns for individual portions, paired wine, serving suggestions, and preparation guides.

Ten international chefs, a winemaker, Westin's international foodservice director, and a registered dietitian met at Westin's corporate kitchens. In just three days, all the recipes for the cookbook were prepared, analyzed, paired with wines, and photographed. In addition to their culinary responsibilities, the chefs attended seminars that explained how to use the exchange systems and how to select healthy ingredients.

The resulting work was a 200-page cookbook with photos and nutritional analyses. Dessert and pastries were amazing, almost all under 250 calories, including spiced tea morning loaf, pumpkin date muffins, apple crumble currant coffee cake, mountain berry meringue, blueberries in Kahlua cream, lemon cheesecake (made with non-fat ricotta cheese and non-fat yogurt), and chilled citrus consommé. Breakfast was even more creative, with shiitake mushroom and tomato omelet (made with egg whites), hominy hash with chilies and smoked turkey, seven-grain almond granola pancakes, millet crepes with dried fruit compote and toasted pecans, almond crepes with wild berry compote, and vegetarian soufflé with tahini sauce

INGREDIENT SELECTION

What about ingredients? Traditional foods are grown or processed in traditional ways, which means with chemical pesticides or fertilizers. Until recently, organic foods, foods grown and processed without chemicals, were not regulated by the federal government. States and private farming consortiums self-regulated agriculture and processing plants. We'll go into more detail about organic foods in later chapters.

The popular definition of organic food continues to be food grown or processed without chemicals, such as hormones, antibiotics, chemical additives and preservatives, artificial colors and flavors or coating agents, such as paraffin. The debate continues about whether bioengineered foods can be considered organic. Another debate is how long it takes a farm to convert from traditional (with chemicals) to organic. It takes a certain amount of time for ground water, trees, soil, etc. to be free of chemicals that have been used over the years. Prices for organic foods have tended to be higher, as there is usually a lower yield per acre. Organic foods are not as "pretty" as traditional foods, with apples that may not be uniform in color or squash that are not uniform in size. If your customers request organic foods, you'll need to take this information into consideration.

Raising food organically does not ensure more nutrition. An orange can only contain so much vitamin C. The issue with organics is not necessarily the nutrient content but the safety factor.

Are organic foods safer? Scientific reasoning would tell us that something that doesn't have chemicals or hormones should be safer to eat. But could there be remainders of foodborne-illness microorganisms remaining from natural fertilizer used? There may still be chemical residues from air or water drift. The debate about organics continues on.

Organic foods are handled just like traditional foods in the kitchen. When purchasing, don't be as picky about appearance and try to buy locally, like at area farmers' markets. Budget more for organic foods. You may have to raise menu prices to meet the costs. As with traditional produce, wash organic produce thoroughly. Processed organic foods will have shorter shelf lives, as they do not have chemical preservatives. Plan your purchasing and preparation calendars accordingly.

FOOD ALLERGIES: ARE THERE ANY PEANUTS IN THE SAUCE?

Beyond good nutrition, a food professional needs to be aware that people may refrain from eating foods because they are allergic to them. It is very important that the people serving the food know all the ingredients in the dishes they are serving. People may be allergic to wheat, certain kinds of fruits and vegetables, certain herbs and condiments, nuts, fish and eggs, to name a few.

Watch Out for Those Strawberries:

Food allergies or **intolerances** are a point of discomfort for nearly everyone at some point in their lives. You eat something and have an unpleasant or uncomfortable reaction and wonder, "Was I allergic to something in the food?"

In reality, there are lots of food intolerances around, but not as many food allergies as people believe. In the United States, only about 3 percent of children and about 1 percent of adults have true food allergies.

A NUTRI-BAR

Allergy or Intolerance: What's the Difference and How Do They Work?

An *allergy* is an abnormal response to food that is triggered by the immune system. It is very important for people who have true food allergies to identify them and avoid the foods or ingredients that cause them. True food allergies can cause very serious illness and can even be fatal. The human intestine is coated with antibodies that protect against food allergy development. Depending on genetics, normal diet, etc., the body sometimes ignores these antibodies and treats certain foods, almost always proteins, as the enemy. When this happens, a person may experience swelling that narrows the lips, throat, and windpipe, making it hard to breathe, and possibly causing death. Less severe allergic reactions can be gastrointestinal distress or hives or rashes. Foods that commonly cause allergies include peanuts, wheat, nuts, some preservatives, shellfish, eggs, and soy.

An *intolerance* is an undesirable reaction to a food that is not caused by the immune system. This reaction may be caused by the lack of an enzyme (such as lactase), asthma (certain food chemicals, such as sulfites, trigger asthma attacks), psychological triggers (eat your broccoli or you'll get it for breakfast!), or overindulgence. Intolerances are not generally as severe as allergies, but they can cause great discomfort. Intolerances sometimes mimic food poisoning. Foods that commonly cause intolerances include dairy products, beans, some fruit, and finfish.

Lobster: Alien Life Form?

In adults, the most common foods that cause allergic reaction are shellfish (like shrimp, crayfish, lobster and crab), peanuts (which are a legume), tree nuts (such as pecans or walnuts), fish, and eggs. In the small fry, eggs, milk, soy, and peanuts are the most common triggers.

The foods that cause allergic reactions are the ones that are eaten the most frequently (oh no, is there a pizza allergy?). For example, rice allergies are frequent in Japan, cod allergies in Norway, and wheat allergies (from pasta) in Italy.

There are many theories as to why certain foods cause certain people to react badly and don't affect other people at all. In the 1800s, there was a commonly held belief that lobster and shrimp caused "reactions" because these ocean delicacies were actually from another world (we're talking planet here, not the soap opera)! There is very little agreement among the scientific community about allergies, but one thing is for certain: Food allergies must be taken very seriously, as they can have serious consequences.

The good news for kids is that they can outgrow allergies to milk, soy, and fruit; peanut and shellfish allergies tend to hang in there. Unfortunately for grown-up kids, an adult-acquired allergy is generally here to stay.

Food intolerances may come and go and can be more or less severe depending on the amount of food eaten, the time of day or even food combinations. Food intolerances are commonly caused by dairy products **(lactose intolerance)**, sulfites (added to foods as a preservative and antioxidant and also naturally occurring in many fruits and vegetables), wheat, and fruit (especially strawberries and oranges). In fact, some people may not realize that they have a food intolerance. They may not relate that queasy feeling every time they have a grilled cheese sandwich to a dairy intolerance.

Gluten intolerance, or gluten-sensitive enteropathy, is actually a food allergy and is caused by the lack of certain enzymes in the body. When gluten (found in all wheat products) is eaten, severe reactions can occur, which, over time, can cause serious disease. People who are gluten intolerant have to avoid foods made with wheat, rye, barley, and any other products that may contain gluten.

Phenylketonuria (say that ten times fast) is a serious food allergy. People born with phenylketonuria cannot synthesize the amino acid phenylalanine. Phenylalanine is found naturally in most protein foods and is also an ingredient in some artificial sweeteners. Perfectly harmless to the majority of people, phenylalanine intake can actually be fatal to those born without the ability to process it. The next time you have the opportunity, look on the label of a diet soda can; you'll see the warning label for phenylketonurics.

Hold the Cheesecake

A food intolerance that is attracting a lot of attention is that of lactose intolerance. The enzyme lactase is necessary to digest lactose, the "sugar" found in milk and dairy products. Some children are born with an inability to produce a sufficient amount of lactase and are given soy substitutes; this intolerance sometimes disappears with age. On the other hand, lactose intolerance may develop with age. One theory is that, as we get older and drink less milk, the body "forgets" how to produce lactase. Lactase deficiency may be hereditary and is also seen in people of similar ethnic background, such as Asian and Mediterranean groups.

Whatever the cause of lactose intolerance, the person who has it can be extremely uncomfortable when dairy products are eaten. Symptoms run the spectrum of a mild stomachache all the way to full-fledged flu-like conditions. Some lactose intolerant people can handle all dairy products in very small quantities, some can handle only several products (yogurt and aged cheeses are typical), and some get faint at the sight of a milk carton.

There are several products designed for lactose intolerant people. **Acidophilus**-infused milk (also called "sweet acidophilus") is regular pasteurized milk which has had lactose-eating bacteria added to it. The bacteria perform the lactose digestion that lactose intolerant people can not. Acidophilus milk can used be wherever you would use regular milk. There are enzyme preparations that people can take before eating lactose-containing foods; these aid in digestion.

Of course, you as the food-service person can experiment with milk replacements. Soy milk or soft tofu can be used in sauces, soups, puddings, and dessert preparations. If there is a soy allergy in addition to lactose intolerance (food service is always a challenge!), then try rice, almond (oh no, check for nut allergies!), or grain milks. Try making a tofu cheesecake—many people can't tell the difference!

Detective Work

Diagnosing food allergies is not an easy task. Very few definitive and simple blood tests cover the spectrum of items that may cause allergic reactions. The doctor has to play detective, taking detailed histories of food eaten, reactions to food, how people who shared the food reacted (to rule out contamination or food poisoning), time of day food was eaten, etc. Skin tests may be used that expose small areas of skin to the proteins extracted from suspected allergens.

There are some controversial methods used to diagnose allergies, such as cytotoxic blood testing and sublingual challenge tests. The cytotoxic test includes adding a food allergen to a blood sample and seeing how the blood reacts. Sublingual testing includes administering dilute food allergens under the tongue and observing if a patient reacts adversely to them.

A Little of This and a Little of That

An established way to diagnose food allergies is by controlling and observing a person's diet. Two of the most accepted methods for diagnosing food allergies are the challenge diet and the elimination diet. The challenge diet is designed to get a response from a person, and the elimination diet is designed to prevent responses.

With a challenge diet, the doctor or dietitian will ask that certain foods or ingredients be served to the patient to see what type and what severity of response is caused. For example, if a patient feels that dairy products cause

A NUTRI-BAR

Sample Elimination Diet

Here is a sample two-day initial elimination diet; this is the most basic form of the diet and is not meant to be used for extended amounts of time or without the supervision of a health-care professional

Day One

Breakfast	*Lunch*	*Dinner*
Apple juice	Grape juice	Puree of carrot soup
Rice cereal	Baked potato	Steamed rice
Peach slices	Grilled zucchini	Braised green beans
Rice crackers	Poached chicken	Grilled steak
	Pears with syrup	Peach sorbet

Day Two

Breakfast	*Lunch*	*Dinner*
Pear nectar	Apple pear juice	Celery mushroom soup
Rice cereal	Steamed potatoes	Baked yam
Grapes	Peach slices	Applesauce
Rice cracker	Grilled turkey	Poached chicken
	Baked apple	Pear slices

an allergic reaction, a meal will be designed to include a dairy product in measurable amounts. In this way, it can be determined if dairy is the allergen. Challenge diets have to be carefully monitored and will not be used to determine allergies where severe reactions have already occurred. Shellfish and peanuts can cause very severe allergic responses and are rarely used in challenge diets. Challenge diets should always be overseen by medical personnel.

With an elimination diet, the most neutral diet possible is devised for the patient. In fact, as much variety is removed as possible. This is so the cause of allergic food reactions can be pinpointed. Elimination diets are highly personalized and may not be nutritionally adequate if used for any length of time. In the first phase of an elimination diet, dairy products, caffeinated products, alcohol, eggs, nuts, peanuts, citrus fruit, tomatoes, wheat, spices, and artificial color are removed from the menu—quite a challenge. The patient is asked to keep a detailed food diary, noting all reactions. After an initial four to six days on the very simple diet, one food is added. If there is a reaction, then a food allergy has been found. Only one food can be added at a time so reactions can be monitored. Elimination diets take a lot of commitment from both food-service personnel and from the patient, as extensive records must be kept and meals carefully planned.

So Now That We Know, What Do We Do?

Food allergies are treated by food avoidance. This is not as easy as it sounds. If you provide made-from-scratch menus, then you know where the flour, eggs, tomatoes, soy, peanuts, shrimp, phenylalanine (found in artificial sweeteners, such as Equal™ or Nutrasweet™), and the like are hiding. If, however, you use any prepared products, then you need to become a label expert. Soy products, such as soy flour, soy analog (used as a meat extender), and soy protein can show up in cheese, snack foods, baking and dessert mixes, ready-to-use entrees, and beverage mixes. Monosodium glutamate (MSG), a common food allergen, is not just found in Asian foods or in salty foods. Used as a flavor enhancer, MSG is found in baking mixes, pudding mixes, ice cream and sherbet and frozen desserts, as well as in salad dressings, canned soups, canned and frozen vegetables, gravy mixes and prepared meats. Wheat can be found in corn chips, peanuts in non-peanut–flavored snack mixes, and flour and soy can be in in canned tuna! Polish up those reading glasses.

Training food staff to be sensitive to food allergies is an imperative. At the least (and not very wonderful), an ignored food allergy can cause extreme discomfort. At the worst, it can be fatal. A daily production meeting is a way to explain "what's in what," that the seafood chowder has both fish (generally okay) and shrimp (a big wheel in the food allergy world) and the chocolate cake has eggs.

Does Food "Cure" Arthritis?

The Baby Boomers and the athletes in your customer base may be feeling the twinges of **arthritis.** As more and more people look to their food to cure or prevent certain conditions, you need to be one step away on your menu design and your marketing. Although no one is sure what causes arthritis and there are no absolute cures for it, some food modifications have been found to help some people. Here are the facts:

Arthritis has plagued humankind for as long as there has been humankind. Despite centuries of study, the cause and the cure are still unknown.

A NUTRI-BAR

If You Can't Eat That, Then Try This

Here are some suggestions foods to substitue for common food allergens.

If Allergic to This. . . .	*Try This*
Peanuts	Cookie or cake crumbs (for dessert toppings), shredded coconut, fruit purees (think peach or grape), apple butter, chopped raisins
Eggs	Egg Replacer™ (a dry vegan mix which can be used in baking), cottage or ricotta cheese, vegetable oil, tofu (if no soy allergy)
Tomatoes	Basil (as in pesto sauce), pureed carrots, onions and garlic (for flavoring)
Milk	Soy or rice milk, grain beverage, tofu, cream of wheat or rice (for cooking), mashed potatoes (for "creaminess")
Shellfish	Grilled or baked tofu, fin fish, grilled chicken, turkey, or vegetables

A NUTRI-BAR

Wanna Learn More?

Food Allergy Network
10400 Eaton Place, Suite 107
Fairfax, VA 22030
www.foodallergy.org

Asthma and Allergy Foundation of America
1125 15th Street, N.W., Suite 502
Washington, DC 20036
www.aafa.org

United States Department of Agriculture
Food and Nutrition Information Center
(301) 436- 7725
www.nalusda.gov/fnic/index.html

There has been some link between arthritis and the health of the immune system. Good nutrition is important for a healthy immune system, so food does play an important role. Arthritis is one of those conditions where every type of diet has been tried, with little to no success. This does not prevent people from making phony claims about the benefits of eating ten pounds of grapes or eliminating dairy from your diet to "cure" arthritis.

In rheumatoid arthritis, the immune system mistakenly attacks the tissue that covers the bone, causing inflammation, pain, loss of fine-motor skills, and decreased strength. No one can give a definitive answer as to why the immune system turns on itself or how to control these attacks.

Since people with arthritis have weakened bones and joints, there is a connection between arthritis, nutrition, and obesity. Since excess weight strains bones and joints, weight loss and/or the maintenance of appropriate weight can help control some of the pain from arthritis. It's not known why, but weight loss even affects arthritis in the hand, alleviating some of the discomfort and pain.

Some food allergies stimulate the immune system and tend to aggravate arthritis (causing even more "attacks"). People with arthritis need to be aware of which foods cause allergic reactions and avoid them as much as possible.

There are no medical cures for arthritis, but pain relievers can alleviate some symptoms. Some pain relievers may cause gastric distress, so be aware that some people with arthritis may require soothing foods from time to time.

Nutrition Concerns

If you can think of it, it has been tried as an arthritis-preventing diet. Over the years, it has been recommended that arthritis patients eat no meat, no milk, and no acid-containing foods. It has also been suggested that diets consist of

A NUTRI-BAR

Truth or Dare

Over years, the following have been offered as "cures" for arthritis, to no avail:

- alfalfa
- molasses
- cod liver oil
- fruit
- garlic
- honey
- lecithin
- megadoses of vitamins
- wheat germ
- brewers yeast
- injections of gold salts
- copper bracelets

only raw foods, fruit only, liquid foods, and many other variations too weird to mention. As far as is known, none of these diets offer any kind of relief or help and can be dangerous. To date, a well-balanced diet is the best type of diet for arthritis patients (and for just about everyone).

Allergic reactions may aggravate arthritic conditions, as stated before, so if foods that sometimes cause allergic reactions are eaten, such as shellfish, eggs, soy, milk, and peanuts, the person should be watched to see if there are any responses.

A healthy immune system is important to decreasing arthritis symptoms and good nutrition is important for a healthy immune system. Think balance (you can use the Food Guide Pyramid, the ADA Exchange Lists, etc.), five servings of fruit and veggies per day (a serving is approximately half a cup of juice, a cup of raw veggies, or a small apple or banana, for example), lots of fluids (forget the caffeine and keep alcohol to a minimum).

Taken from another perspective, poor nutrition is almost a guarantee of a depressed immune system. Poorly functioning immune systems can almost guarantee a worsening of arthritic conditions, so start pushing the fruit, veggies, whole-wheat products, and sparkling water.

As mentioned above, excess weight stresses joints that are already stressed by arthritis, so your clients may be concerned about weight loss. Take a reasonable approach to weight loss, remembering that it takes about a 3,500-calorie reduction to lose one pound (sigh!). Weight loss should not be more than one or two pounds per week. Offer a good selection of low-calorie beverages (iced and hot herbal teas, sparkling water with a splash of juice, etc.) and crunchy, lo-cal snacks (fresh fruit, baked potato or apple chips, unsalted pretzels, etc.), and menu selections that are baked, broiled, steamed, poached, braised, grilled, barbecued, or stir-fried rather than deep-fried or sautéed.

FALSE OR DECEPTIVE NUTRITIONAL CLAIMS: SPEAKING OF SNAKE OIL—GRAND PROMISES WITH FOOD

Many different types of food and the nutrients they contain have been sold over the years as "cures" for anything from "woman's complaint" to cancer to impotence. To understand how the truth gets twisted, let's establish some basic nutritional truths:

1. Calories in = calories out. If you need 2,000 calories to meet your daily energy needs and you eat 2,000 calories, you will maintain your weight. If you eat more than 2,000 calories, then you will gain weight. And if you eat less than 2,000 calories you will lose weight.
2. One pound of weight = approximately 3,500 calories. To gain a pound, you have to add 3,500 calories to your diet. To lose a pound, you have to take away 3,500 calories.
3. Weight cannot be lost in the spot you select. You can tone an area or tighten up some muscles, but you can't pinpoint a spot where you decide to lose weight.
4. As far as we know, there are no out and out nutritional cures for cancer, AIDS, hepatitis, or other severe diseases. Good nutrition is very important in helping the body combat any disease. No one food has been shown to be a "cure."
5. Herbs are medicine, too. Just because a product is advertised as "all natural from herbs" doesn't mean it can't make your blood pressure rise or cause kidney damage.
6. There is no one food that will reverse or prevent aging, get rid of wrinkles or cellulite or whiten your teeth. Good nutrition is a combination of lots of different types of food and fluids. If someone has found the fountain of youth, he or she is keeping it a secret.

But Can I Lose Ten Pounds in a Weekend?

Refer to numbers 1 and 2 above. Many, many different products on the market guarantee weight loss. Our favorites are grapefruit juice or vinegar preparations that will "burn" fat away. Not only is this not possible, it could be dangerous to drink acetic acid (the acid contained in vinegar) over extended periods of time.

Not only is it impossible to quickly lose real weight, as in fat, it can be dangerous to lose more than one or two pounds per week. Certain pharmaceutical and **herbal preparations** can induce the loss of fluid in the body, called the **diuretic effect.** Along with water, you lose essential minerals, such as potassium and magnesium. Lose enough of these minerals and your blood pressure can rise, your heartbeat can become irregular, and your kidneys can fail. Every year people are seen in emergency rooms after taking certain weight-loss formulas. In the past several years, some deaths have been associated with some of these products.

How to Separate Fact from Fiction

Any plan that guarantees that you can "lose all the weight you want and eat everything you want" is obviously false advertising. It either doesn't perform the way it promises, or it's so dangerous no one should use it.

But what about products that seem reasonable? Many years ago, a "diet bread" was very popular. You were to eat a slice of this thin bread before meals and follow the diet plan that came with the bread. People lost weight on this plan, crediting the bread for having special properties.

How did it work? If you replaced the bread with a glass of water, you could save money and lose weight. If you take a small portion of a low-calorie food before you sit down to a meal, you are already partially full. This will usually let you eat less and still feel full. The diet plan that came with the bread was a reasonable, low-fat menu. Was this product false advertising? No. Just a way to make the wallets of non-nutrition–savvy people a little lighter.

No foods burn or absorb calories. No single foods will enhance athletic performance or guarantee an "A" on your next exam. The only way to lose weight is to take in fewer calories than you need. The only way to enhance performance, scholastic, athletic, or otherwise, is to eat a balanced diet, drink lots of fluids, and get reasonable amounts of exercise and rest.

But, you say, I feel better when I take the herbal study aid, or I lose weight when I make my favorite diet soup. The mind is a wonderful thing! The power of suggestion makes many things possible. If you think and believe that that herbal study aid will help you concentrate, then it probably will. That diet soup you make is probably low in calories and fat and you probably are careful about the other foods you eat with it. If it works and does no harm, then go with it!

Whatever you do, use scientific reasoning when assessing nutritional or diet aides. If it seems too good to be true, it probably is!

BACK TO REALITY: KEEPING RECIPES HEALTHY AND INTERESTING

Is all this talk about eating healthy, nutritious foods getting you nervous? Afraid you'll never see a plate of nachos again? Don't worry. That's not where we're going with this.

Unless people are very ill, they do not need severely restricted fat or salt diets. Unless you are a culinary professional working in health care, you probably won't need to supply severely restricted diets. However, your customers who are interested in nutrition will appreciate menus that offer lower-fat items that are interesting and high in flavor.

Does this mean you have to get rid of the butter and the bacon? No, it just means that you need to decrease the amount that goes into each portion. Perhaps you can crumble the bacon on a turkey club sandwich, using one slice

The following is a partial listing of Web sites that provide good health and nutrition information.

Name of Organization	Web Address
USDA Food Data	*http://www.usda.gov/cnpp*
Berkeley Wellness Letter	*www.berkeleywellness.com*
Tufts University Nutrition Navigator	*www.navigator.tufts.edu*
Harvard University Health Information	*www.intelihealth.com*
National Cancer Institute	*www.cancernet.nic.nih.gov*
American Cancer Society	*www.cancer.org*
American Dietetic Association	*www.eatright.org*
American Heart Association	*www.americanheart.org*
Government Healthfinder	*www.healthfinder.gov*
International Food Information Council	*www.ifi.cinfo.health.org*
Mayo Clinic Oasis	*www.mayohealth.org*
Quackwatch	*www.quackwatch.com*
Communicating Food for Health	*www.foodandhealth.com*

Figure 2–4 Working the Web

instead of three. Serve the sandwich on a seven-grain bread and pile on the sliced cucumbers, tomatoes, shredded lettuce, sprouts, and even shredded carrots. You've added extra nutrition, extra taste, and extra crunch and removed some of the fat.

Can you bake with butter? Of course! What would oatmeal cookies be without it? Just replace some of the butter with applesauce or apple juice concentrate. Add chopped raisins or dates and some chopped nuts to increase the fiber content and the unsaturated fat amount. It's not the ingredient; it's the amount.

Many chefs produce great chocolate cakes with a minimum amount of fat from shortening and eggs. The secret? Believe it or not, they use fruit purees, especially dried plum. Before you say "ick," you should know that some of the top pastry chefs in the country are doing this.

Fried foods are great, but there are other ways to prepare food that are just as, if not even more, tasty. You can barbecue, grill, roast, sauté with stock, oven poach with parchment, stir fry or smoke foods rather than stick them in a tub of fat.

In addition to thinking about the types of foods you might reduce when designing menus, you will also want to consider which foods add more nutrition. By adding more nutrition, you can also add more color, texture, and interest. For example, a creamy white wine sauce looks good on broiled fish. But so does a tri-colored pepper coulis. Three different colors of bell peppers are roasted, peeled, pureed, and seasoned. Arrange a stripe of yellow, green, and red pepper coulis on a dinner plate, and then place a serving of golden broiled red snapper on top of the coulis. Lots of color and flavor, no fat.

Wines and **fruit and vegetable purees** can be reduced to the texture of a glaze and served as a sauce for entrees, vegetables, rice, pastas, and grilled vegetables. Beans are available in every color of the rainbow. Use them as a garnish for entrees, tossed into raw and cooked salads, pureed for sauces or dips, or used as a main ingredient in a vegetable burger. Lentils can be formed into a paté and black beans can be pureed for a "creamy" full-flavored soup.

Root vegetables add texture and mouth feel without fat or salt. A classic **potage Crecy** (puree of carrot soup) can be updated by eliminating the cream that is used to finish it; instead use low-fat kefir (a Middle Eastern tangy cultured milk). Sweet potato can be used as a pie filling, beets as a crimson puree to form a base for soup or a dramatic sauce. Celery root cooks down to a white, tastes-like-cream-and-butter base for soups.

When you get a recipe that is higher in fat or salt, or lower in nutrients than you'd like, think about swapping ingredients that have the same texture or flavor without the extra fat or salt. Many newstand magazines, such as *Cooking Light* or *Vegetarian Times* have columns devoted to modifying gourmet recipes into sleeker versions.

Have you noticed that many of the methods for healthy food preparation are also more economical than the methods requiring more fat? Healthy menus are not just good for your customers; they're good for you!

Nutri-Words

Acidophilus: a lactose-loving benign bacteria. Added to milk to help drinkers digest lactose. Acidophilus-infused milk makes milk tolerable for lactose-intolerant people.

Arthritis: a very general medical term which covers over 100 illnesses that cause swelling and pain in the joints and connective tissues

Calories: a general term for the amount of energy that can be released with the digestion and absorption of food.

Carbohydrates: carbohydrates should be the primary source of energy in the body and consist of a large group of foods that can be sugars, starch or fiber.

Diabetes: a disorder of the endocrine system in which the body cannot properly utilize insulin. Diabetes can result in circulatory disorders, loss of vision, heart disease, and other syndromes.

Diuretic effect: certain natural and synthetic chemicals trigger the loss of body fluids. Along with water, essential nutrients, such as potassium, are lost. Certain diet preparations contain diuretics, causing dangerous water loss.

Energy: the fuel needed to do chemical, electrical or physical work. Sometimes used interchangeably with the term "calorie."

Energy-giving nutrients: the energy obtained from carbohydrates, fats and proteins. Carbohydrates and proteins yield four calories per gram and fats yield nine calories per gram.

Fat: the energy-giving nutrient with the highest amount of calories per gram. Fat is essential for body temperature regulation, synthesis of many hormones and body chemicals and for energy.

Food allergy and intolerance: allergies are adverse reactions to food or environment and are longer lasting than intolerances, which tend to be transient. Food allergies are the immune system's reaction to a food protein, which it identifies as a danger. Symptoms of food allergies can consist of wheezing, sneezing, skin rash, swelling of the throat, diarrhea and cramps, heartbeat irregularities, and shock. The foods most commonly causing allergic reaction include peanuts and nuts, shellfish, wheat, and eggs. The foods most commonly causing food intolerances are dairy, fruit, and spices.

Food technology: the science of food, which can include package engineering, research and development of new flavors and products, and quality-control analysis.

Fruit and vegetable purees: fruits or vegetables that have been peeled, chopped, and processed to a smooth texture.

Gluten intolerant: an inability to digest, absorb or tolerate one of the protein components of wheat, called gluten.

Health: balance of mental and physical well-being with an absence of disease.

Heart disease: a group of diseases that may involve the heart muscle or the veins and arteries feeding into the heart.

Herbal preparations: teas, pills, capsules, and powders containing roots, leaves, stems, flowers, and seeds of plants thought to have health-giving properties. Chamomile tea or Gingseng capsules would be examples of herbal preparations.

High blood pressure: blood pressure which measures above 120/80. Also called "hypertension." High blood pressure may be an indication of underlying disease, such as heart disease, diabetes, or kidney disease.

Lactose intolerant: an inability to digest, absorb, or tolerate one of the carbohydrate components of diary products, a dairy sugar called lactose.

Macrobiotic: with origins in Buddhist philosophy, a macrobiotic diet is a primarily vegetarian diet with ten increasingly exclusive stages. The highest stage consists of only brown rice and water. Macrobiotic diets have come to be thought of as whole-foods (whole grains, fresh fruits, and vegetables) diets, sometimes used to "cleanse" the system.

Nutrient dense: foods that have high levels of "good" nutrients, such as protein, vitamins and minerals, and low levels of empty calories. For example, a baked potato would be considered more nutrient dense than French fries.

Organic: organic foods are raised and processed without chemicals and meet the standards of the USDA National Organic Program.

Osteoporosis: a "thinning" of the bones caused by a combination of poor diet and hydration, lack of exercise, and disease.

Potage Crecy: a classical pureed soup with the main ingredient of carrots.

Protein: proteins consist of strands of amino acids. Different arrangements of amino acids result in different proteins. Proteins are important in many body functions, including integrity of muscle tissue and skin.

Spa cuisine: a term originally coined at *Le Pyramide,* in Paris, by renowned chef Ferdinand Point. Spa cuisine has come to mean gourmet cuisine which accentuates the flavor of regional foods in season and uses very little fat or salt.

Sucrose: a sugar built from glucose and fructose. Is also known as table sugar and is commonly used to sweeten beverages, candy and bakery products.

Vegetarian: a person who excludes animals or animal products from the diet. A vegetarian generally does not eat meat but will eat dairy products and eggs. A vegan excludes all animal products from the diet, eating only plant-based foods.

Whaddaya Think?

1. What types of healthy carbohydrates, proteins, and fats do you regularly include in your diet?
2. Which do you usually follow for distribution of calories, the USDA's recommendation or the American Heart Association's?
3. Where do you get your eight glasses of non-caffeinated, non-sugared, non-alcoholic fluids every day?
4. How is it that a baked potato is more nutrient dense than French fries?
5. Which is more nutrient dense: soft-serve frozen yogurt or nonfat soy milk; carrot cake or buttermilk biscuits; vegetable omelet or cheddar cheese omelet; roast turkey thigh or broiled red snapper?
6. What's your definition of health?
7. Can you see at least six good reasons to concentrate on good nutrition?
8. If you wanted to see how healthy you are, what types of tests or tools would you expect a health-care professional to use?
9. Give some entree suggestions for several spa cuisine dinners, a la Ritz Carlton or Westin.
10. Do you see an advantage for food-service operators to use organic foods when possible?
11. How would you train your front-of-house staff about handling customers with food allergies?
12. What's the "best" arthritis diet?
13. Suggest several decadent desserts for lactose-intolerant customers.
14. You have an unlimited budget. Design the ultimate healthy fast-food operation.

Critical Application Exercises

1. Review the concept of "nutrient dense." Select the more nutrient-dense items from the list below, explaining why you made the choice:
   a. Cole slaw or shredded iceburg lettuce
   b. Banana split or fresh orange
   c. Raisins or brownies
   d. BLT or cheddar-cheese omelet
   e. Nachos with cheese or baked potato with salsa

2. Outdo the Ritz Carlton. Think of an upscale healthy breakfast promotion that you can market to Ritz Carlton–level chains.
3. Field trip! Visit a natural foods store and check out the fresh and processed organic foods. Compare prices with traditionally grown and processed foods.
   a. Which type of food was more expensive? Was the price difference appreciable?
   b. Are both types of food esthetically appealing to customers? If you taste-tested any of them, how do flavors compare?
   c. Prepare an argument, pro and con, for both sides: Why I use traditional food products in my restaurant. Why I use organic food products at my restaurant.
4. Suggest ways to train front-of-the-house staff to handle customers with food allergies.
5. How might you offer suitable alternatives to the following menu items, for customers who have to cut back on fat, salt, or calories, but don't want to lose all the flavor:
   a. Guacamole (avocado dip) and nachos
   b. Pizza, extra cheese, extra sausage
   c. Philadelphia cheese steak (nice, greasy beef with cheese sauce, fried onions, and peppers)
   d. Two scoops of chocolate ice cream with hot fudge, whipped cream, and chopped nuts

References

Squires, Sally. "When it comes to long-term weight loss, there's no magic bullet," *Los Angeles Times,* January 15, 2001, pg A24

Chapter 3

The First and Last Anatomy Lesson

Chapter Overview

Chapter Objectives

After reading this chapter, the student should be able to:

1. *Detail the anatomy of taste*
2. *Suggest how to develop the palate*
3. *List the components of flavor and suggest how to maximize each one*
4. *Trace the breakdown of nutrients through the digestive tract*

5. *Explain the role of ancillary digestive organs*
6. *Plan menus that cater to people with various nutrition related conditions*
7. *Explain how digestion and absorption is affected by stress*
8. *Suggest how to improve personal kidney health*
9. *Detail how over the counter medication and supplements can affect nutrition*
10. *Offer alternatives to caffeine in daily fluid intake*

ANATOMY OF TASTE

Pre-Tasting: Scratch and Sniff

Before you start digesting and absorbing, you gotta eat. And before you eat, you gotta see and smell. Taste builds into **flavor,** and before you know it, that mango sorbet is gone.

Your nose and **mouth** are the gateway to culinary paradise. Just think, as a food-service professional, you'll have at least ten-thousand **taste buds** per customer to tantalize. You know that your tongue is able to perceive four taste sensations: sweet, salty, bitter, and sour. It is also proposed that there is a fifth taste—*umami*—or savory. This is described as the taste from soy sauce or roasted meats.

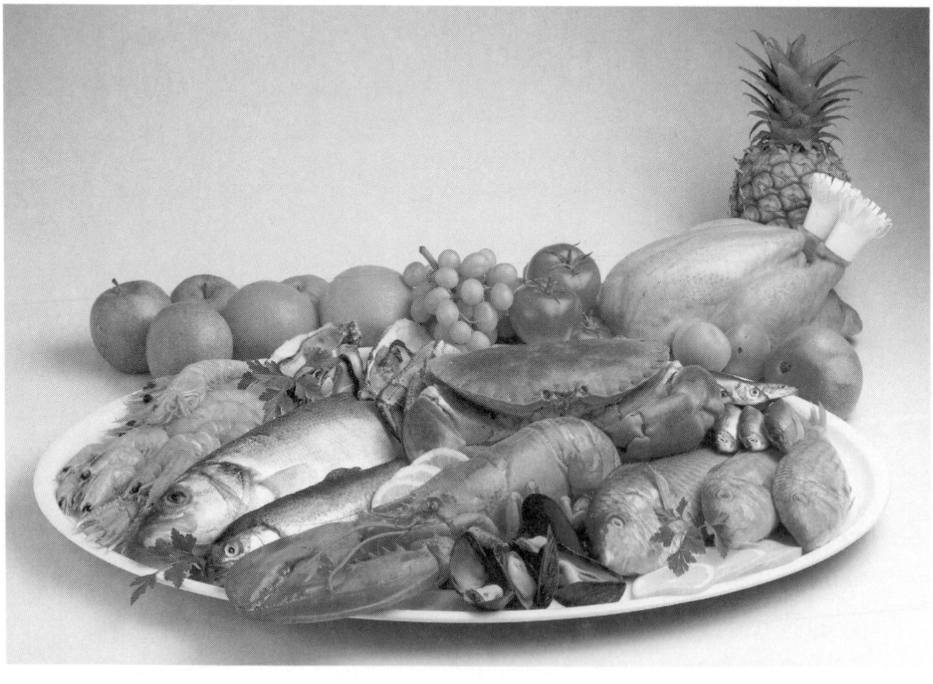

"See" and "smell" are an important part of "eat". Start with fresh ingredients.

Not Just the Tongue

Taste does not begin or end on the tongue. The back of the throat, the lining of the mouth, and the tonsils also have taste buds. Approximately 90 percent of taste relies on your ability to smell. Think about it. When you have a cold, your tongue is not affected, but you still can't taste very much. If your nose is stuffed up, you can't get the amplification you need to taste.

FLAVOR

Components of Flavor

Tastes are airborne aromas before they hit your mouth. Think about that freshly brewed coffee or that baking bread. Inhale. Cells at the top of the nose sense these aromas and translate them into messages for the brain. The brain receives the messages and sends down an "ahhhh!" When you take a sip of coffee or a bite of bread, you release the taste-making chemicals in the food. Between the chewing and sipping, you bring in air and pump these tastes past lots of taste receptors. The more air and more taste buds, the more messages that can get to the brain. This is why you can't taste very well when you have a cold. Your sinus passages are probably swollen or stuffed, preventing air from getting in. Your taste buds are not "sick," but without air, they can't sense what's passing over them.

Flavor Testing: Coke™ or Pepsi™

The classic test to prove this is to close your eyes, pinch your nose closed and allow someone you trust to feed you several unknown pieces of fruit. With just texture to go on, you can't distinguish between an onion or an apple.

Taste is an important part of nutrition and survival. Bitter is sensed way at the back of your tongue. The position in which bitter is situated is considered a built-in survival technique. In nature, few sweet things are poisonous, but many bitter things are. If you happen to toss something into your mouth with very little chewing, it bypasses the sweet, salty, and sour sensors. Everything has to hit the back of your tongue before being swallowed. So, if you toss a bitter, poisonous berry that requires little chewing into your mouth, the bitter sensors at the very back of your tongue will send a fast message to the brain, asking for assessment before swallowing.

Tasting as a Survival Mechanism

If food is tasteless, people tend to not want to eat it. On the other hand, if food has an exciting, interesting taste, people will take extra portions. Nowadays, many people wish food didn't taste so good to them, so they can cut back on calories. In the good ol' cave-people days, if you didn't eat what was available, you starved. People with acute tasting abilities could sense subtle flavors that sparked their appetite. You taste, you like, you eat, you live another day to chase that sabre-tooth tiger.

In modern times, people at both end of the lifecycle have many nutritional needs. Small children and seniors need to eat nutrient-dense varieties of foods. Without taste, their intake suffers, as does their health. Although you may not be attempting to coax your restaurant clients to improve their nutritional intake, by making them roasted garlic asparagus or the savory orange-glazed broccolini, you're performing both a culinary and nutrition service.

Look and See: Developing a Palate

Taste, smell, touch, sight, and sound are all part of flavor. So are temperature and texture. **Visual perception** (what something looks like) and **textural perception** (how something feels in your mouth) are important components of taste acceptance. Consider this. If you serve people a cola drink that is clear, rather than brown, they'll probably tell you that it does not have much flavor. Limp, pale celery has a strong celery flavor, but no color or crunch; most customers will tell you it has no flavor. If you like crisp bacon, you'll probably perceive that lightly cooked bacon doesn't have much flavor.

Try this experiment: Purchase a large bottle of clear, lemon-lime soda. Pour the soda into five identical clear glasses. Place a drop of red food coloring in one glass, yellow food coloring in another, green in another. Leave two glasses free of food coloring. Place all the glasses but one in the refrigerator and allow to chill. Allow friends or family to sample all five of the sodas. Explain only that these are samples of citrus sodas. It's almost guaranteed that the yellow-colored soda will be identified as "lemon," the green as "lime," and pink as "cherry-" or "berry-" lemon, the cold, clear sample as "boring" or regular lemon-lime soda and the warm sample as "too sweet" or "no lemon flavor." Your participants won't believe you when you show them that all the samples came from the same bottle. Remember this experiment when you are attempting to feed a three-year-old child or trying to merchandise a new menu item. Perhaps you've heard that English beer doesn't "taste good." It tastes just fine. It could be the same brand of beer. It's usually served at room temperature, and you're used to drinking it iced cold! In reality, you can taste more of the beer at room temperature.

Temperature affects flavor in a big way. You perceive flavors best when they are close to body temperature (98.6°F). Foods that are superhot or supercold can't be properly tasted. Your taste buds, which are made of protein like the rest of your skin and muscles, don't function well at extreme temperatures.

Try this. Take several spoonfuls of your favorite ice cream. Now let some melt. Try it again. You'll probably get a more intense flavor, which could be a good thing or a bad thing. There's a reason that inexpensive red wine, such as sangria, is served chilled and expensive red wines are allowed to come to room temperature. The colder the product, the less your taste buds can sense. The warmer the product, up to 98.6°F, the more you can taste.

Behavior Modification

Flavor and taste are also influenced by age and environment. Babies prefer sweetness when they're born and progress to saltiness in about six months. Babies and young children experience bitter flavors more intensely than adults do, so they tend to dislike bitter-tasting foods. This may be nature's way of protecting children, as many poisonous substances found in nature have a bitter taste. Kids don't turn up their noses at Brussels sprouts or broccoli because they just hate them. These vegetables genuinely can be too strong for a child's palate and can taste very strong and unpleasant to them.

We also "learn" our **taste palate.** If not given salt, you don't miss having salt on your food. If you are given a lot of salted foods, then your taste buds learn to rely on the "BAM!" of salt rather than more subtle natural flavors. When's the last time you tasted the potato in your French fries? The salt generally overpowers the flavor of potatoes. With the right texture, you could serve salted cardboard to some people, their palates have become so "salted out."

Behavior modification can influence your taste palate. Maybe you always got mild chicken soup when you had a fever, ginger ale when you had an upset **stomach,** or a chocolate cake for every birthday. You will taste these foods and associate them with special events. This could be a good thing or a bad thing. The taste of chicken soup could remind some people of comfort and caring and some people of being sick. So take the safe way out when designing a recipe and rev up your chicken soup with lots of seasonings, like peppery chicken tortilla soup or Thai hot and sour chicken soup.

Super Taste Bud

Some people have super tasting ability. It's thought that these people are born with more taste buds. Genetics help, as do early culinary experiences and the state of oral health. Some expert tasters can sip a cup of coffee and tell you at which elevation the coffee beans were grown. Wine connoisseurs with developed palates can identify the year, growing area and bottling technique of still (uncarbonated) and sparkling wines.

Smoking = No Taste

Aging does not mean that people will lose all sense of taste. However, smoking, coffee, cola and tea, allergies, and some medications can exert enormous influence on taste. Heavy smokers lose most of their tasting ability pretty early on. Some medications influence the way taste buds function. Other medications leave an off-taste in the mouth, making everything taste odd. For example, potassium supplements, given to people taking high blood pressure medication, have a strong, metallic taste and make everything taste "rusty."

DIGESTION OR RIGHT TO THE GUT

As unromantic as it sounds, food is ultimately about **digestion** and **absorption.** A decadent, twelve-course Escoffier meal and a bag of chips both break down to carbohydrates, fats, and proteins somewhere between your mouth, **esophagus,** stomach, **small intestine** and **large intestine,** with some help from your **pancreas, kidney, liver** and **gallbladder.**

Simply put, digestion is the breakdown of the nutrients in food, and absorption is the transport of the nutrients around the body to where they're

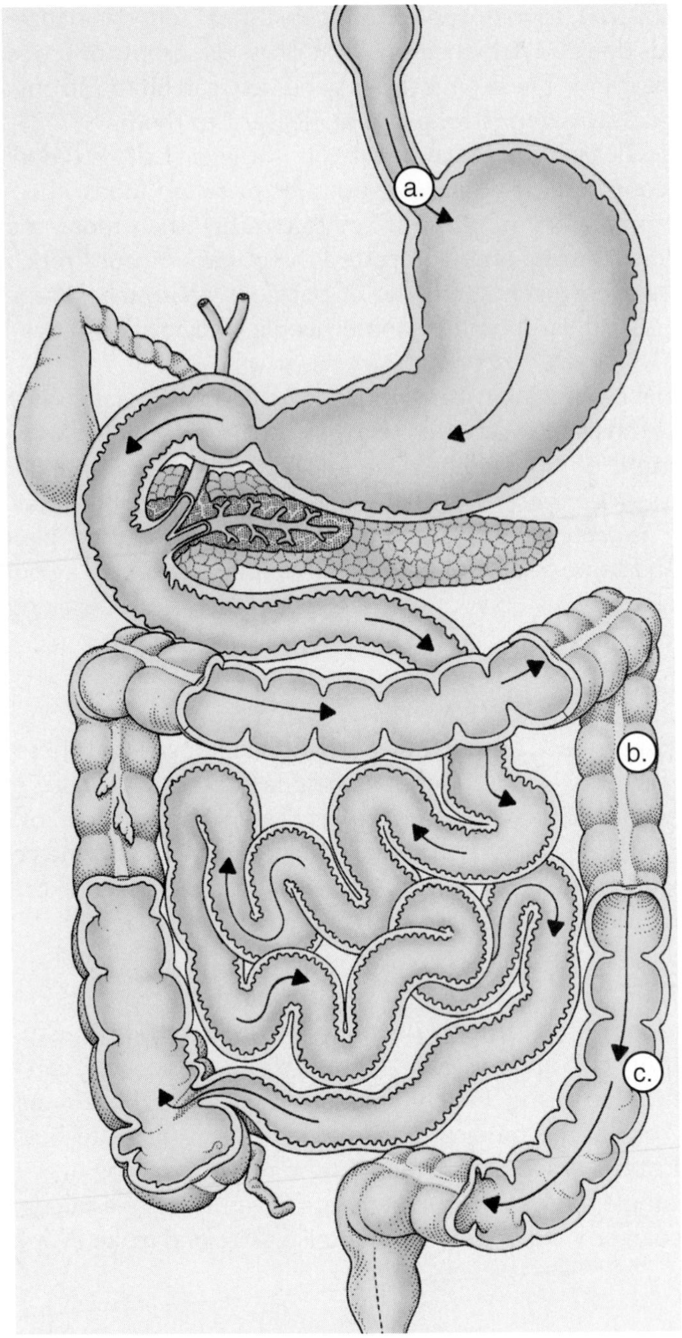

Figure 3–1 A short tour through the digestive system: a) stomach, b) small intestine (portions of), c) large intestine

needed. Chewing up food is not enough to extract the nutrients from it. Your body needs to do a little chemistry, a little ripping and tearing, before you can turn that popcorn into usable energy.

Your body is at one level a very sophisticated and advanced machine, and on another level it's pretty primitive. Digestion and absorption are a bit of both. Once you've chewed and swallowed, your body performs an intricately choreographed dance of interacting muscles, passageways and personally autographed chemicals. Your brain tells your small intestines to start ebbing and flowing, your pancreas to start brewing the insulin, and your large intestine to prepare to synthesize some vitamins. You couldn't design machinery that worked so smoothly, especially on autopilot, since everything we just described is done unconsciously, as reaction and reflex.

As we've discussed, your palate is a finely tuned instrument. Once that freshly squeezed blueberry-guava juice or that buttery cranberry-lemon scone has been swallowed, the "touchy-feely" part is over. Your body doesn't care how much you've spent on ingredients or how long it took to prepare a meal. It's looking for **glucose,** a breakdown product of any carbohydrate you ingest; **amino acids** from protein, whether from lobster or beans and rice; and **fatty acids** from olive oil or cheddar cheese. Vitamins, minerals, and water are broken out from food and sent to where they're needed.

Breakdown of Nutrients

All carbohydrates are broken down to glucose, all proteins to amino acids, and all fats to fatty acid. Some foods are easier for your body to tear down. This means you get more energy from foods that are easier for your body to get at. A good example is the protein from eggs versus the protein from rice and beans. Both are high in protein, but egg protein easily falls apart, whereas rice and beans have lots of fiber and make the body work to get at the contained protein. When you eat an egg, you get close to 100 percent of the protein it has. When you eat rice and beans, you get closer to 75 percent. Just as an aside, eggs are considered by scientists to be the perfect protein, utilized by the body better than any other kind of protein.

> FOOD FOR THE MIND
> During digestion, the body attempts to break all carbohydrates to sugars, all proteins to amino acids, and all fats to fatty acids and glycerol.

Anatomy of Digestion

Before you can use the nutrients (absorption) you have to get at them (digestion). Digestion is your body's way of breaking protein into amino acids, carbohydrates into simple sugars, and fats into fatty acids and glycerol. Your body does not know how to use a piece of fried chicken. But it does know how to digest the protein (from the chicken), the carbohydrates (from the flour or bread crumbs used for the coating) and the fats (from the cooking oil), and absorb the amino acids, simple sugars, and fatty acids from that lovely piece of chicken.

Mouth

Digestion is a team effort. Muscles, hormones, **enzymes,** beneficial bacteria, fluids and internal organs cooperate to break that pizza into a usable format. Digestion begins in the mouth. **Saliva** contains specific enzymes that begin to break down carbohydrates. Carbohydrates begin to be digested in the mouth and are finished off in the small intestine. Chewing breaks the food into smaller pieces, making it easier to moisten with saliva, and exposing it to more digestive action. The smaller the pieces of food, the more efficiently digestion works throughout the entire process. So there is truth to the rumor that you should chew your food twenty times before swallowing. You'll wind up doing the work one place or another.

> FOOD FOR THE MIND
> Feed those Fillings (Cavities) Sugar is not your teeth's enemy, it's the enamel-leeching bacteria that live on sugar that are the enemy. You remember from your food-safety classes that bacteria need time, temperature, air, water, the correct acid level, and food to grow. Sound like someplace in your body? Yes! Your mouth! You can't do anything about the temperature, or the water or air in your mouth, but you can do something about the food. You have a certain amount of bacteria in your mouth at any one time, no matter how much you brush and floss. Some of those bacteria would love to break down your tooth enamel. If you don't feed the bacteria, it won't grow. Since carbohydrates are the only thing that begin to digest in the mouth, keep your mouth free of carbohydrates and the enamel-corroding bacteria won't grow. Sugar does not "rot" your teeth—it's the uninvited guests in your mouth that do.

Esophagus

Once you've swallowed, it's all downhill from there, literally. The food travels down the esophagus. The esophagus is no more than a conducting tube, known for its propensity to bulge out and cause heartburn and **hiatal hernias** (more about that later). Just remember that the esophagus needs gravity to work. If you have a huge meal and then sack out on the couch, the esophagus has to get five brownies down a narrow tube, working against gravitational pull—an almost impossible task. Think about stuffing a couple of sandwiches and a supersize soda down a tube with the diameter of a garden hose (at best). This is the very good reason for you to eat reasonably slowly and chew your food thoroughly. Every once in a while, there will be an emergency room case of someone who gets a large piece of hot dog stuck at the bottom of his or her esophagus. This has to be surgically removed. Don't overcrowd your esophagus, and it will be nice to you. And just in case, be sure everyone knows the Heimlich maneuver. Technically, the Heimlich maneuver is used to dislodge substances blocking the trachea, prior to reaching the esophagus.

Stomach

The esophagus empties into the stomach, where some real digestive action begins. This two-pint (or four cups or one liter) holding tank is the bus station for carbohydrates and fats. Only protein is digested in the stomach with **hydrochloric acid** and other fun substances. Carbohydrates and fats are just traveling through, getting broken into smaller pieces. It takes about two to three hours for a meal to leave the stomach. At this point the food exits into the small intestine.

Small Intestine

The small intestine is small only in diameter. If you uncoiled the small intestine and measured it (do not try this at home), it would measure anywhere from ten feet to twenty-two feet in length. The small intestine is a big deal when it comes to digestion. Fat, carbohydrates, and leftover protein are digested along its length, assisted by muscular contractions, enzymes and absorbed by lots of **villi.** Villi are microscopic fronds in the intestinal wall, looking like coral waving in the ocean, that increase the absorbing area of the intestine look like lots of minuscule fingers, or a live coral bed, attached to the walls of the small intestine. Food stays in the small intestine for four to ten hours, depending on the size of the meal and the physical condition of the eater. So much for waiting an hour after you eat to go swimming.

> FOOD FOR THE MIND
> So what about waiting an hour before swimming? As you can see from the description of digestion and absorption, you'd have to wait about four to ten hours for complete digestion. Waiting an hour allows food to clear the esophagus (which takes only seconds) and get to the stomach and intestines. However, depending on the type of meal eaten, food will remain in your system for much more than one hour.

Large Intestine

After the small intestine comes the large intestine. The last part of the large intestine is called the colon, and it is about five feet long. The colon is not a digestive organ. It helps to absorb fluids and may even assist in the production of some vitamins (with the help of beneficial bacteria and certain nutrients). Food may stay in the colon for one to three days, after which it is eliminated and digestion is complete.

Gallbladder, Kidneys, Pancreas, Liver

The mouth, stomach, and small and large intestine are the organs through which food actually passes. Every best actor needs a supporting cast. In the case of digestion, the pancreas, gallbladder, kidneys, and liver never physically touch the food, but they play important roles in helping it to be digested. The liver, gallbladder, and pancreas provide bile. Bile is necessary for digestion of fat. The pancreas also produces enzymes and pancreatic juices important for digestion, as well as the hormone insulin to help in glucose absorption. The kidneys extract certain minerals and maintain proper fluid balance. The liver is the filtering organ for everything that you eat and drink, sending nutrients out to where they're needed and processing toxins to be eliminated from the body. Be good to your liver. Without it, no more you.

> FOOD FOR THE MIND
>
> Enzymes are like mothers-in-law. A scientist would tell you that enzymes are "protein-containing catalysts that enter and leave a reaction unchanged in form." Sounds good, but what does that mean in English?
>
> Most reactions need a little push or a boost to get going. In the good old days, cars needed to be hand-cranked to get them started. The crank would be a good example of an enzyme. It starts a reaction, gets it going, and leaves, without changing itself in any way. Another way to look at enzymes is to think of them as a mother-in-law. You and the spouse are hanging out, watching TV. Mother-in-law pops in, starts yelling about the floors need vacuuming, the dishes need washing, and how about painting that door? You start running around like crazy, busting suds, sweeping rugs—you're really going. Her job done, mother-in-law, like the true enzyme she is, puts on her hat and leaves, no worse for wear.

ABSORPTION: SURROUND AND CONQUER

There are different types of absorption. Remember that the purpose of absorption is to make nutrients available where they are needed. Absorption allows some amino acids to get to that burn on your left index finger so that the skin can start to repair. Or to move some glucose (the major simple sugar the body likes to use) over to those leg muscles to fire up some energy and get them running.

Nutrients can be absorbed with the help of electrical charges that your body generates. Scientists like to sound important and call this "active transport." Translated into English, it means that some energy is required to move particular nutrients. Passive diffusion is the opposite of active transport. That is, no energy is required, the nutrients just sort of go along for the ride. Another type of transport is called "endocytosis" and it resembles a bad science fiction movie. Nutrients are surrounded and enveloped by cell walls and moved along in the cell this way. Rent a copy of the 1950s movie, *The Blob,* and you'll see endocytosis on the big screen. The point is, glucose, amino acids, and fatty acids don't just float around until they accidentally find somewhere they're needed. The body has mechanisms to haul nutrients around to exactly where they need to go.

Nutrients are absorbed in different parts of the body. Different parts of the small intestine have cells specific for absorbing fats, carbohydrates, and proteins. Good guys like vitamins, both fat-soluble and water-soluble (see Chapter 7 for a discussion on vitamins), and bad guys, like cholesterol, are absorbed in the small intestine as well. Minerals and water are absorbed by the colon, which is located at the end of the large intestine.

A Quick Review

Every part of the human digestive system plays an important part in processing the food you eat. When you eat a piece of pizza, you become a seething mass of chemicals, enzymes, and muscle contractions.

Digestion and absorption are two distinct functions. Digestion is the breakdown of foods into nutritional components the body can utilize. An example of this is the breakdown of cheese in your pizza. Your body can't use the cheese, but it can use the breakdown products of the cheese, amino acids, fatty acids, and monosaccharides, done by the process of digestion. Absorption is the transport of the digested foods to where they are needed, and ultimately used, by the body.

Take a bite of pizza. Digestion begins in the mouth. As the teeth and jaws grind and chew the pizza, saliva from the salivary glands moistens the pizza and supplies enzymes that begin to break down some of the crust (carbohydrate digestion). The saliva moistens the food, making it easy to transport. You swallow, sending the pizza down the esophagus towards the stomach.

The esophagus is the connecting tube between the mouth and the stomach. Once the pizza hits the stomach, you'll begin protein digestion. Pepsin (a stomach protein enzyme) breaks down the protein. Peristalsis (muscle contractions which resemble the movement of clothes in a washing machine) keeps the rest of the pizza-mass moving along. The stomach is lined with epithelium, a substance that contains literally millions of gastric glands. Cells in the gastric glands secrete the equivalent of hydrochloric acid to digest protein. In the presence of stomach acids, the pizza cheese "melts" and breaks down from its whole protein form into its component amino acids. Why doesn't the stomach, which is made of protein, digest itself? One reason is that specialized stomach cells produce alkaline substances which neutralize stomach acids.

The unrecognizable mass that was your pizza flows from the stomach into the small intestine. The small intestine is the workhorse of digestion. Digestion is completed in the small intestine. Chemical digestion is performed in the first part of the small intestine, the duodenum. Chemicals are secreted by the liver and the pancreas to help digest fat. Fat is broken down into fatty acids and glycerol and any leftover proteins are broken down into amino acids. Carbohydrates are broken down into monosaccaharides (very simple sugars). After digestion has been completed in the small intestine, food flows to the large intestine.

The liver has many responsibilities, including detoxifying everything you swallow. The liver secretes bile, which helps break down fat. That extra olive oil on your pizza is assisted in digestion by the liver. No food every reaches the pancreas, but the pancreas is essential for digestion and absorption. The pancreas produces enzymes and hormones which help digest fats and carbohydrates.

Water and minerals are extracted and stored in the large intestine, some vitamins are synthesized, and undigested food is concentrated into a form that can be eliminated by the body. The large intestine is divided into the ascending colon, the transverse colon, the sigmoid colon, the cecum, and the rectum. The area of the large intestine called the "colon," from the cecum to the rectum, is the area where colon cancer can develop. Colon cancer is a leading form of cancer in the United States.

So, digestion begins in the mouth and ends in the small intestine. The mouth, esophagus, stomach, and small intestine actively process food with chemical assistance from the liver and pancreas. Carbohydrate digestion begins in the mouth, protein digestion begins in the stomach, and all digestion is completed in the small intestine.

Once digestion is complete, nutrients are processed for storage or energy use, and waste materials are eliminated through the large intestine.

NUTRITION-RELATED CONDITIONS: WHAT'S IT TO YA?

What does this all mean for the food-service professional? Believe it or not, because you work with food, many of your clients will expect that you know all about it, including the nutrition and health aspects. Many more people than you realize have to watch what they eat because of health conditions. And if they come to your property, they are going to expect you to accommodate them, to a reasonable degree. This is good business for you.

This means that if a customer has problems with the stomach, small or large intestine, pancreas, gallbladder, or colon, you may hear about it. Remember that many customers will expect that if you work with food, then you know about food. Be prepared to amaze them with your knowledge (but don't play junior medical person and dispense advice—not unless you've got malpractice insurance).

Here's a rundown of some diseases and/or conditions associated with digestion and absorption.

Dental Cavities

In the mouth, dental problems may be the starting point for nutritional problems. If you can't chew certain foods, then you'll avoid them. This is okay for beef jerky or beer nuts, but not so okay for fresh fruits and vegetables. A lot of the malnutrition seen in senior citizens is caused by the inability to chew particular foods.

Dental cavities, also called dental caries, can be caused by poor dental care. You now know that carbohydrate digestion begins in the mouth. And to what are carbohydrates broken down? Sugars! And what do the bacteria that grow on your teeth enamel like to eat? Sugars! Does this mean don't eat carbohydrates? No, it means get rid of the sugar that's hanging around your pearly whites. If you can't brush your teeth after you eat, then use "on the road" solutions, which can include rinsing your mouth vigorously with clear or salted water or chewing sugar-free gum.

By the way, if you don't want to feed enamel-eating bacteria, stick to complex carbohydrate–containing foods, such as popcorn, whole-wheat bread and cereal, raw or cooked vegetables, fresh fruit, and other whole-grain foods. Foods that contain simple sugars, such as hard candy, soda, and syrups, are more quickly broken down in the mouth and more easily used by the bacteria.

Hiatal Hernia and GERD: The Esophagus or May the Force of Gravity Be with You!

The esophagus has muscular valves (called sphincters) that prevent the backflow of food and acid from the stomach. If they don't work properly, a portion of the stomach and its contents flow into the esophagus. The tissue in your stomach was meant to withstand acid, but the esophagus was not. When acid backflows, heartburn results. Severe heartburn, officially known as GERD or gastro-esophageal reflux disease, can cause symptoms that feel very close to a heart attack. Depending on your genetics and lifestyle, you can prevent heartburn or GERD. Remember that the esophagus is a tube with a very small diameter, about the size of a hot dog. Everything you stuff down your gullet has to slide down the esophagus. So don't eat huge meals. Get into the habit of "grazing" with small frequent meals. Small meals are easier for the esophagus to accommodate and also require less acid to digest. Don't lie down after a meal. Gravity is your esophagus' friend, assisting the food to flow downstream. Alcohol, **caffeine,** and smoking (oh no, attacking the holy trinity of students!) irritate the stomach, causing more acid production. Finally, you'll have to decide on fashion or GERD. Really tight clothing can press on the stomach and force it up into the esophagus—how's *that* for a fashion statement!

If the esophagus is continually stretched out of shape, as a result of overeating, inherited tendencies for weakened tissues or improper lifting techniques for example, then a hernia, or pouching out may result. A hiatal hernia can feel like having an inflated balloon inserted under your rib cage. Although there are new surgical techniques to correct hiatal hernias, lifestyle change is still the treatment of choice. Changes can include losing weight, if overweight, and following the guidelines for preventing GERD, listed above. Hiatal hernias and GERD can be very painful and annoying. People with GERD or hiatal hernias will be looking for light-in-volume and light-on-the-spice types of menus. Chilies, Tabasco, coarsely ground pepper, or any ingredient that causes fire in the mouth will feel even worse once it slides down the esophagus of someone with GERD. Fresh or dried mild herbs, such as basil, oregano, thyme, and tarragon, should be fine.

Stomach Upsets

Hydrochloric acid is great if you've got to digest half a prime rib. However, if you are under a lot of stress, overdo it on the caffeine or alcohol or tend to take a snooze after eating a three-course meal, you may be plagued with "acid stomach." The lining of the stomach can handle small amounts of acid, which is generated when there is some protein digestion to do. If acid is secreted when there's no protein to work on, as in the case of too much caffeine or stress, then the stomach acid looks for some other protein to break down. This could be the stomach lining, which is made of protein. An "ulceration" is a type of burn. What would happen if you spilled some acid on the skin of your hand? A burn, or ulcer. Think of **stomach ulcers** as acid burns, which is what they are. Stomach ulcers can range in severity from mild discomfort to life threatening.

Many people turn to **antacids** to neutralize, or disable, stomach acid. As we've noted in this chapter, antacids can interfere with the absorption of some nutrients. If taken in large amounts over long periods of time, antacids can cause health problems. To decrease the need for antacids, follow the information given about keeping a healthy esophagus. Don't eat big meals, eat slowly, cut back on caffeine and alcohol, don't lie down after you eat, and lose the spandex. In the meantime, the recovering ulcer sufferer needs mild, but flavorful meals, such as fresh spinach pasta tossed with a light dusting of grilled mushrooms, petite pois (baby green peas) and Pecorino-Romano cheese (5).

Diverticulosis and Diverticulitis

The large intestine is a real workhorse and generally works away without letting the owner know that it is there. The intestinal wall is lined with small pouches, called "diverticula." The presence of diverticula in the colon is called "diverticulosis," and is almost universal in people over forty years old. Diverticulosis is not a disease.

The diverticula are kept healthy, partially by a high-fiber diet. This keeps food moving along in the intestine. Diverticula can become inflamed when irritants, such as seeds, lodge in them. If a diverticula becomes inflamed, diverticulitis can result, causing cramps, gas, indigestion, and constipation and diarrhea. If a diverticula ruptures, surgery may be necessary.

Diverticulitis can be prevented by eating a reasonably high-fiber diet and drinking lots of fluids. This means at least eight glasses of water or the equivalent and five to six servings of fruit and vegetables per day. Whole grains and other fiber-containing foods, such as oatmeal, fresh salads, and whole-grain pasta, should be included as well.

People in the recovery stages of diverticulitis need mild diets. Once they are fully recovered, bring on the grilled vegetables with a balsamic reduction and fresh herbs and assorted melon with fresh, seasonal blueberries.

Constipation, Gas, and Colon Cancer

The colon, the end of the digestive system, can really let you know that it's there. Constipation, although not a dinner table topic is on the minds (and other parts) of Americans. Americans spend over 2 billion dollars a year on products that promise to prevent or solve constipation. We can let you in on

Food	Interaction
Dairy, high in calcium	Antibiotics and iron
High fiber	Reduce pain relievers, such as acetominphen (Tylenol)
High protein	Increase aspirin
Caffeine	May increase heart rate in some people
Alcohol	Combined with aspirin, can cause ulcerations, with antihistamines acts as depressant
Antacids	Iron
Diuretics	Potassium

Figure 3–2 Food and Drugs

a hint: fiber and fluids. Your large intestine requires the right amount of fiber and fluid to work properly. So stock up on the apples, baked potatoes and sparkling water and save your money from all those "magic" cures. **Laxatives** can be habit-forming, and pretty soon your system can't work on its own. Some people with eating disorders abuse laxatives as a weight-loss method. So, they ruin their entire digestive system. They may need to take some form of laxatives their entire life because their system doesn't work right anymore. They don't lose weight, but they do lose minerals and nutrients.

There are other problems that involve the large intestine that can be serious, sometimes life-threatening diseases. Irritable bowel syndrome, colitis, Crohn's disease, and colon cancer affect many Americans each year. People need to modify their fiber and nutrient intake with some of these conditions.

The gallbladder and pancreas work both independently and in team situations. The pancreas secrete substances that help the body to absorb fat, and the gallbladder helps to store these substances. If one or both of them are not working properly, then it may be difficult for a person to handle foods with fat in them. The pancreas is a very important part of carbohydrate metabolism. People who have problems with their gallbladder may need foods that are light in fat, as they have problems digesting fat. See the discussion about the pancreas, insulin, and energy in Chapter 4 for details about its functioning. If the pancreas malfunctions in one way, a person may be unable to digest fats. If it malfunctions in another way, a person may not metabolize sugars properly, leading to diabetic diet restrictions.

You should be nice to your liver, as it is both the detoxification capitol and the chemical manufacturing plant for your body. Just about everything you ingest winds up eventually in your liver, where it is transformed to a usable form. It is then sent to the area of the body where it is needed. Whether you think of them as so or not, many of the foods you eat contain substances that your body identifies as toxic. It is the liver's role in life to take harmful substances, such as alcohol, ingested remnants of tobacco toxins, and some preservatives, and make them harmless. You can give your liver a break by drinking lots of non-alcoholic, non-caffeinated beverages, such as water and fruit or vegetable juice. This helps flush out some of the toxins. You can also attempt to avoid large amounts of toxins. The liver is a real trooper and can hold its own against most toxins for a while. Taken in large amounts over long periods of time, however, the liver becomes hardened, called "cirrhosis," and can no longer function.

MICROBES AND THE GUT

Your body is a condominium for microscopic beasties. It is estimated that there are ten times the number of beneficial bacteria in the digestive system than the number of all the other cells in the entire body. There are at least 350 species of bacteria in the digestive tract, constituting over 100 trillion (that's 100,000,000,000,000 or more than the U.S. national debt) cells. Don't worry, there's lots of room. About 400 lactobacillus, good-guy bacteria, found in yogurt that can help the digestion, can fit on the dot of the "i" in "fit." You have a mixture of good and not-so-good bacteria in your gut at any one time. Some of those bacteria are actually used by your large intestine to synthesize vitamins. Other bacteria are trying to invade your stomach and make you feel seasick. As long as the good guy bacteria outweigh the bad, you're in good shape.

Gas or bacteria doing what they do naturally can cause flatulence, or it can be caused by swallowed air. So shut up and eat. You'll take in less air so your body will produce less carbon dioxide (a mixture of carbon and oxygen that resembles the bubbles in soda). If you haven't got much carbon dioxide in your system, then you won't have much gas.

Eating small quantities of foods containing sulfer, such as beans, cruciferous vegetables, like cabbage or broccoli, instead of massive quantities, will give your gut time to digest them slowly and completely. When the bacteria in your gut break down these types of sulfur-containing foods, the results can be particularly socially inappropriate.

Flatulence and belching can also be caused by carbonated beverages, such as soda and beer, chewing gum, and by smoking (since air is inhaled). Reconsider your habits if you sound like an internal combustion engine after drinking a liter of soda.

Lactose Intolerance

For a more detailed discussion of **lactose intolerance,** see Chapter 4. The enzyme lactase is needed to digest milk sugar, that is, lactose. If you don't have enough of this enzyme, then you cannot break down the sugar portion of dairy products. Some people with lactose intolerance can eat small amounts of solid dairy products, like Swiss cheese or yogurt, but can't tolerate fluid dairy products, like milk. Others can't tolerate any dairy products. There are specialty milks sold with lactose-eating bacteria, such as acidophilus, that make dairy products easier to digest. Yogurt and other cultured products are also lower in lactose because of their good-guy bacteria. And there's always soy or rice milk to use in the Béchamel or the cream of mushroom soup.

STRESS AND THE GUT

Why does mental stress physically affect us? There are very strong connections between the brain and the gut. The stomach, liver, small intestine, gallbladder, esophagus, and large intestine have nerves that are directly connected to the brain. You know that when you smell good food cooking, you may salivate or your stomach may contract or secrete acid in preparation for eating and digesting. This is beneficial nervous activity.

Stress causes excessive nervous activity, which can result in overproduction of stomach acid, tightening of the muscles in the stomach or esophagus, etc. This is harmful nervous activity. This kind of activity can make you feel hungry when you are not, leading to eating more calories than you need, which ultimately can lead to excess weight and its related issues. It can cause acid burns, or ulcerations, to form in your stomach, as a result of acid overproduction. It can cause malabsorption syndrome, where the gut empties itself of partially digested food, causing cramps and diarrhea. The moral to the story is to learn how to decrease the amount of stress in your life and how to accommodate the inevitable daily stress so you can have a healthy digestive system and a reasonably happy life.

FOOD AND DRUG INTERACTIONS

Nutrition does not function in a vacuum. The foods you eat and drink and the medications you take and in what combination will determine how much you nutritionally benefit. Some interactions are beneficial. Vitamin C, obtained from food or supplements, and iron are best buddies. Ingested together, they improve the body's absorption of both nutrients. Iron and calcium, two essential nutrients, can cancel each other out when taken together. They bind together in such a way that the body can't get at either of them. So have your calcium-containing yogurt smoothie for breakfast and your fresh spinach salad for lunch.

Chemicals and medications can interfere with the body's ability to absorb nutrients. Caffeine, that magic substance, might be great for a lift, but it's bad news for calcium, potassium, and other minerals. Caffeine decreases the body's ability to absorb and retain these minerals. Is this a suggestion to give up caffeine? Don't be ridiculous! How else will you get through reading this book? If you "gotta have it," then make dietary adjustments. Have a double cappucino in one hand and a fruit smoothie, made with bananas, orange juice, mango, melon, and other fruit of your choice, in the other hand.

Antibiotics are very important to cure some diseases; they can be true lifesavers. Just make a note that calcium can interfere with the body's ability to absorb antibiotics. Read the label and ask questions. Some medications are meant to be taken on an empty stomach so they will do what they're supposed to do. By the way, "empty stomach" translates to taking medications two hours before eating or four hours after eating so plan your menu accordingly (Fauci).

Some hypertensive (high blood pressure) and cardiac medications are in a group called "diuretics." Diuretics can also be found in over-the-counter weight loss medications and in herbal preparations and teas. Diuretics assist the body in getting rid of excess fluid. Getting rid of the fluid is fine, but the minerals lost with the fluid are not so fine. As with caffeine, if you take diuretics (and you should do this only under medical supervision), you should plan on compensating for the loss by adding more minerals to your diet. More on this in Chapter 7.

Oral contraceptives can decrease the absorption of folic acid. Folic acid is known to prevent many birth defects, as well as being essential for healthy blood formation and protein absorption. An increase in folate-containing foods or a nutritional supplement might be in order.

Antacids can decrease the absorption of iron, a nutrient essential throughout life. If you can't avoid taking antacids, then adjust your iron intake accordingly. Just remember, don't take the antacid and the iron-containing food or supplement at the same time (James, p. 4)!

THE FOOD PROFESSIONAL'S ROLE

As food-service professionals, you are not qualified to diagnose diseases (hey, chef, I got a pain right here . . .) or provide therapeutic diets. You can, however, understand some problems your customers may have and provide foods that they can enjoy.

What we mean is, if a customer comes into a restaurant and demands that a meal be prepared with under 50 milligrams of cholesterol or is 5 on the glycemic index, no can do. You definitely do not want to get involved with the "I am a brittle diabetic and if my meal exceeds 500 calories I'll keel over" discussion. As much as you would like to accommodate all customers, the meals you prepare are not meant to be measured with science lab accuracy. Even if you did measure everything as accurately as you could, food is a natural product and has variations. A glass of orange juice could have 80 or 100 calories, depending on the type of orange and the time of year it was harvested.

Without getting into too much special detail or purchasing a lot of specialty foods you can offer menu items that are moderate in fat, salt, and calories and higher in fiber. There are lots of ways to cook chicken or fish. A higher-fat method would be to deep-fry. Lower-fat methods involve poaching, steaming, braising, barbecuing, grilling, stewing, en papilotte (oven steamed in parchment), stir frying, and rotisserie-cooking. These lower-fat methods are not necessarily more expensive, in either ingredients or labor, and would be fairly easy to incorporate into a menu. By doing so, you're a nutrition hero.

Let's continue. Baked potatoes are great, but high in fat and salt when topped with sour cream, butter, cheddar cheese, and bacon. Your health-watching customers will appreciate being able to select from lower-fat potato toppings, such as non- or low-fat plain yogurt, shredded skim-milk mozzarella, non- or skim-milk ricotta cheese, chopped tomatoes, garlic, green onions or chives, radishes, carrots, bell peppers, and chilies. Salsa, chutney, chopped grilled vegetables, grilled mushrooms, vegetarian chili, and grilled onions are low fat but really dress up a potato. Mashed potatoes can be mashed with olive oil, plain yogurt, garlic, and rosemary for a lower-cholesterol potato. And who said potatoes had to be white? Yukon gold potatoes look creamy and buttery without any extra fat, and Peruvian purple potatoes look so weird people will never miss the sour cream. Fresh sweet potatoes can be baked, roasted, grilled, and mashed. They are more colorful and more moist than white potatoes and require little in the way of fat or salt to make them taste good. As an added perk, sweet potatoes are higher in fiber and beta-carotene than white potatoes. Your industrious intestines and liver will convert beta-carotene to vitamin A.

A Word from the Master

Customers who have to watch their salt and fat intake will flock to restaurants that cater to them. Take your cue from Master Chef Victor Giselle, current president of the Culinary Institute of America and coach for the Culinary Olympics, among some of his accolades. Working with dietitians, he created Cuisine Actuelle, a high-end cuisine that shouts "Fresh," "Wonderful,"

"Enjoy," and barely whispers "low in fat and salt." Chef Giselle created such menu items as roasted pepper soup, smoked salmon steaks with celeriac and cucumber relish, marbled lemon cheese cake, and tomato risotto. Doesn't sound like punishment, does it?

FOOD FOR THE MIND
Victor Gieselle's Books

Cuisine Actuelle (1992), Taylor Publishing (Dallas, Texas)

In Good Taste (1999), Prentice Hall (Upper Saddle River, New Jersey)

KIDNEY HEALTH

Your kidneys are hard workers and you should treat them nicely. These fist-shaped organs shaped like, well, kidneys (where do you think kidney beans got their name?) are real powerhouses. They know how to keep what your body needs and get rid of the rest of the unnecessary stuff. Without them, you could not get rid of the end products of protein metabolism and could not maintain your electrolyte and fluid balance. In other words, without well-running kidneys, your body does not have a way to rinse away the unusable leftovers from digestion, keep fluid levels where they should be, or maintain the right amount of potassium, sodium, and other important minerals. Pretty important stuff!

FYI: THINK BEFORE YOU DRINK

What Happens

Nephrons are the very small units in the kidney, which are the worker bees of the operation. When there is damage to the kidneys, the number of functioning nephrons decrease, decreasing the ability of the kidney to do what they're supposed to do. As kidney disease progresses, kidneys are no longer able to properly filter protein, fluid, or minerals.

Diabetes and high blood pressure are two of the biggest culprits related to kidney disease. Chronic infections can cause problems, but they can usually be cleared up with antibiotics, plenty of rest, and plenty of fluids. Physical injury can physically damage the kidneys and impair their ability to function, so wear your seatbelt in the car and protective equipment when working out at the gym.

High blood pressure affects the way blood circulates through your body. Since the kidneys rely on good circulation to remove waste products from the body and since high blood pressure affects circulation, the two work against each other to cause both damage to the kidneys and the circulatory system. In an otherwise healthy person, blood pressure control is helped by maintaining proper weight, staying fit, not smoking, eating meals that are moderate in fat and salt and, of course, eliminating stress (yeah, right!).

Diabetes also affects the circulatory system, sometimes damaging the blood vessels. When blood vessels are damaged, the kidneys cannot get rid of fluid, potassium, and sodium effectively. This can make you retain fluid and minerals, resulting in weight gain (from fluid), swollen ankles and wrists. Diabetic renal disease is a very critical disease and must be treated constantly.

According to the Greater Kidney Foundation of Cincinnati, early signs of kidney disease for people with diabetes can be some of the following: high

PLATE I

Dry and Fresh Ingredients for Nutrition-Minded Culinarians

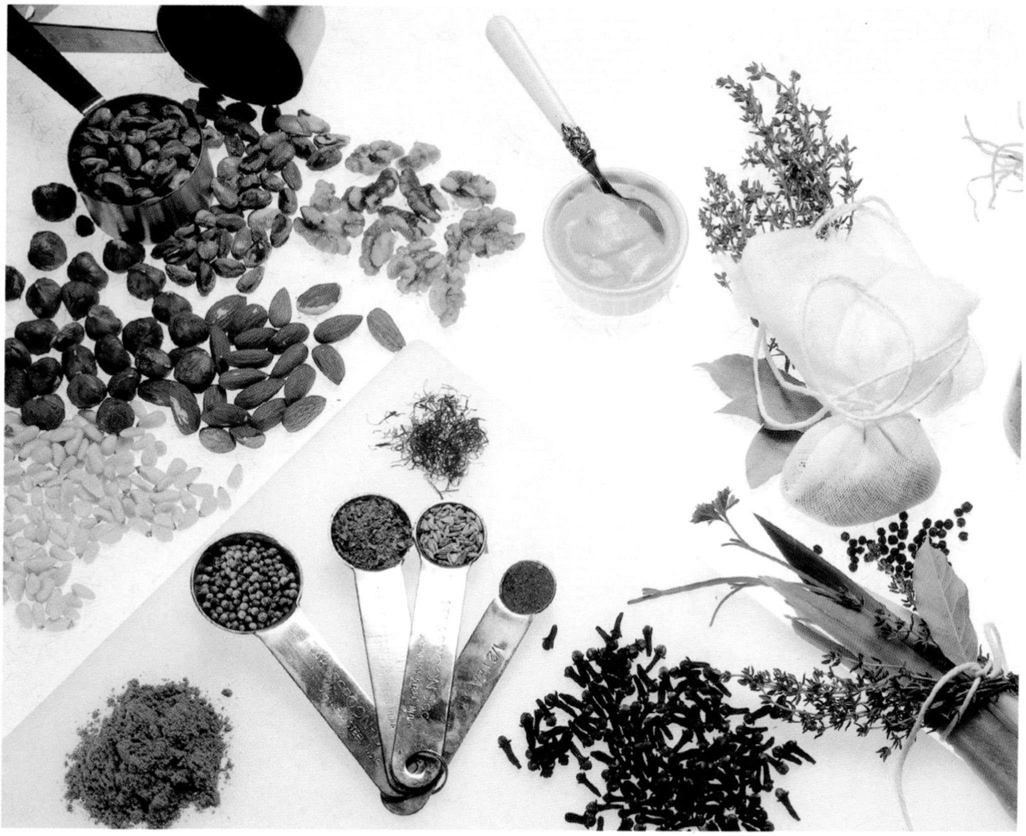

PLATE II

Nuts and Olives

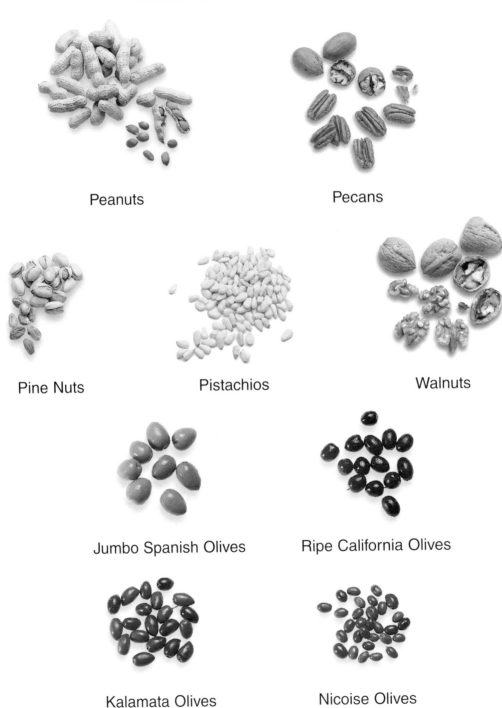

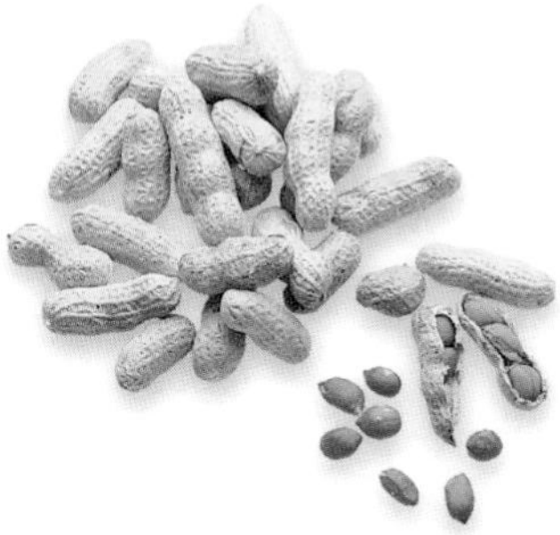

Peanuts

Pecans

Pine Nuts

Pistachios

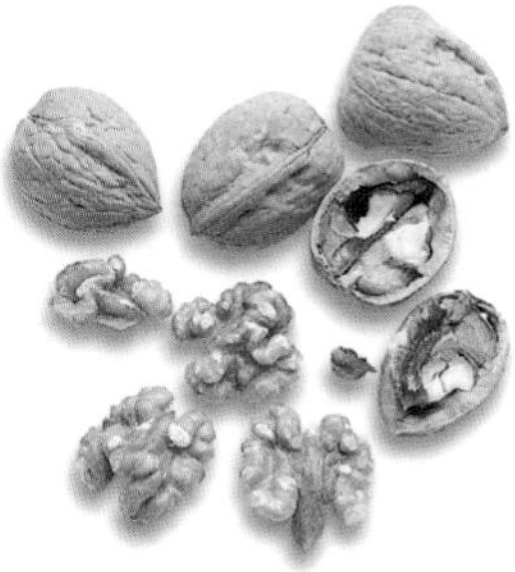

Walnuts

Jumbo Spanish Olives

Ripe California Olives

Kalamata Olives

Nicoise Olives

PLATE III

Fresh and Dry Herbs and Spices

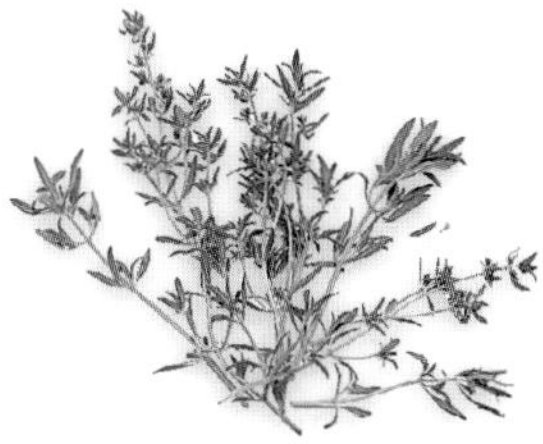

Savory

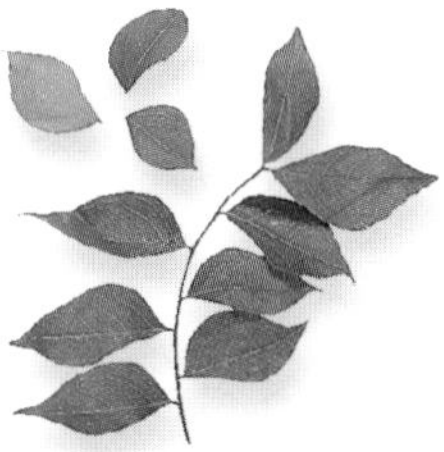

Curry Leaves

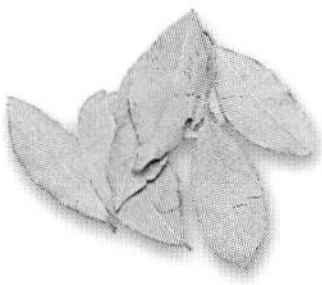

Bay Leaves

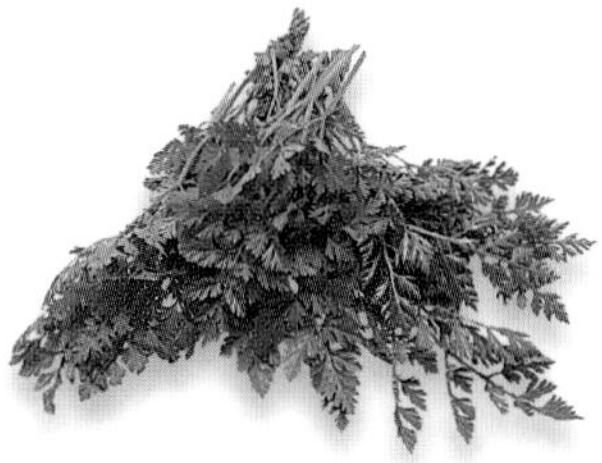

Chervil

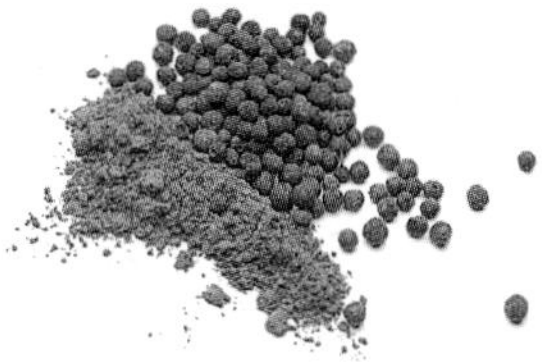

Allspice

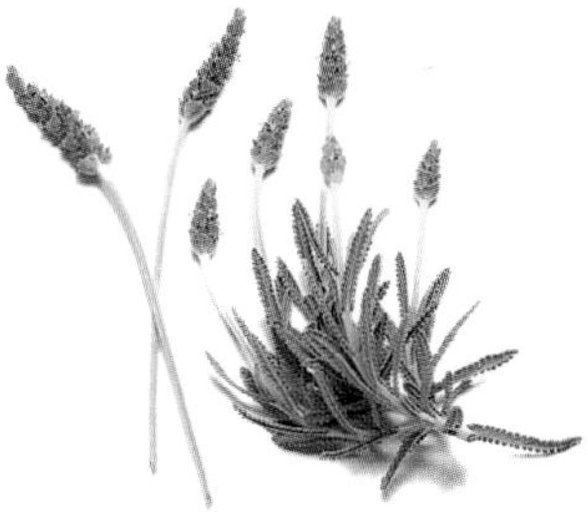

Lavender

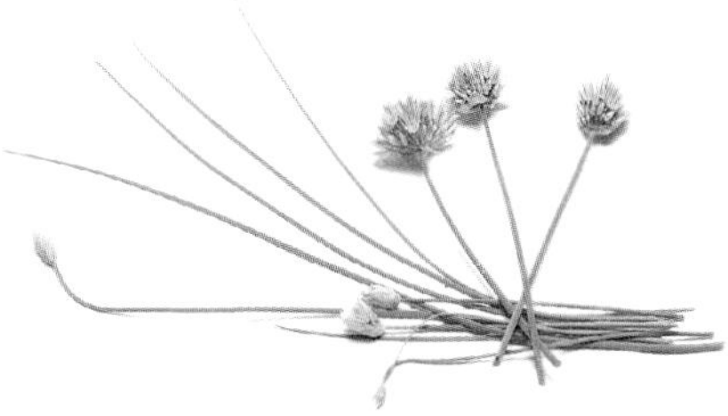

Chives

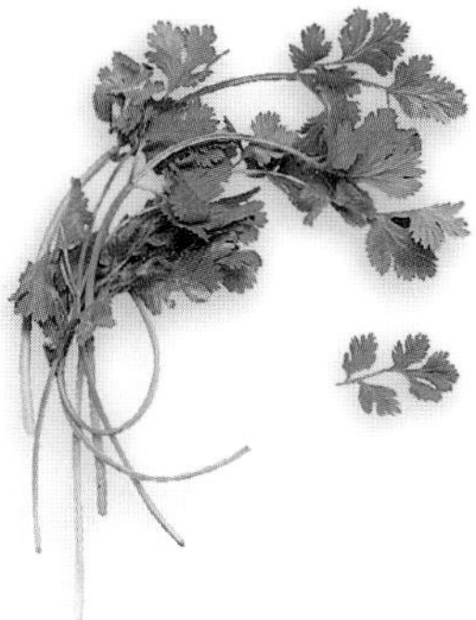

Cilantro

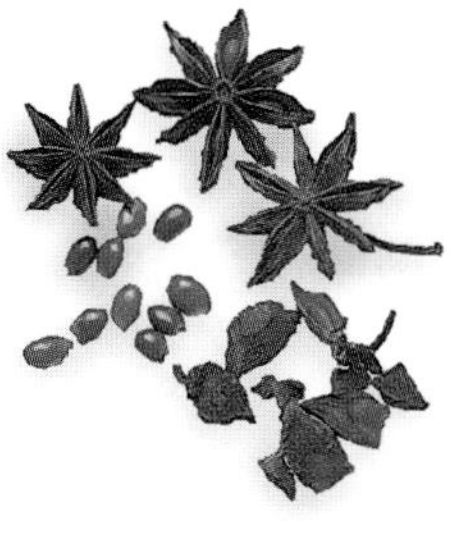

Star Anise

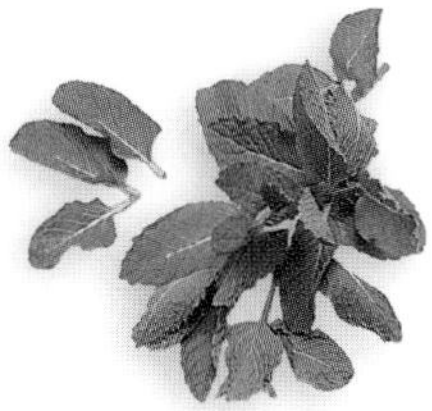

Spearmint

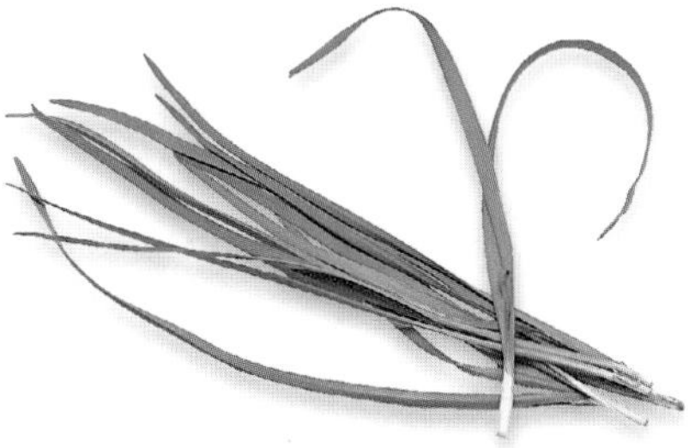

Garlic Chives

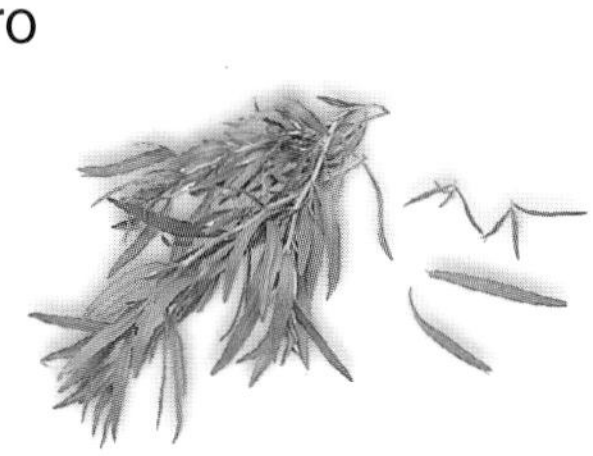

Tarragon

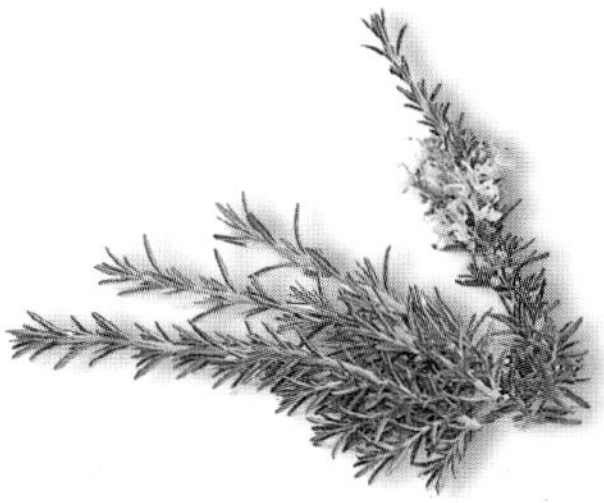

Rosemary

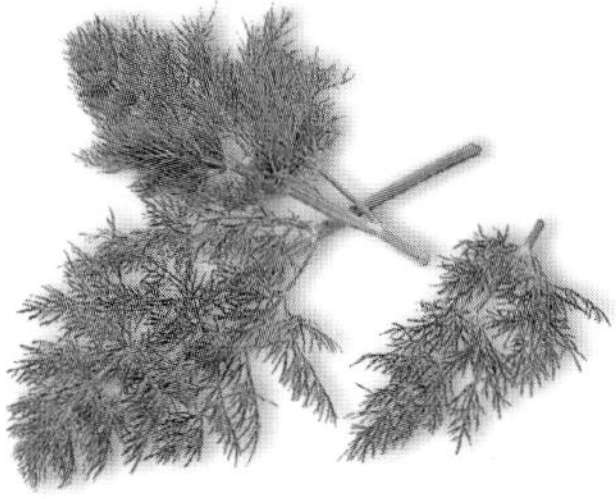

Dill

PLATE IV

An Array of Spices

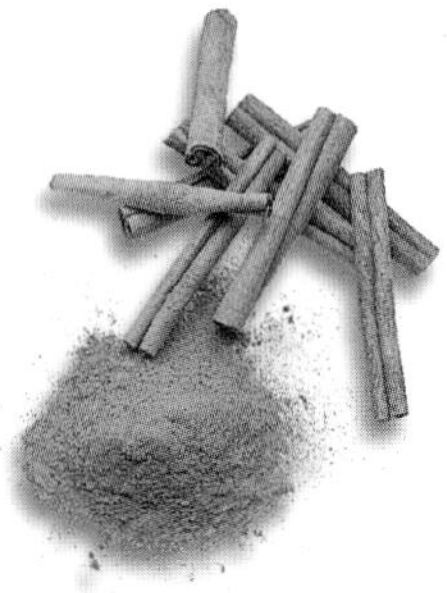

Ground Cinnamon
and Cinnamon Sticks

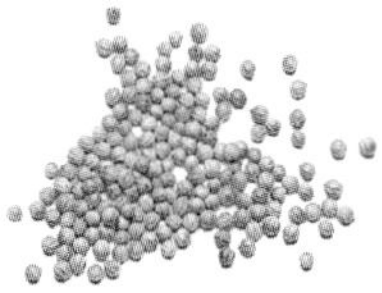

Coriander Seeds

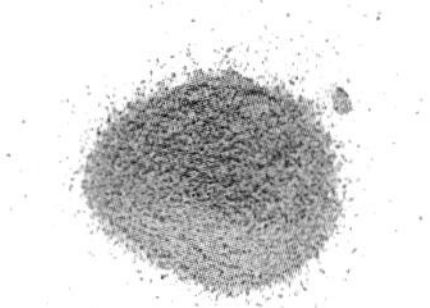

Cayenne Pepper

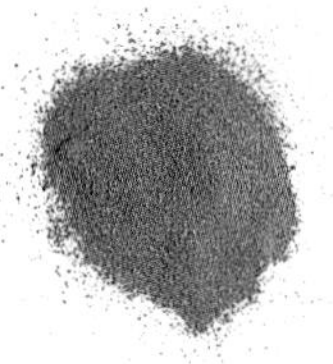

Paprika

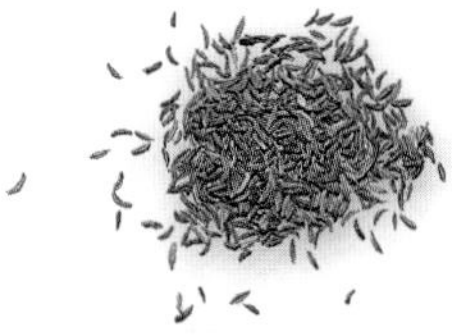

Caraway Seeds

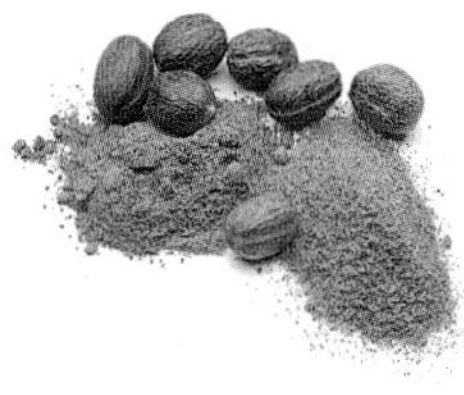

Whole Nutmegs with
Ground Mace (left) and
Ground Nutmeg (right)

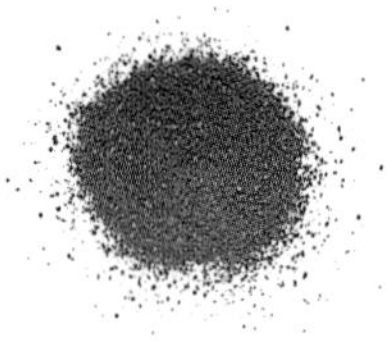

Chilli Powder

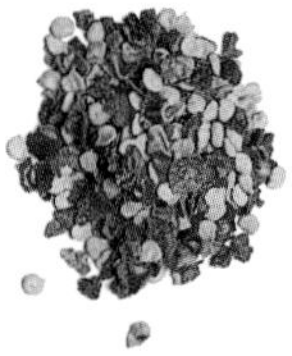

Crushed Chiles

PLATE V

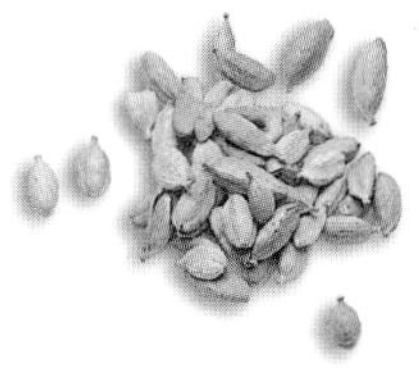

Cardamom Seeds

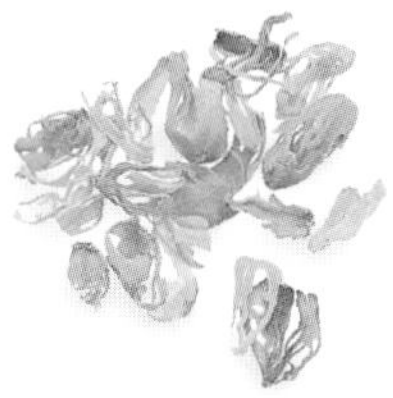

Mace

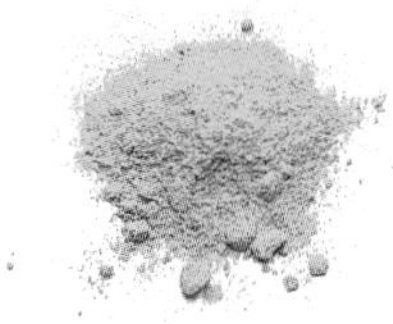

Turmeric

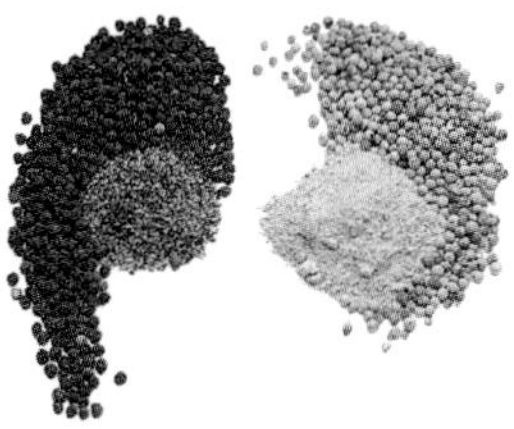

Black Pepper (left) and
White Pepper (right)

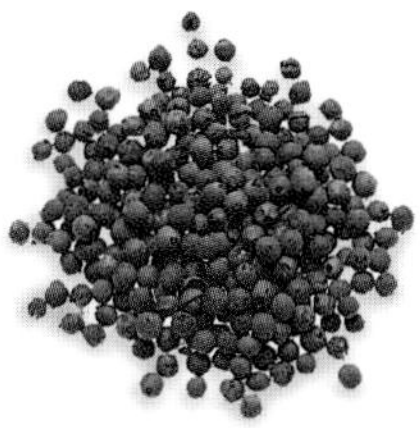

Green Peppercorns

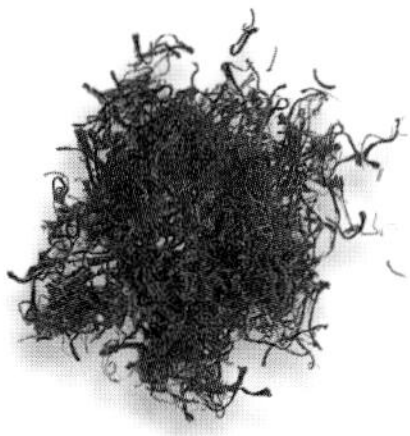

Saffron

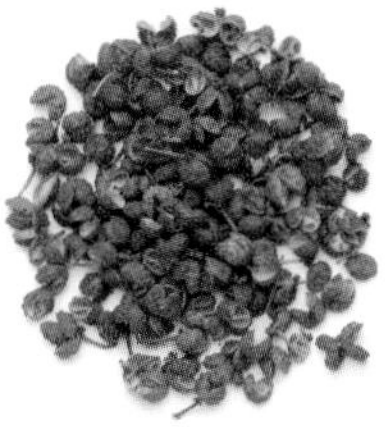

Szechuan Pepper

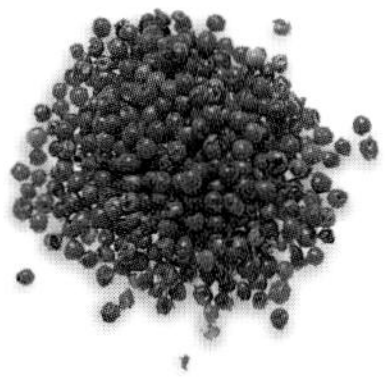

Pink Peppercorns

PLATE VI

Some of the Many Available Mushrooms

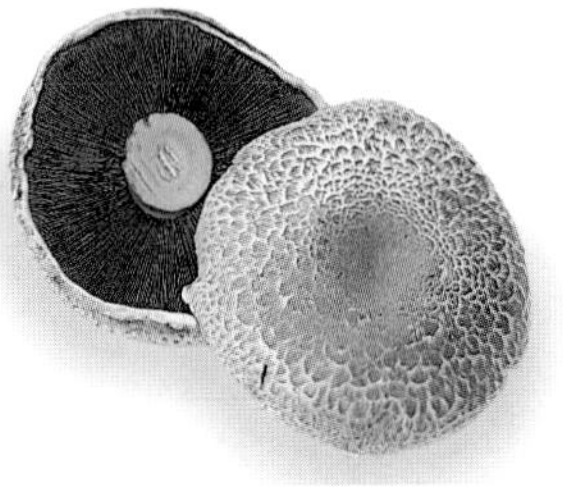

Portabella

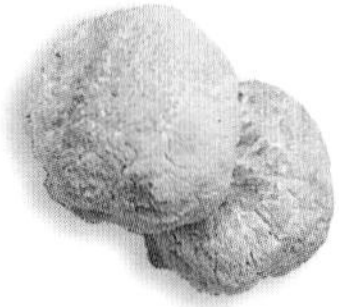

Pom Pom Blanc

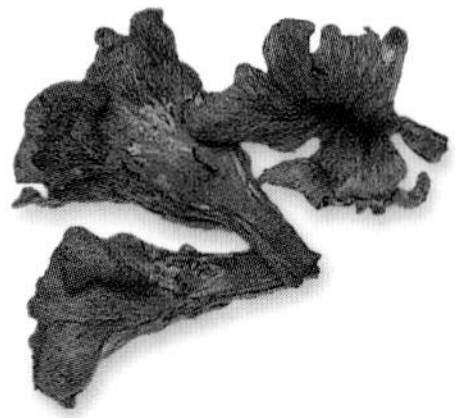

Black Trumpet

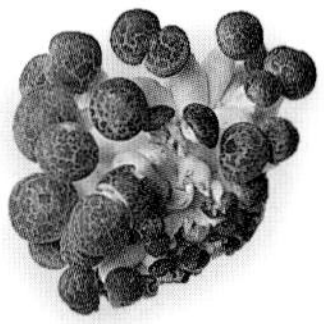

Clam Shell

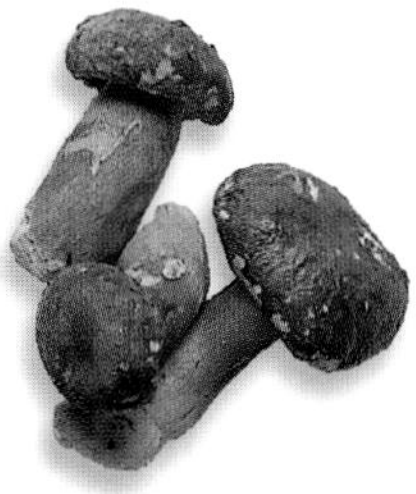

Porcini (cèpe or cep)

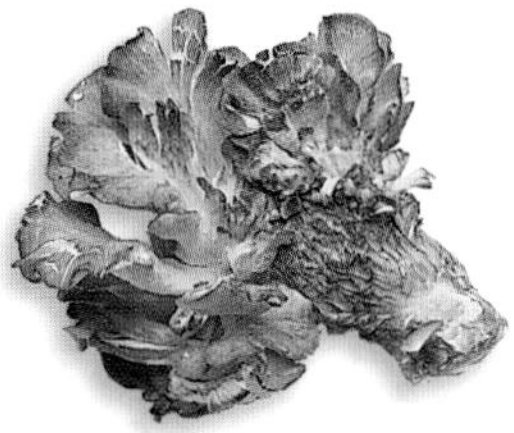

Hen of the Woods

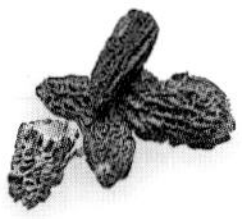

Morel

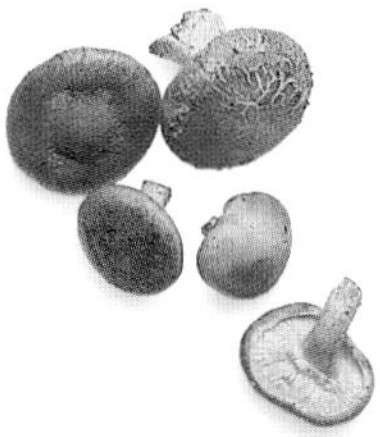

Shiitake

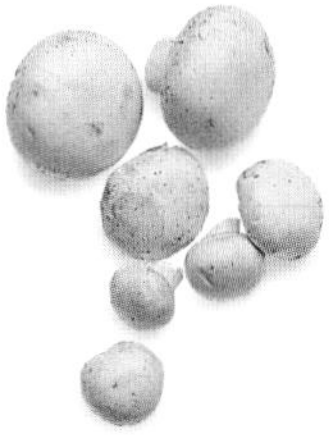

White

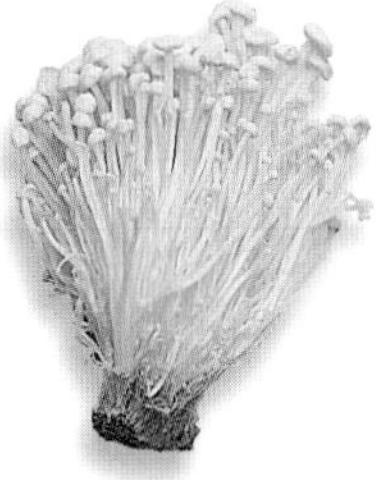

Enokidake

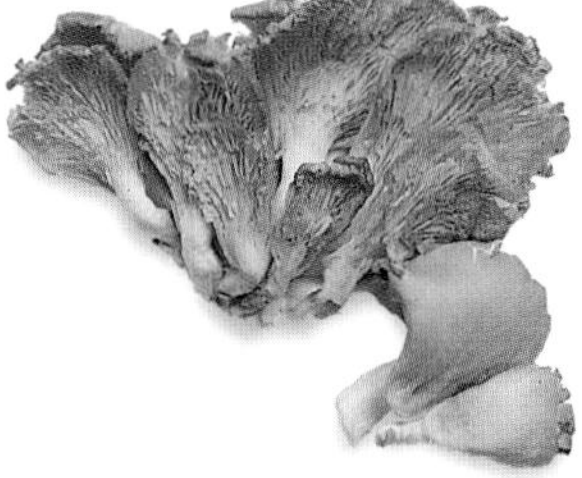

Oyster

PLATE VII

Freida's Herb Wreath: Herbs Are "Interior Decorating" for Food

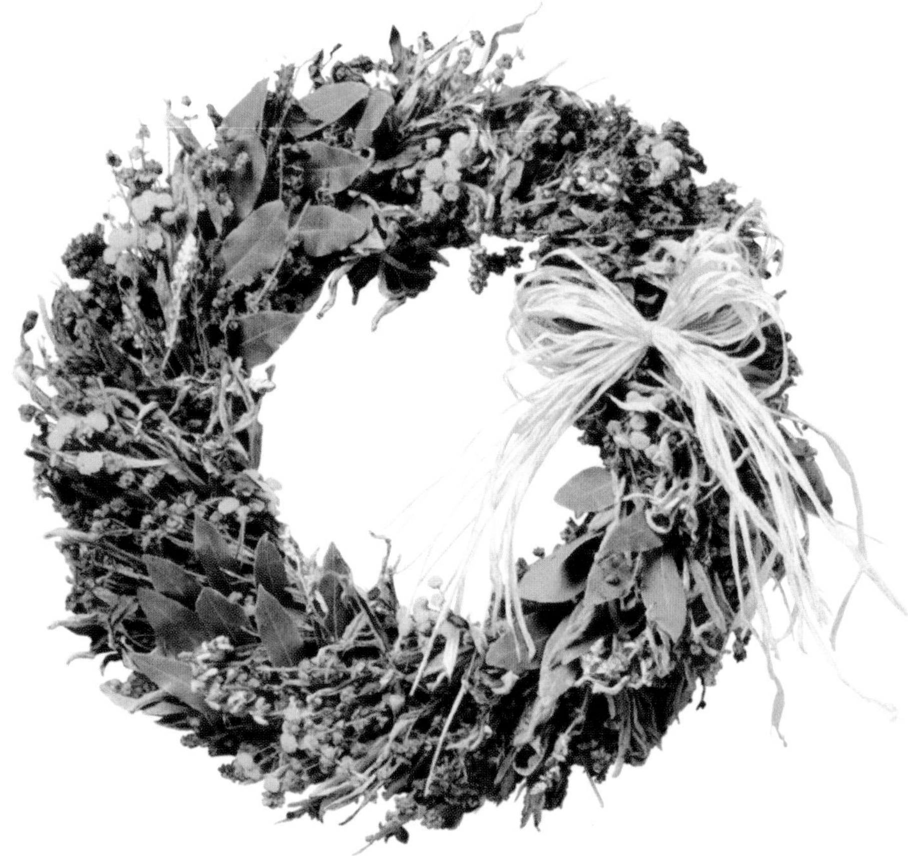

PLATE VIII

Think of These as Salad Ingredients!

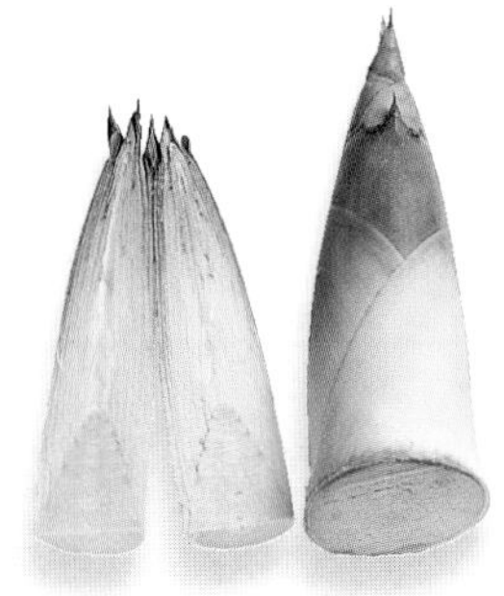

Fresh Bamboo Shoots

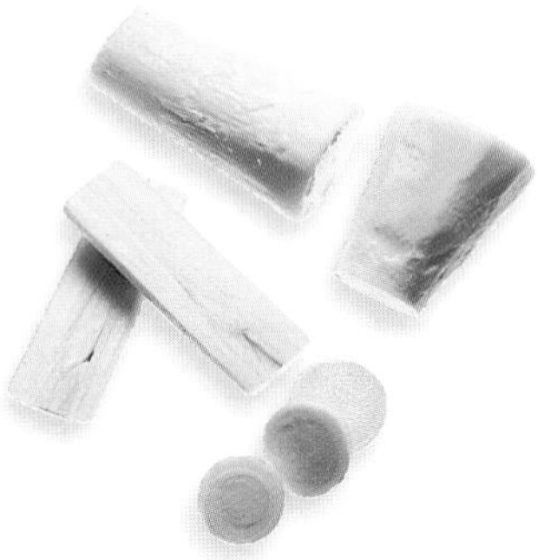

Hearts of Palm

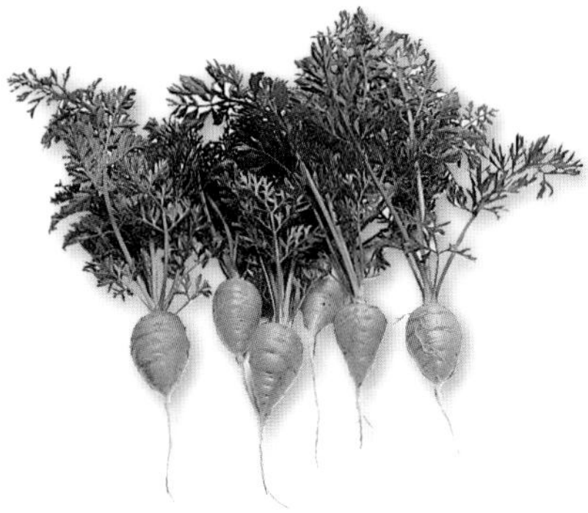

Baby Globe Carrots

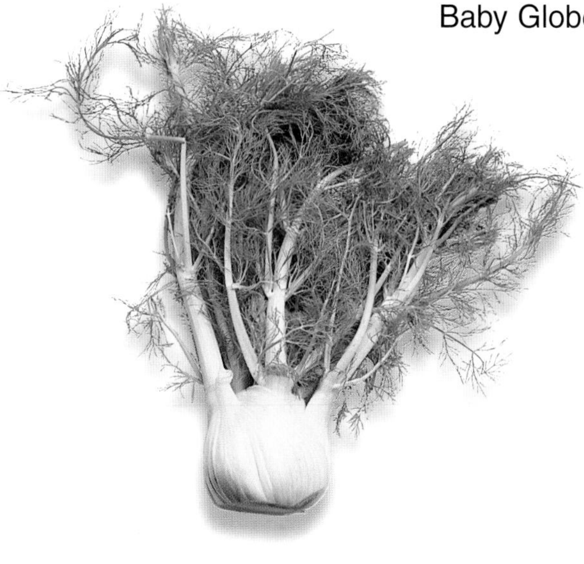

Fennel

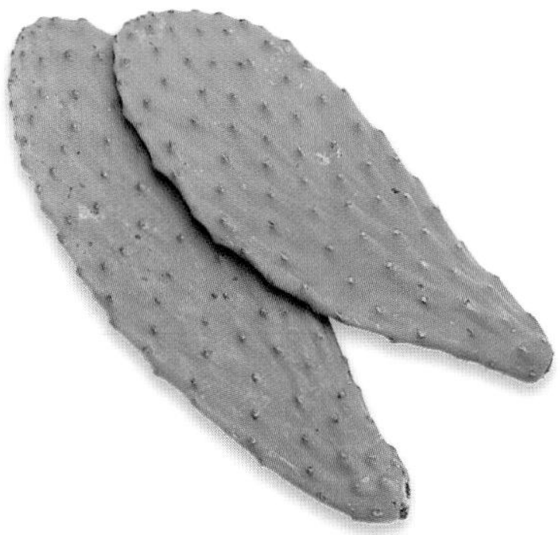

Nopales

PLATE IX

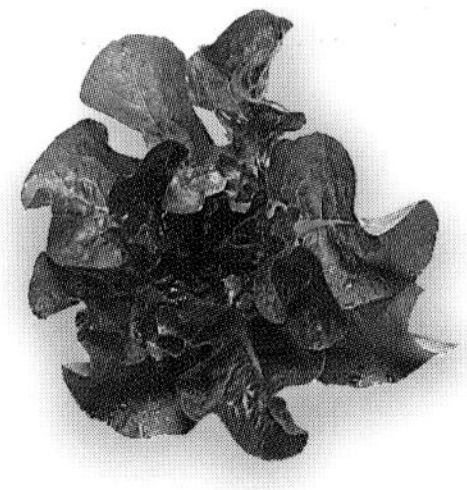

Brune d'Hiver

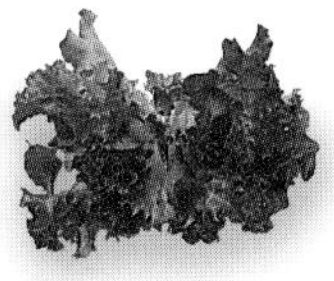

Lola Rosa

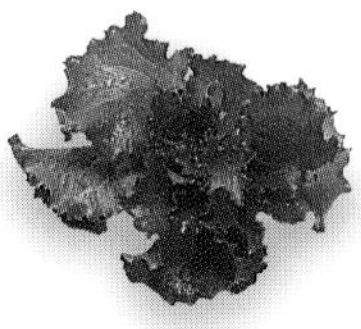

Red Sails

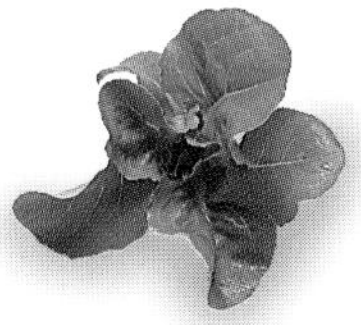

Baby Green Bibb

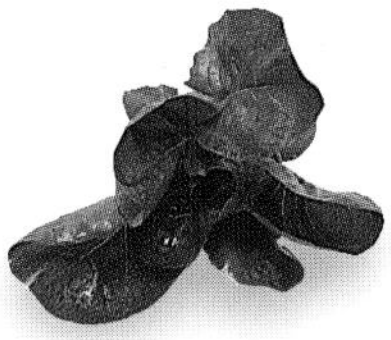

Baby Red Bibb

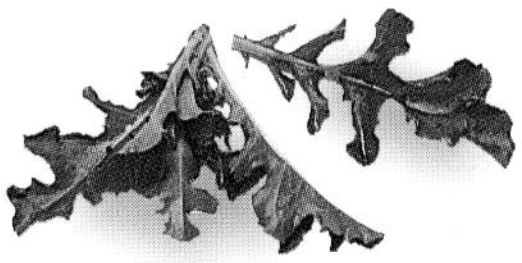

Baby Red Oak Leaf

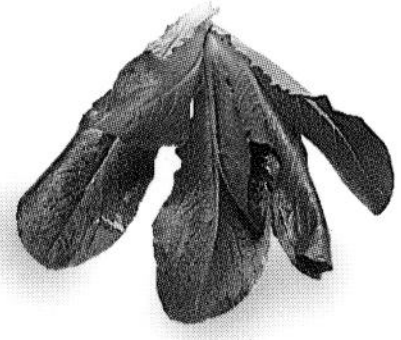

Baby Red Romaine

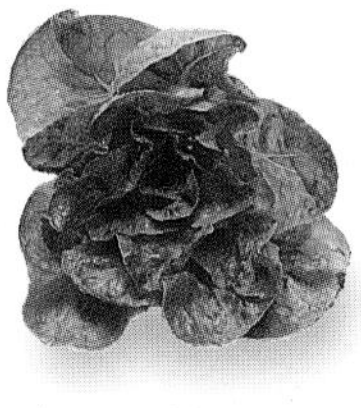

Pirate

PLATE X

Variety of Root Vegetables

Jicama

Fingerlings

Purple Potatoes

Parsnips

Red Potatoes

Russet Potatoes

Daikon

Yukon Gold Potatoes

Rutabagas

Sweet Potatoes

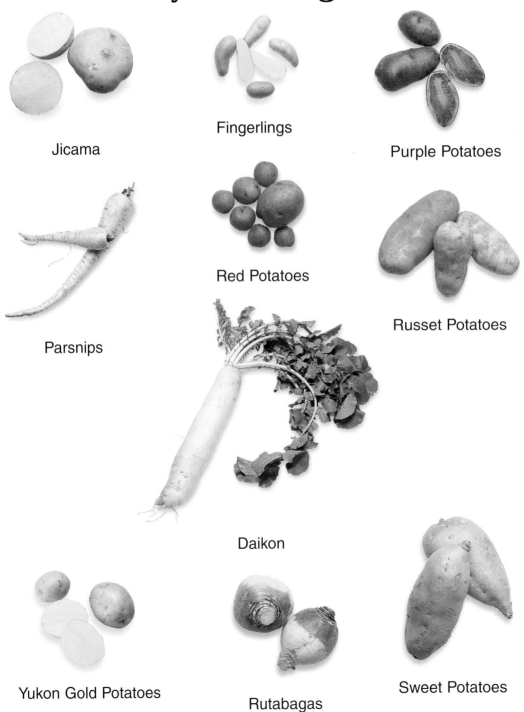

PLATE XI

Assortment of Grains

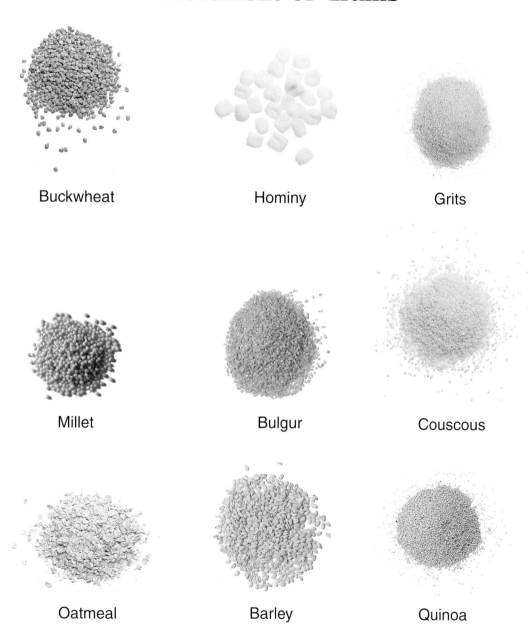

Buckwheat

Hominy

Grits

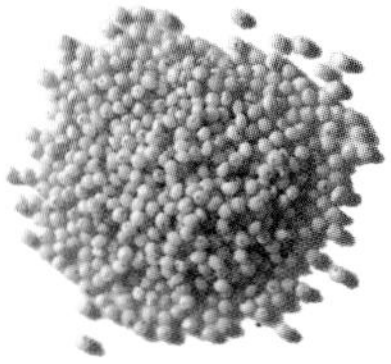

Millet

Bulgur

Couscous

Oatmeal

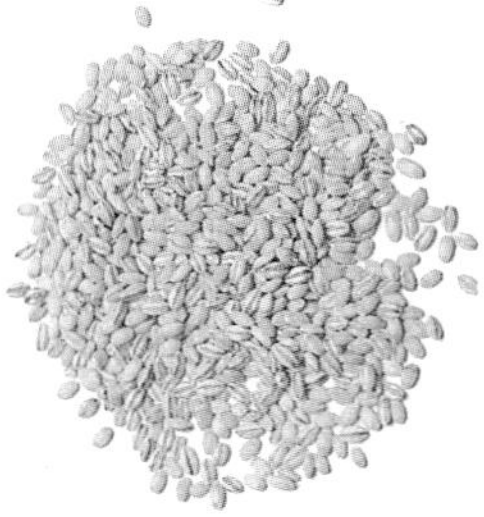

Barley

Quinoa

PLATE XII

A Variety of Seasonal Produce

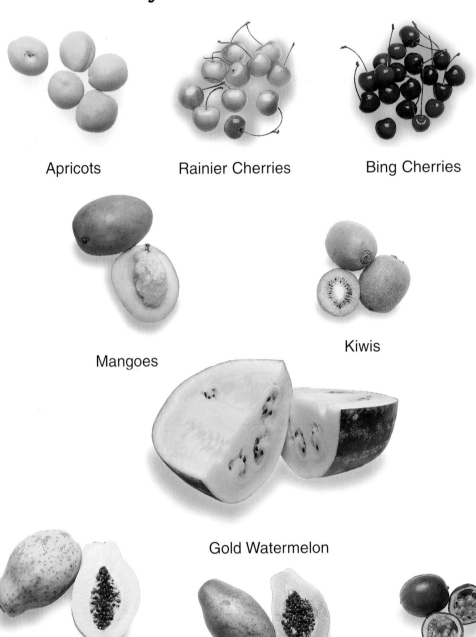

Apricots

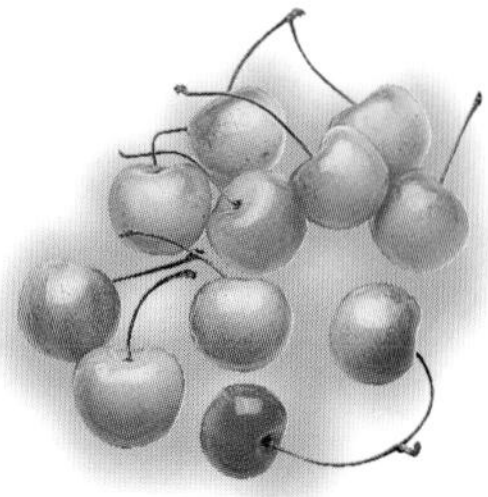

Rainier Cherries

Bing Cherries

Mangoes

Kiwis

Gold Watermelon

Papayas

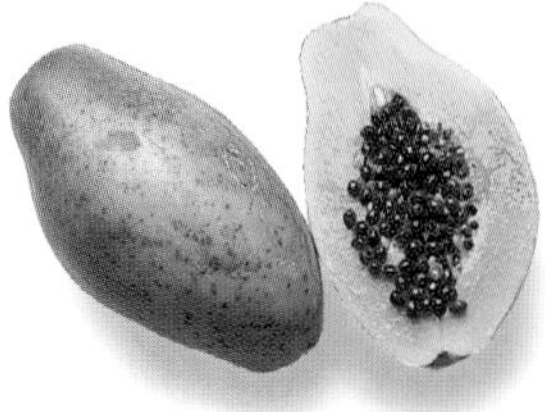

Red Papayas

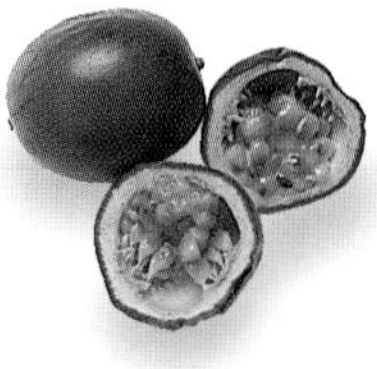

Passion Fruits

PLATE XIII

Colorful Produce

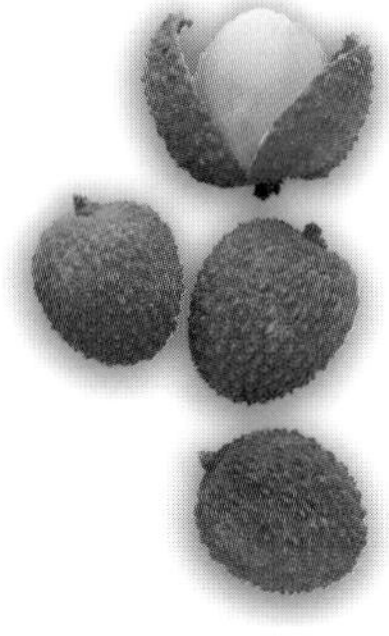

Lychees

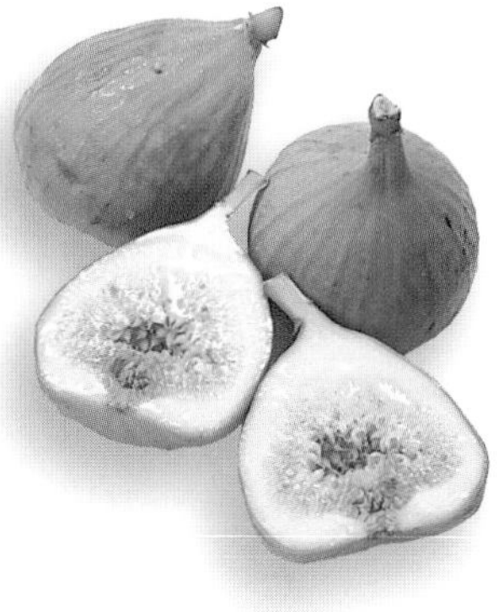

Calimyrna Figs

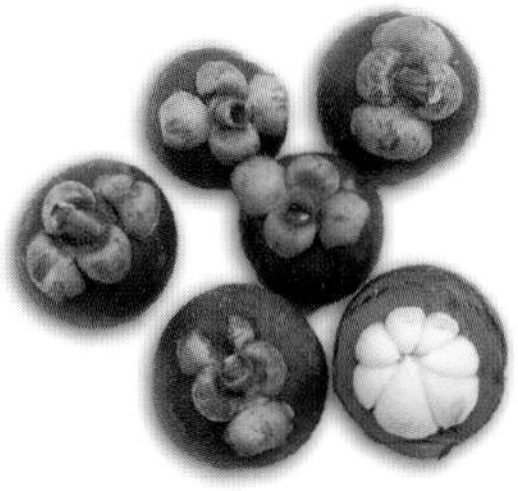

Mangosteens

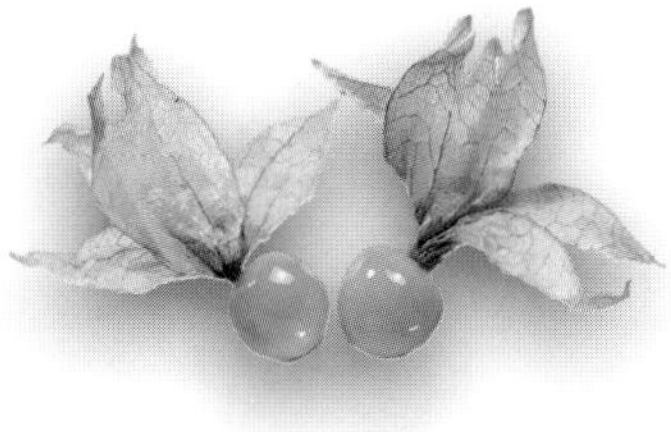

Cape Gooseberries

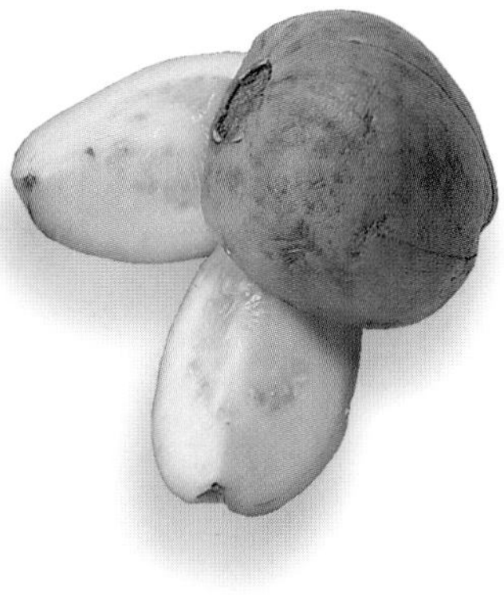

Guava

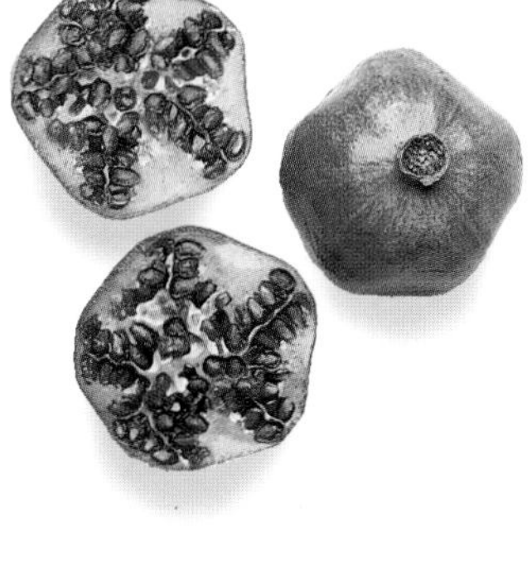

Pomegranates

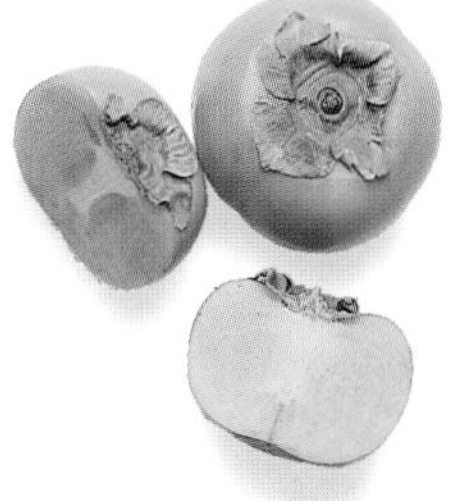

Persimmons

PLATE XIV

Fresh and Dried Produce Add Flavor and Color

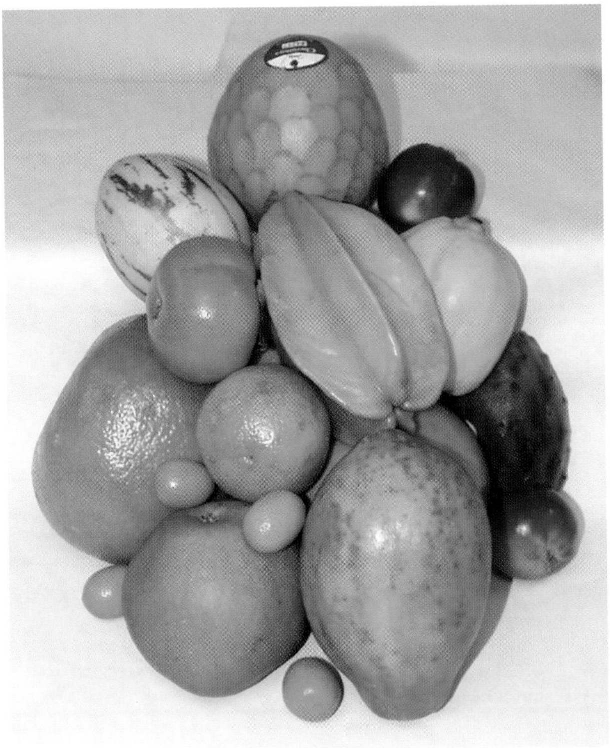

Cherimaya, Pepino Melon,
Fuya Persimmon, Moro Orange,
Oroblanco, and Kumquat

PLATE XV

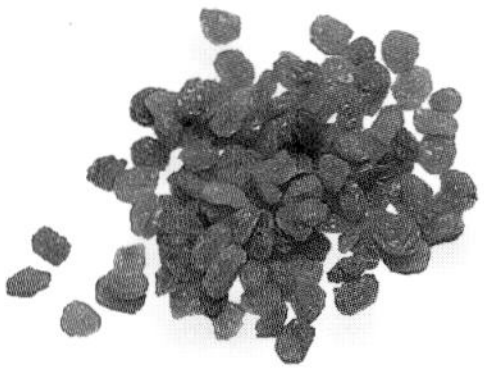

Golden Raisins

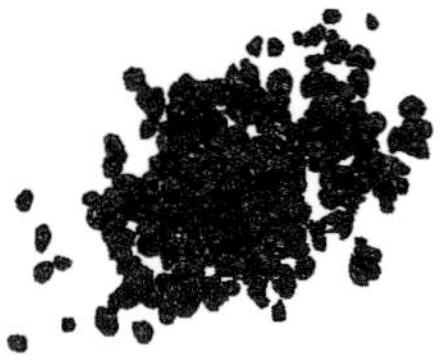

Currants

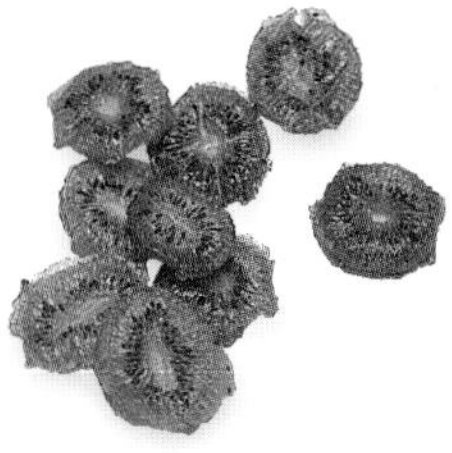

Kiwis

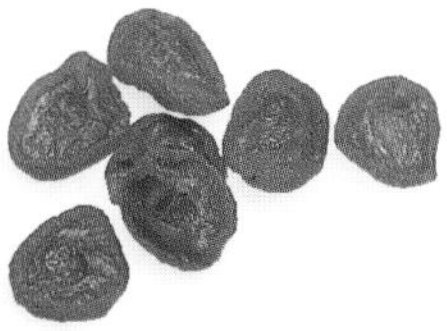

Apricots

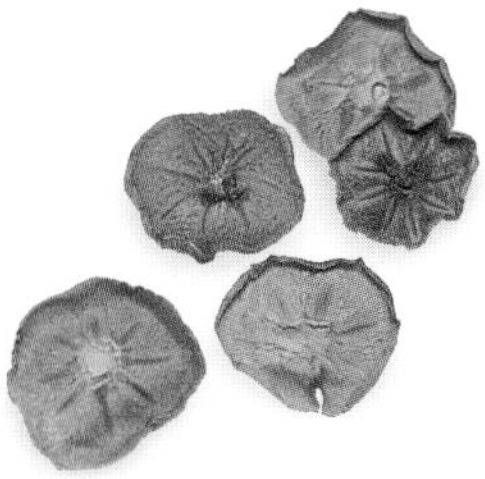

Persimmons

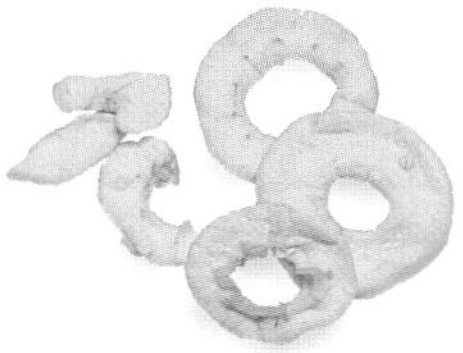

Apples

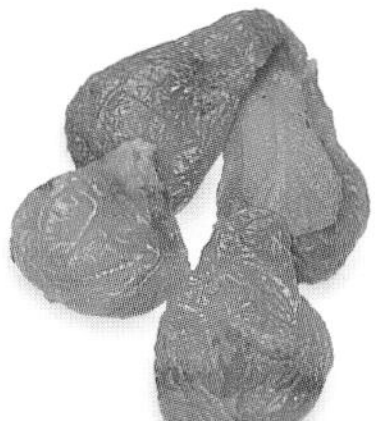

Pears

PLATE XVI

Bring a Bouquet of Flavor to the Table

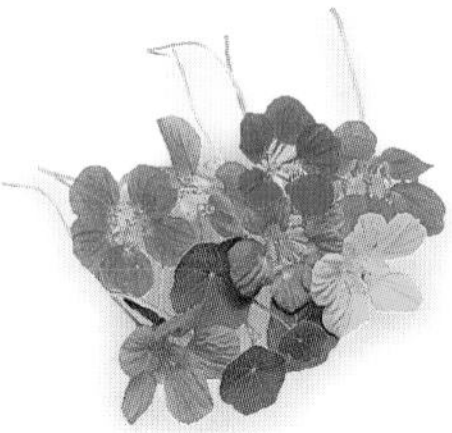

Nasturtiums

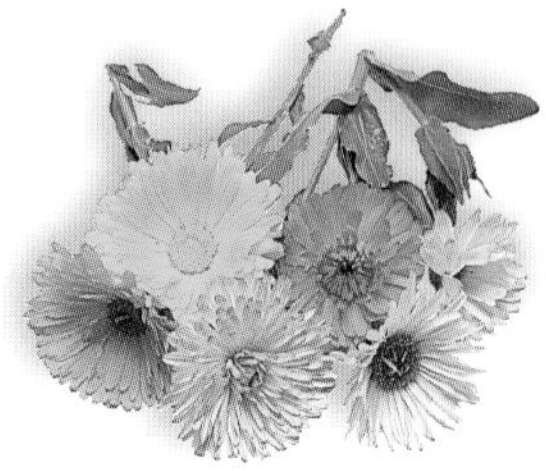

Calendulas

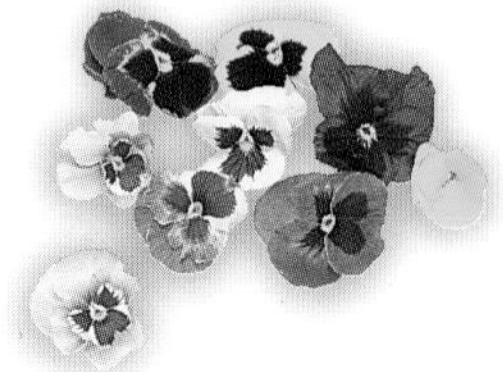

Pansies

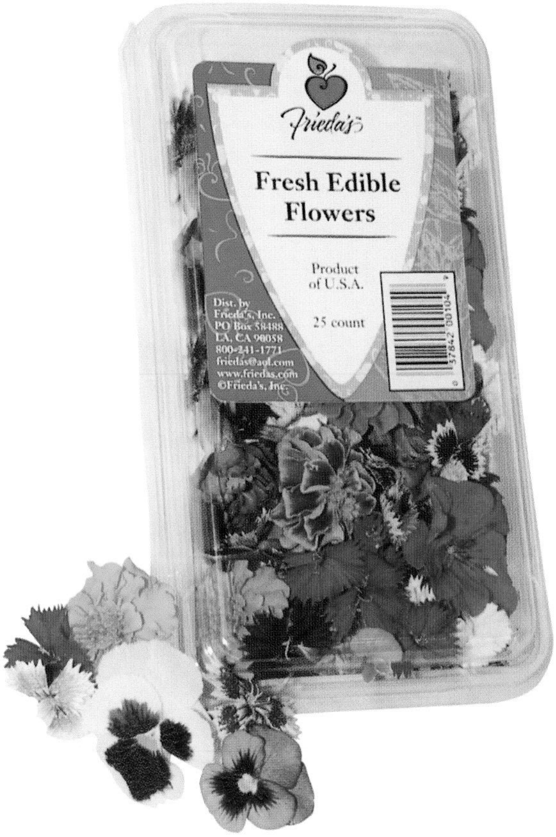

Freida's Edible Flowers

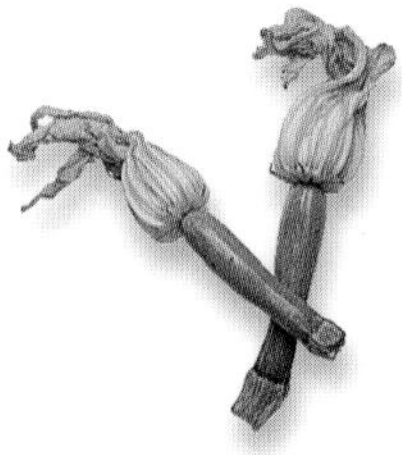

Baby Zucchini with Blossoms

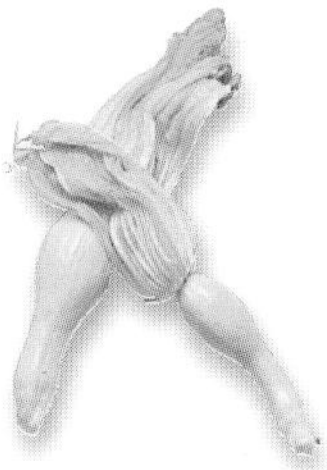

Baby Yellow Squash with Blossoms

blood pressure, ankle and leg swelling, leg cramps, weakness, paleness and anemia, excessive itching (not caused by medication, dry skin, etc.), frequent nocturnal urination, less need for diabetic medication, and protein in the urine. Diabetics must be particularly vigilant about these symptoms.

What, Me Worry?

So, what about people without diabetes or high blood pressure? Should they worry about kidney disease?

Well, worry leads to stress, and stress can lead to high blood pressure, so let's forget about the worrying. Being conscientious about your health is a better way to look at it. Nobody gets extra points for worrying. Most people just need to add a little TLC to their usual routines to keep their kidneys working at the peek of perfection.

Most healthy people won't give their kidneys a lot of thought. Probably an occasional urinary tract infection may remind them that they are there.

Bacteria grow at a fast rate in the bladder. With your fast-paced life, you may walk around with a full bladder more often than you like. The longer the bladder is full, the more time the bacteria have to grow, possibly resulting in infection. Some of these bacteria may infect the kidneys and a full bladder can put a lot of pressure on the kidneys, causing some damage.

The moral to this story is to avoid having a full bladder for a prolonged amount of time and to drink plenty of fluids, to give the bladder and kidneys fuel to rinse themselves out.

Cranberry Truth

E. coli is responsible for many urinary tract infections (estimated 8 to 10 million per year in the United States). There are natural ingredients in cranberries that stop the growth of *E. coli* (Busch). Available as juice and pills (that claim to concentrated cranberry extract), dried fruit, and even power bars, cranberries are becoming a popular ingredient, both for their supposed health properties and for the color and tang they add to foods. It's not been established if cranberry juice or other cranberry products truly enhance kidney and bladder health. However, fluids are very important for keeping the kidneys and bladders happy, and cranberry juice is definitely high in vitamin C—a proven good thing!

Just about any kind of fluid will make your kidneys smile *except* those with excessive sugar, salt, or caffeine. Sugar can encourage the growth of bacteria in the bladder. The kidneys must filter salt, so the more you take in over what you need every day, the harder your kidneys have to work. Caffeine plays a number on your circulatory system, and encourages your body to get rid of fluid it really needs. You can drink quarts of fluid, in the form of coffee or iced tea, and wind up dehydrated because of the caffeine. So go easy on the coffee, tea, soft drinks, and sports drinks (a little is okay, just take it easy) and think: fresh, refreshing fruit juices (blueberry-ginger lemonade and iced passion fruit herbal tea come to mind) and clear, sparkling water.

Here are some fluid ideas:

1. Water (yes, water)—iced, with a twist of lemon, lime, orange or tangerine, sparkling, flavored.
2. Fruit juice—mixed with sparkling water blended with yogurt or nonfat milk, frozen and served as slush. Try blending fresh watermelon and adding it to lemonade; mix orange juice, apricot nectar, and mango nectar together; freeze white grape juice and serve in a tall glass of cranberry juice.
3. Herbal and decaffeinated teas: try iced green tea with a twist of ginger, hot green tea with lemon and mint, hibiscus tea with orange slices, herbal tea blends mixed with clove and nutmeg.

Mother Nature's Plan B

Fortunately, kidneys were designed to have a lot of reserve. Even if 60 percent of the kidney's nephrons are destroyed, kidneys still function reasonably well. Usually, symptoms don't show until kidney function is down to 30 percent.

You can function well with only one of your two kidneys. Some people are born with only one functioning kidney, some lose a kidney to disease or injury, and some people choose to donate a kidney to help someone in need. Mother Nature was really thinking when she designed the kidneys.

Some forms of kidney disease can be controlled with a carefully planned diet. This is a diet with limited amounts of protein, sodium, potassium, and fluids. These nutrients are processed by the kidneys. By limiting them, you make life easier for the diseased or damaged kidney.

Healthy people do not benefit from limiting these nutrients, so don't consider this as a "preventative." Watch your health, have regular check-ups, got lots of rest and exercise, don't smoke, drink lots of healthy things, and your kidneys will be good to you.

CAFFEINE: FRIEND TO THE STUDENT, FOE TO THE BODY

All right, prepare for some bad news. While caffeine is getting you through those long study nights and through those interminable nutrition lectures, it is also raising the bad cholesterol in blood and hollowing out your bones. Bummer.

How can this happen, you say? That wonderful, aromatic, energy-stimulating hot beverage, made lovingly by your favorite barista, how could it be bad? Drinking coffee has been associated with heart disease and osteoporosis (thinning of bones).

The studies found that it was the type and the amount of coffee consumed that made the difference between health and disease. People, who drank more than five to six cups of unfiltered coffee, like espresso or cappuccino made from espresso, had lower bone density and more incidence of heart disease.

A NUTRI-BAR

*Foods High in Potassium**

The following have 300 or more milligrams of potassium per serving:

8 ounces whole, lowfat, nonfat, and buttermilk

3 ounces cooked beef, liver, pork, canned salmon, chicken, and veal

4 ounces dried apricots, raisins, and prunes, 1 medium banana, ½ small cantaloupe or honeydew, 2 ounces dried dates and figs, fresh peaches and apricots, ½ medium avocado

4 ounces cooked beans

10 fresh mushrooms

3 tablespoons peanut butter

1 baked potato

1 baked sweet potato

1 medium tomato

6 ounces canned tomato juice

1 cup cold all-bran cereal

*This information can be used in two ways: to increase the amount of potassium in a healthy person's diet or to decrease the amount of potassium in a renally-impaired person's diet.

A NUTRI-BAR

Kidney Quiz

Courtesy of the National Kidney Foundation

1. True or False: When uncontrolled, very high blood pressure is up to twice as likely to result in kidney disease.
2. About 5 to 30 percent of diabetic patients will eventually have kidney failure.
3. One of the six warning signs of kidney failure is puffiness around the eyes.
4. Kidneys help stimulate white blood cell production.
5. Kidneys are the size of your fist and are shaped like kidney beans.
6. A person can only live with two kidneys.

Answer Key: 1. F 2. T 3. T 4. F 5. T 6. F

It's not just the caffeine in the coffee that causes heart disease. A study that looked at how switching from caffeinated to decaffeinated coffee affected people with high blood cholesterol found that people's cholesterol actually increased with decaffeinated coffee (James, p. 4). This showed that it wasn't just the caffeine, and that high volumes of either regular or decaf can do some damage.

Further research showed that natural substances found in arabica coffee beans, which accounts for over 75 percent of all coffee in the world, caused cholesterol to rise. These substances do not pass through paper filters, but do pass through wire and nylon filters. Even coffee filtered through paper contains some of these substances. Five to six cups seems to be the magic amount. Under five or six cups per day did not seem to increase cholesterol. More than five or six cups significantly increased the risk of heart attack. These cholesterol-raising compounds were not found in Robusta beans, the other major type of beans grown in the world. Okay, you say, then why don't we just use Robustas? Because Robustas are very, very strong in flavor and acid and because they are in short supply. Even if you could afford pure Robustas all the time, you wouldn't have to worry about bacteria destroying your tooth enamel. The Robustas would dissolve it first.

To add insult to injury, while you're poisoning your heart, your bones are heading out of town. Several studies have shown that women who regularly had more than five to six cups of coffee a day had thinner bones. In addition, they tended to have more calcification in their arteries. Calcification of arteries is an indicator of heart disease. It's a sort of circular reaction. Substances in unfiltered coffee tend to raise the level of cholesterol in the blood. The extra cholesterol starts to stick to the walls of the arteries and becomes hard, or calcifies. The more cholesterol, the less calcium in the bones and the more hard stuff, useless calcium, in the arteries.

What's the moral of the story? Filter your coffee when you brew it. Don't drink five cups of coffee a day on a regular basis. Save that French-pressed coffee or espresso for special occasions. As hard as it is, attempt to arrange your schedule so that you don't need to rely on coffee to keep your heart beating.

Nutri-Words

Absorption: utilizing the components of digested food for energy, growth, repair and other reactions necessary in the body.

Amino acids: the breakdown product of protein digestion; important for many functions in the body, including build up and repair of skin, tissue and muscle, and maintenance of the immune system.

Antacids: natural or chemical products used to suppress the production of hydrochloric acid by the stomach. May interfere with protein digestion and the absorption of certain vitamins and minerals.

Caffeine: a stimulant found naturally in coffee, tea and cocoa. May elevate blood pressure and affect the ability to perform tasks that require concentration.

Digestion: the physical and chemical act of breaking down food to useful components.

Diverticuli: the finger-like protrusions on the surface of the small intestine responsible for the absorption of nutrients.

Enzymes: protein-containing catalysts that enter and leave a reaction unchanged in form; necessary for the process of digestion.

Esophagus: the tube that links the mouth and the stomach.
Fatty acid: the breakdown product of fat digestion; an important component of many chemicals in the body.
Flavor: the inherent quality of food that makes it either enjoyable or not enjoyable.
Four natural tastes on the tongue: taste buds naturally perceive sweet, salty, bitter and sour.
Gallbladder: an ancillary digestive organ that secretes bile, necessary for fat digestion.
Glucose: the breakdown product of carbohydrate digestion; an important source of energy in the body.
Hiatal hernia: a pouching out of the esophagus that can be caused by poor eating habits.
Hydrochloric acid: the digestive fluid secreted in the stomach necessary for protein digestion.
Kidney: a filtering organ, important for the body's fluid balance.
Lactose intolerance: an inability to digest and absorb the sugar found in dairy products.
Large intestine: the organ at the end of the digestive tract, responsible for the absorption of fluids and the fermentation of certain nutrients. The end of the large intestine is called the colon.
Laxatives: natural or chemical products that relieve constipation by irritating the intestine. Can become addictive.
Liver: a filtering organ, responsible for detoxifying ingested chemicals.
Mouth: the organ that is the beginning of the digestive process.
Pancreas: an organ responsible for supplying bile, necessary for fat digestion, and for the hormone insulin, necessary for carbohydrate metabolism.
Saliva: the fluid secreted in the mouth by the salivary glands to assist with digestion.
Small intestine: the organ responsible for the completion of and commencement of certain nutrients.
Stomach: the organ responsible for digestion of protein and for preparing food to enter the small intestine.
Stomach ulcer: a "burn" in the stomach caused by excessive hydrochloric acid secreted in the absence of food.
Taste buds: small, finger-like protrusions on the surface of the tongue that are flavor receptors.
Taste palate: the collection of flavors that one is most accustomed to.
Textural perception: in regard to taste, the feeling of food on the tongue. such as found in the smoothness of ice cream or the crunchiness of a fresh apple.
Villi: microscopic fronds which increase the absorbing area of the intestines.
Visual perception: in regard to taste, the appearance of food allows for prejudgement of taste, or " you eat first with your eyes."

Whaddaya think?

1. What is your impression of the fifth taste on the tongue, unami?
2. Can you explain the interplay between aroma and taste?
3. What type of taste test would you set up to prove the link between visual perception and taste?
4. What is your personal taste palate?

5. What environmental, psychological, and physical factors influence taste?
6. Take a "fantastic voyage" through human digestion and absorption of food
7. How would you suggest that someone avoid acquiring a hiatal hernia?
8. Do you think that stress affects digestion?
9. What's the bad news about caffeine and nutrition?
10. Suggest some low-fat dessert items that will intrigue your customers.
11. What's the deal with alcohol? Why is it considered to damage the body?

Critical Application Exercises

1. Obtain a piece of poster the same height as you. Tape it to a wall:
   a. Outline all the organs involved in digestion and absorption.
   b. Label the organs and list all the enzymes and chemicals each needs to complete digestion and absorption.
   c. List all the "jobs" that the organs have.
2. Taste-test time:
   a. Collect a green apple, peeled onion, head of elephant garlic, and a peeled, raw potato. Cut them all into quarters.
   b. Have someone you trust blindfold you. Clamp your nose closed.
   c. Have your trusty assistant give you a sample of each product. See if you can identify them without being able to see them or taste them.
3. Do a little kitchen science—perfect for entertaining at parties:
   a. Prepare your favorite flavor of gelatin and let it set. Slice and drain some fresh and canned pineapple. Place the fresh slices on one side of the gelatin and the canned slices on the other side. Record your observations.
   b. Place a small piece of fresh beef, chicken, or firm tofu in a dish. Soak one side in vinegar and the other side in orange juice. Record your observations.
4. Addictions aside, concoct at least five ideas for hot and cold beverages to replace caffeinated coffee beverages, such as lattes or cappuccino.

References

Busch, Felicia (Ed.) (2000). *A Taste of Life.* Boston, MA: Ocean Spray Cranberries, Inc.

Cataldo, C. B., Nyenhuis, J. R., et al. (1989). *Nutrition and Diet Therapy Principles and Practice,* 2nd ed., New York: West Publishing Company.

Cramer, T. (1992). "A burning question: When do you need an antacid?" *FDA Consumer,* 26:1, 18.

Fauci, A. S., Braunwald, E., Isselbacher, K. J. et al. (1998). *Harrison's Principles of Internal Medicine.* New York: McGraw-Hill.

James, C. T. (1991). "Food and drugs: Do they mix?" *Health Sciences Review,* Spring p. 24.

Postgate, J. (1992). *Microbes and Man* (3rd ed.). Cambridge: Cambridge University Press.

Chapter 4

Carbohydrates

Chapter Overview

Chapter Objectives

After reading this chapter, the student should be able to:

1. *Explain how including carbohydrates on the menu will improve the customer's health and the operation's bottom line.*
2. *Describe the various types of carbohydrates and how they are metabolized and used by the body.*
3. *Explain the difference between sugars, starches, and fibers, offering menu examples.*
4. *Suggest how to construct menu items for gluten intolerant customers.*
5. *Describe the mechanism of enzymes in digestion in reference to lactose intolerance.*
6. *Detail the difference between Type I and Type II diabetes, especially in reference to menu selection.*
7. *Offer alternatives to honey and sugar for vegan customers.*
8. *Describe the metabolic damage caused by excess alcohol use.*
9. *Define soluble and insoluble fiber.*
10. *Compare current popular nutrition theory to that of Dr. Kellogg's or Graham's.*
11. *Suggest how to include sugar substitutes in a food service operation.*

NUTRITIVE VALUE OF CARBOHYDRATES

Carbohydrates are what makes the world go 'round. Carbohydrate crops are the most plentiful on earth. Rice, wheat, corn, beans, potatoes—all carbohydrates. Most nutrition authorities agree that carbohydrates should be the larger part of your intake every day. The USDA Guideline for Americans suggests that carbohydrates should be at least 55 to 60 percent of your daily caloric intake.

Profit Margin for the Food Professional: Good For the Waistline and the Wallet

This suggestion is good for the health of your body and your pocketbook. Carbohydrates are easily digested and absorbed and are a good and efficient source of fuel for your body. Most carbohydrates are very low in fat and

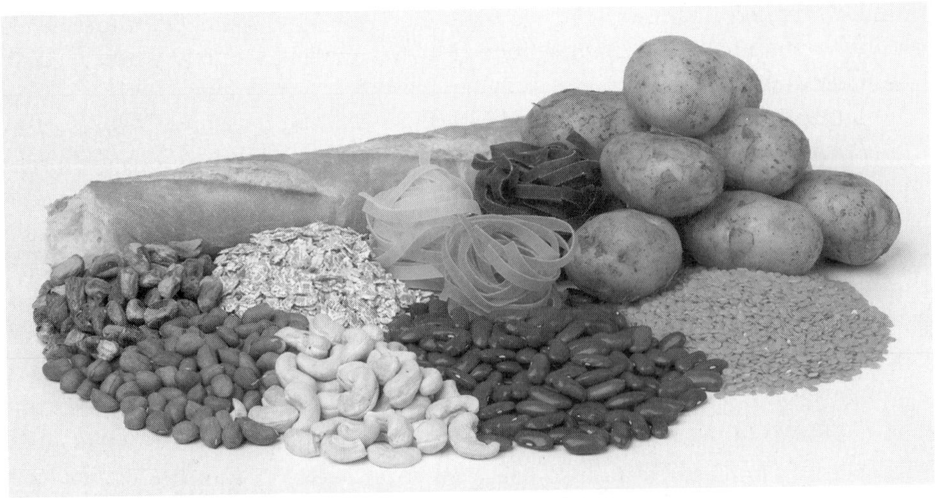

Do ingredients such as these make up 55 to 60 percent of your menus?

sodium. Minimally processed carbohydrates, such as whole-wheat bread, brown rice, and dried beans are high in fiber, vitamins and minerals.

Menu Design with Carbohydrates

Carbohydrates are relatively inexpensive and usually easy to prepare. A baked potato can be an elegant side dish or even a fast entrée, easy on the labor and the cost. A chef can look like a real hero for only pennies when sending out plates heaped with steaming angel hair, fettuccini, or spaghettini. Most people like some type of carbohydrate. Who do you know that absolutely hates every type of potato, pasta, corn, rice, hot or cold cereal, bread, grains, or beans?

GLUTEN INTOLERANCE

Causes

Now that you mention it, there are some people who need to avoid wheat and some grain products. Some people are born without the ability to digest gluten, the protein found in wheat. They can eat rice, corn, beans, potatoes, and some other grains, such as soy and amaranth, but have to stay away from gluten-containing products. There are more people who have this condition than you might think. Just search the web or cruise the cookbook selections at a bookstore. There are many organizations and support groups for people who are gluten intolerant. Be prepared to answer questions from gluten-intolerant customers about the menu.

Products to Avoid

Wheat-free eating takes some planning. "Wheat-free" means that no wheat flour ingredients are used in a food. These would include whole-wheat flour, all-purpose flour—any flour made from wheat. Flours made from other ingredients, such as barley, rye, corn, or potato are usually okay. As usual, when it comes to people you can't make generalizations. Some gluten- and wheat-intolerant people can eat everything but wheat. Others have sensitivities to other grains. It's the food professional's responsibility to inform customers what is in the food. It is the customers' responsibility to know what they can handle. Wheat allergies are among the most common food allergies.

Gluten-free is much more restrictive. Gluten is the protein component in many grains, including wheat, barley, rye and oats. Gluten-free means that there are no ingredients from these grains used in a food. People who have celiac disease (the old-fashioned term for this was "sprue") are borne with an inability to tolerate glaidin, which is contained in gluten. Gluten or gliadin is toxic in their small intestines, damaging the intestines in such a way that nutrients cannot be absorbed. For a celiac person, the smallest trace of gluten can be harmful.

A person with a wheat-allergy could eat a gluten-free product, but a person with celiac disease or gluten intolerance could not eat just a wheat-free product, because other grains contain gluten. Some common foods that contain gluten include bouillon, some soy sauce, vinegar, dessert mixes, snack foods, such as roasted peanuts or potato chips, and some extracts that

Commercial chocolate beverage and other drink mixes

Malt powder

Cooked or dry pasta made with wheat, rye, oat, and barley; also macaroni and noodles

Cooked or dried cereals made from the grains listed above

Bread or bread products (crumbs, croutons, bread sticks) made from grains listed above

Convenience items (soups or soup mixes, cake mixes, pudding mixes, salad dressings, frozen entrées, etc.) which may have the grains listed above as an ingredient

Commercial vinegars

Commercial salad dressings and other condiments, such as ketchup and mayonaise

Beer and ale, cereal beverages (such as Postum or grain milk, like rice or oat milk), root beer

Figure 4–1 Some Gluten-Containing Food Products

contain alcohol. Gluten is added as an ingredient to enhance the flavor or texture of these products.

Menu Suggestions

If you are preparing foods from scratch, using unprocessed ingredients then you will know if a menu item is gluten- or wheat-free. Arrowroot, cornmeal, soy, rice, tapioca, and potato products should be okay for most gluten-intolerant people. If you use any processed items, such as spice blends, mashed potato mix, soup bases, etc., then you will need to read the labels very carefully or even contact manufacturers about their products. This issue may not come up often, but it's always important to be prepared.

SUGAR, STARCH, AND FIBER

For most people, the health and cost benefits of carbohydrates are good business. You can feed your customers on the cheap! All carbohydrates are plant-based, so vegetarian customers as well as those looking to cut back on their

A.M.: assorted fruit or fruit or vegetable juices, rice or corn cereal with milk, muffins made with rice or corn flour, butter or peanut butter (check the label for gluten; some peanut butter has it), fruit preserves

P.M.: Chicken or tofu stir-fried with seasonal veggies, potatoes steamed with fresh herbs, green salad with raspberry vinaigrette, fresh fruit slices, sorbet (Check labels on soy sauce for stir fry and vinegar for vinaigrette)

Snack: Rice cakes with salsa and guacamole or seasoned cheese popcorn with vegetable sticks

Figure 4–2 A Sample Gluten-Free Menu

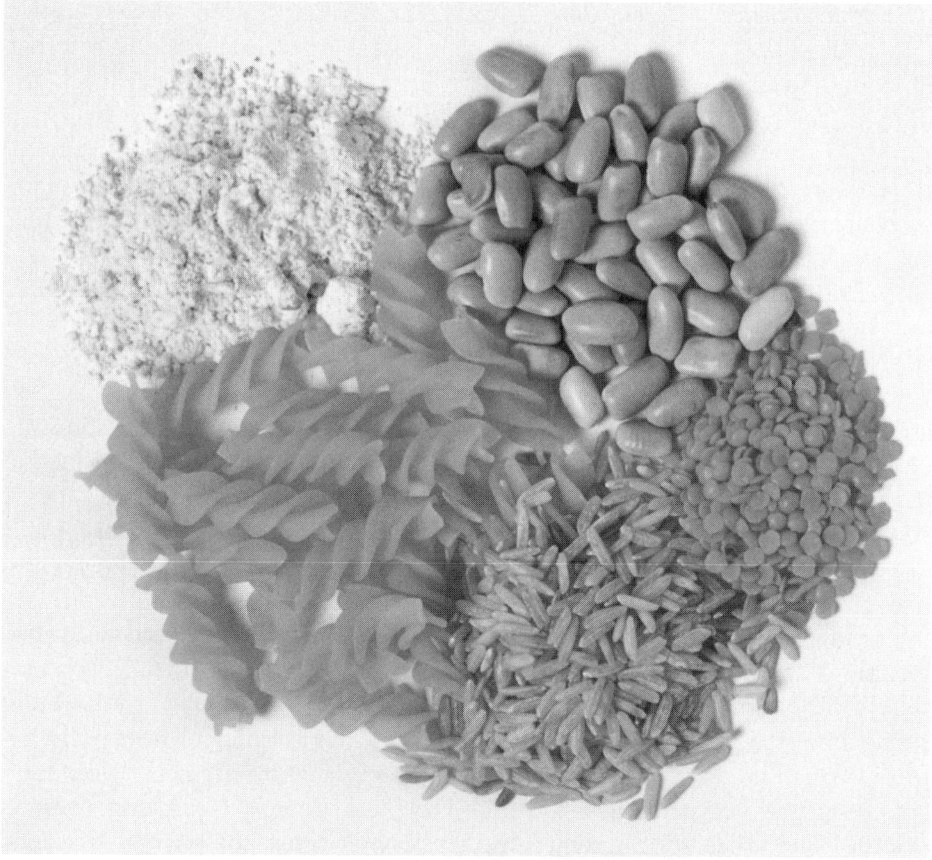

Which of these ingredients are acceptable for gluten-intolerant customers?

animal protein intake will be happy. Think about pasta primavera prepared with carrot and spinach fettucini, yellow, red and green bell peppers, baby green peas and carrots, or an herbed gnocchi (potato pasta) with a ragout of smoked chanterelles. Roasted sweet potatoes with a pineapple-orange glaze or six-bean firehouse chili are just a few ways to attractively showcase carbohydrates on the menu.

All carbohydrates contain 4 calories per gram. Carbohydrates are divided into three categories: simple carbohydrates, also called "sugars" or **"simple sugars"; complex carbohydrates,** also called **"starch";** and fiber. Just to confuse issues, scientists call simple carbohydrates "monosaccharides" and "disaccharides" and complex carbohydrates "polysaccharides."

Just remember that sugar, starch, and fiber are the three main categories of carbohydrates. Those will be the terms you'll use most often. Keep the other terms in the back of your mind, in case they ever come up.

HOW CALORIE AMOUNTS FROM FOOD ARE DETERMINED

We told you that all carbohydrates contain 4 calories per gram, and they do. Whether or not your body can get to all the calories or not is another story. Ever wonder how food technologists figure out how many calories a food contains? One of the methods they use involves burning a food completely to ash. Special ovens called bomb calorimeters can measure the amount of heat the food gives off while it is burning. Remember that energy equals calories. If you can measure the amount of energy something gives off while it is being burned, you are measuring the amount of calories it contains.

You know that you "burn" calories when you use energy. That's one of the reasons you get so hot when you are doing a heavy workout or running up stairs while carrying twenty pounds of books. Your body acts like an oven, burning food to release calories.

Some food is more easily burned for calories than others. The less fibrous, or the less complex a food is, the more easily it can be burned for calories. By the same token, the less complex a food is, the less energy is required to break it apart. Simple sugars contain very little or no fiber and have no structure to speak of. So, if you eat a couple of spoonfuls of sugar, as in soda or a Popsicle, your body can obtain almost 100 percent of the energy found in them. It requires hardly any energy to burn up sugar. Unfortunately, since sugar is so easily burned, you use it up very quickly, creating those sugar "rushes" and then corresponding lows. This is not a comfortable feeling and makes it very difficult to sustain a consistent energy level.

However, if you give your body some oatmeal to tackle, you won't get exactly 4 calories per gram of oatmeal. Oatmeal contains both starch and fiber. Both starch and fiber have a lot of structure, and it takes your body some time and energy to break these foods down in order to obtain energy from them. The downside? You have to wait a while for energy and you don't get everything you paid for. The upside? You have energy over a longer period of time, as it takes your body a while to slowly release the energy. No highs and lows, just a consistent amount of energy available over a long period of time, probably two or three hours, depending on your activity level. Because it takes energy to get energy from oatmeal, you can eat a little more, as you are burning a little more. In addition, oatmeal contains vitamins and minerals, while table sugar contains nothing but calories.

Food professionals use different types of sugar for different types of cooking. See Figure 4–3 for a sugar glossary. The type of sugar used may depend on what's available, what the region is known for, or what flavor or color the chef is looking for. Molasses and honey give deep, rich tastes and flavors to food. Great for gingerbread, not so hot for angel food cake. Fructose may have a slightly sweeter taste than sucrose. Brown sugar adds texture to baked products. Selecting different sugars does not influence the nutritive value of the dish, just the taste, flavor, and color.

HOW THE BODY USES ENERGY FROM CARBOHYDRATES

Ever wonder why you can eat all the salad you want? Salad vegetables, such as lettuces, spinach, radishes, celery, onions, cucumbers, and bell peppers are made up largely of fiber. Although fiber contains four calories per gram, humans lack the ability to break down most fiber. If you could get at it, you could have the energy. But you can't get at it. The downside? Very little energy from very high-fiber foods. The upside? Since you can't obtain very many calories

Brown rice syrup: syrup expressed from cooking brown rice. Has the taste and consistency of honey. Used by vegans who want to avoid processed white sugar.

Brown sugar: white sugar with added molasses. No, brown sugar does not have additional nutritional value.

Confectionary sugar: (also called 10X sugar or powdered sugar). This is sucrose that has been pulverized into a fine powder.

Corn syrup: a breakdown product of cornstarch containing mostly glucose.

Dextrose: molecules of glucose.

Fructose, galactose, and glucose: simple sugars that are the end product of carbohydrate metabolism.

Granulated sugar: good old table sugar, also called sucrose.

High fructose corn syrup: extracted from cornstarch, very inexpensive to produce. Mostly fructose with a little glucose added in. Used in many food products.

Honey: mostly glucose and fructose made from the sucrose in flower nectar. Honey should not be given to children under the age of one year, as it contains some bacterial spores that a child's immature digestive system can't handle. Want to know more? Visit *www.honey.com*.

Mannitol and sorbitol: sugar alcohols produced from the glucose in fruit. Bacteria in the mouth cannot use mannitol and sorbitol, so they are not associated with tooth decay. Mannitol and sorbitol are more difficult to absorb, so even though they physically contain the same number of calories as glucose, they do not release the same numbers of calories.

Maple syrup: sucrose syrup harvested from maple trees.

Molasses: a byproduct of sucrose processing. Blackstrap molasses absorbs iron from the equipment used to process it.

Raw sugar: the first step in extracting sucrose from sugar cane. It takes the form of crystals. Usually not sold in the United States, as it can contain high concentrations of dirt and bug parts.

Stevia: an extract from a tropical plant, stevia is available as a powder that looks like sugar and as a syrup. Because it is a natural product, the degree of sweetness can vary from product to product. Very expensive and in limited supply at this time.

Turbinado sugar: raw sugar that has been cleaned of dirt and bug parts.

White sugar: sucrose. Processed by concentrating and recrystallizing raw sugar.

Figure 4–3 How To Make It Sweet

from high-fiber foods, you can eat more of them. More on the health benefits of fiber later in the chapter.

SUGARS AND ENZYMES (-OSES AND -ASES)

You know something is a sugar if it ends in "ose." So, **glucose,** fructose, **lactose,** and maltose are all sugars.

The big-deal simple sugar is glucose. It is the most basic sugar. Glucose is what the body is looking for when it breaks down bread, potatoes, fruit, and any carbohydrate-containing food. It is the basis for fuel in the body and the only fuel that the brain will use. Whenever you digest carbohydrates, the bottom line is the glucose.

You'll want to review Chapter 3's basic digestion and absorption. Remember that carbohydrate digestion begins in the mouth. The salivary glands secrete enzymes that help start carbohydrate metabolism. Carbohydrates are washed down the esophagus and through the stomach. Carbohydrate digestion is completed, and absorption is begun in the small intestine. The pancreas and the liver help in the absorption of carbohydrates. The pancreas secretes insulin, a hormone that enables cells to absorb glucose. This is the ultimate use of all carbohydrates. The liver releases glucose into the bloodstream as needed and also acts as the body's savings account for glucose. For efficiency, the liver changes glucose into a storage form, called glycogen. We'll talk more about glycogen in Chapter 8, when we cover menus for athletes.

Lots of different enzymes are needed to digest all the different types of carbohydrates you eat. Just as anything that ends in "-ose" is a sugar, anything that ends in "-ase" is an enzyme. If you want to digest the sugar sucrose, then you need the enzyme sucrase. No problem. The brain triggers the body to produce enzymes when it figures out what you ate.

LACTOSE INTOLERANCE

If you grab some yogurt for breakfast or add a slice of cheese to your sandwich, you are eating dairy products. Dairy products contain lactose, or milk sugar. You need the enzyme lactase to digest lactose. Perhaps you've heard of people who are lactose intolerant? Many people think that means you are "allergic" to milk. Not so. You can handle the protein, the fat, the minerals, and the vitamins in milk. You just don't have a way to break down the milk sugar.

Some people are born without the ability to produce **lactase.** Particular ethnic groups, especially African Americans and Asians, have a tendency to be **lactose intolerant.** This is thought to be an evolutionary matter, since diets in the country of origin had very little dairy. The body is very efficient. If something is not needed, the body doesn't develop it.

Some people lose their ability to produce lactase. This is a matter of "use it or lose it." If you don't ingest any dairy products for many years, the body thinks, "Why should I keep this knowledge around? It's just cluttering up the brain." When you reintroduce dairy products back to your diet, the body says, "What's this? I don't remember this!" Sometimes lactase production returns, and sometimes it doesn't.

People who are lactose intolerant vary in their ability to handle dairy products. Some can eat very small amounts of solid dairy products, such as cheese or sour cream. Others can't handle any type of dairy product. Some people cope with lactose intolerance by avoiding dairy products. They substitute fortified grain, rice or **soy milk,** and cheese for dairy products. They'll select sorbet (sherbet has some dairy in it), fruit ice, or soy or rice frozen desserts instead of milk-based items.

Some lactose-intolerant people will ingest lactase in the form of pills or liquid before they eat dairy products. This adds back what the body doesn't have. There are also specially modified dairy products for lactose-intolerant people. Acidophilus is a lactose-loving good bacteria. If you put some acidophilus in milk or yogurt, the bacteria will digest all the lactose for you. This solves the problem for people who can't digest lactose on their own; the bacteria do it for them. The next time you go to the grocery store, check out the dairy section of acidophilus-containing milk or yogurt.

SELECTING SUGARS FOR FOOD PREPARATION

Simple sugars are simple sugars. Some people believe that "natural" sugar, such as honey, is "better" for them than corn syrup or white sugar. Not so. Your body does not distinguish between sugar from maple syrup or sugar from granulated white sugar. Most all sugars are "natural," as they are processed from beets, sugar cane, corn and dates. Remember, your body is looking to take every type of carbohydrate it can get its hands (or diverticuli) on and break it down into glucose. If it makes you feel better to get your sugar high from "natural" sugars, such as turbinado or date palm sugar, so be it. Your gut doesn't care.

However, there is a difference between sugars gotten from syrup or honey and sugars gotten from milk (lactose) or fruit **(fructose).** Maple syrup, honey, or corn syrup are sugar, nothing else. No redeeming nutritional value. When you obtain sugar from an orange or from yogurt, you are also getting protein, minerals, and vitamins, fiber and all those other good nutrition things. In addition, when you obtain sugar from what nutritionists like to call "whole foods," such as fruit or juice, it takes your body a little longer to extract the sugar. This means that there is a steady, gradual release of sugar into your bloodstream, giving even amounts of energy over a decent period of time. As we've mentioned before, when you get sugar from concentrated sources, such as soda or candy, you get the "soar and crash" effect. Lots of sugar is released into your bloodstream all at one time. It is used quickly and then disappears. Anyone who's ever had a sugar rush and the ensuing sugar "low" knows what we mean.

DIABETES

Speaking of selecting different types of sugar, we should talk about one of the health conditions that affects how much and what type of sugar people can ingest. **Diabetes** is becoming more and more prevalent in the United States. In 2000, diabetes reached an all-time high among the under-thirty population. Linked to both genetics, lifestyle, and obesity, food-service professionals will be seeing more diabetic customers in their operations. You should have a basic understanding of diabetes, so you can decide how or if you will attempt to accommodate diabetic customers.

Food	*Tablespoons of Sugar*
⅛ apple pie	2
½ cup applesauce	1½
2-inch piece frosted cake	3
1 tablespoon catsup	½
2 ounces sugared cold cereal	3
2 sticks chewing gum	½
1 cup chocolate milk	2
12 ounces cola	5
1 sandwich cookie	1
1 glazed donut	2
1 plain donut	1
½ canned fruit (heavy syrup)	2
12-oz Kool Aid™	6
½ cup Jell-O™	2
1 cup fruited yogurt	3

Figure 4–4 A Spoonful of Sugar

History

Diabetes, whose full name is "diabetes mellitus," is not a modern disease. In fact, ancient Egyptian and Chinese writings dating back to 1500 B.C. describe diabetes in full detail. The word "diabetes" comes from the Greek word which means, "to flow through," and "mellitus" comes from the Latin word for honey; referring to the spilling of sugar into the urine of diabetics.

Ancient physicians could diagnose diabetes, but they had little or no treatment for it. Ancient treatments including withholding fluids, using various herbs believed to "absorb" sugar. Leeching, a procedure in which a doctor would attach leeches, small water animals that are cousins to slugs and whose favorite food is blood, to patients' skin and allow them to suck out a certain amount of blood. This was thought to get rid of the "defective" blood. Leeching was used until the mid 1800s.

Type I and Type II Diabetes: The Isle of Langerhans Is Not a Vacation Spot

Only in the past two hundred years have the causes and treatments of diabetes been reliably researched. Remember the "islets of Langerhans," cells found in the pancreas, from your high school biology class? In 1860, a German doctor named Paul Langerhans (surprise!) discovered a cluster of cells in the pancreas that produced insulin. It was not known what insulin did in the body. After observing lab animals who had their pancreas removed, Dr. Langerhans put two and two together and postulated that insulin controlled the body's ability to process carbohydrates. This broke open the way for diabetes treatment.

In 1921, two Canadian researchers discovered the beneficial effects of injecting insulin in animals and people. This discovery greatly improved the life expectancy and the quality of life for diabetics. Prior to the use of injectable insulin, diabetics had an average life span only into their twenties; they were told not to work or exercise and not to marry or have children. At this point, there was little understanding about the relationship between diabetes and diet; in fact, a high-fat, no-carbohydrate diet was often recommended, as it was felt that diabetics must refrain from eating any type of sugar or starch.

Type I and Type II Diabetes

As diabetes research progressed, it was found that diabetes was not always caused by the absence of insulin in the body. It was found that some people with diabetes had normal or even excessive amounts of insulin, leading to the distinguishing of Type I (or **insulin-dependent**) diabetes and Type II (or non-insulin-dependent) diabetes. The identification of Type II diabetes opened the door for research on the link between lifestyle, including diet and exercise, and diabetes treatment.

No one is really certain what causes people to develop diabetes. Some people carry a genetic trait for diabetes, but never develop it. Some people have no genetic trait for diabetes, yet they develop it. Diabetes has been definitively linked to obesity. The United States is experiencing an epidemic of obesity among school-age children. Many of these children are developing Type II diabetes as a result of their obesity. The moral to the story? Treat your body well by maintaining a healthy weight, exercising, getting rest, staying hydrated, eating right and avoiding drugs, alcohol, and smoking, and you'll put yourself at less risk for diabetes.

Just as a fast review. There are two basic types of diabetes. Type I diabetics rely on injectable insulin. In the past, Type I diabetes has been called juvenile diabetes, but that name is no longer used. Type II diabetics can many times be treated without insulin, with diet and exercise being important parts of treatment. In the past, Type II diabetes has been called adult-onset diabetes. Neither type of diabetes limits itself to particular age groups, and so the more appropriate Type I and Type II terms are used today.

Diet and Exercise

If you needed to explain to someone with Type II diabetes how diet and exercise can help them, you might want to use the following explanation: Your body's cells get their energy from a sugar called glucose. Glucose is gotten from many different types of foods, such as potatoes, fruit, breads, pasta, etc. Glucose is stored in the liver. When your body needs energy, your liver releases glucose into the blood. The organs that need the energy grab the glucose and use it. Insulin, a substance released by the pancreas helps glucose get inside cells.

If you are a Type II diabetic your pancreas might not be able to release all the insulin it makes. Insulin is the "key" that opens locked cells to pave the way for insulin use. Without insulin, the body doesn't know how to use glucose. When the glucose can't get inside the cells, it accumulates in the blood. Too much glucose in the blood can lead to many medical problems. The medication that Type II diabetics take is not insulin. It is a substance that says to your pancreas "wake up and make some insulin of your own!"

You can help your body use the glucose it needs by taking diabetic medication properly, exercising, and eating properly. It has been found that just a ten-pound weight loss (in people who need to lose weight) helps insulin work better and that regular exercise also helps your body use insulin.

War is hell but good for diabetes. When looking at the number of people who had diabetes, researchers found that death from diabetes fell during wartime. This was attributed to the lack of fancy food and increased activity during times of rationing of food and fuel. Researchers saw the same thing in populations used to hard work and limited food supply. Diabetes was generally low in these populations until times of affluence. Then, with decreased exercise from work and increased calories the researchers saw a corresponding rise in the number of people diagnosed with diabetes. This pointed to the relationship between diabetes, diets, and exercise (Fauci, p. 3).

After it was understood, in the 1920s, that injected insulin alone was not enough to control diabetes, and that the way diabetics ate affected their diabetes, researchers set out to find exactly what type of diet should be recommended to diabetics.

One theory, in the 1930s, was that diabetics knew intuitively what to eat. In other words, researchers thought that your body would tell you what it needed. That didn't work. Eliminating all sugar from the diet didn't either. After much trial and error, it was found that diabetics did best when they ate a balanced diet that kept them at their ideal body weight.

Resources

Based on the balanced-diet theory, the American Dietetic Association began to formulate diabetic diets. From observation it was found that avoiding certain foods did little to control diabetes, whereas a diet balanced in protein, fat, and carbohydrates seemed to help the condition.

But how to design balanced menus for all diabetics all the time? It couldn't be expected that every diabetic would visit his or her dietitian regularly to pick up menus. It was also not realistic to expect that diabetics could or would adhere strictly to menus for which they gave no input. This is when a great solution was devised—the exchange lists for meal planning.

Exchange Lists for Meal Planning

The exchange lists for meal planning, with variations on a theme, are what many dietitians and health-care workers have used to calculate diabetic diets for the past four decades. The exchanges are arranged into three groups. The carbohydrate group includes starch, fruit, milk, and vegetable exchanges; the meat group includes very lean, lean, medium-fat, and fat meats, seafood, poultry, and meat substitute exchanges, and the fat group includes saturated and unsaturated fat exchanges. Each exchange is assigned a calorie level; for example, one fat exchange is forty-five calories. Each food within the exchange is assigned a portion amount. For example, one slice of bacon, one-eighth of an avocado, and one teaspoon of margarine are all one fat exchange and all worth forty-five calories. People who have worked with the exchanges for a while find they can analyze a recipe or a menu in a matter of minutes.

The exchanges give patients and menu planners freedom of choice. Instead of being told that they must have grapefruit juice at breakfast time, patients are told that they are entitled to one fruit exchange in the morning. This can be translated in the correct portion size of juice, fresh fruit, dried fruit, or canned or frozen unsweetened fruit.

Diabetics are counseled as to the correct calorie level for maintenance of good health. The exchange lists allow them to select types and amounts of food while maintaining a healthy calorie level. For example, if patients are told they could have one fruit exchange, two lean meat exchanges, two starch exchanges, and one fat exchange for breakfast, they might select cantaloupe wedges, steamed tofu, two slices of toast and margarine one day. The next day they might decide on tomato juice, an egg-white omelet, and a toasted bagel. Both meals comply with the assigned exchanges.

Carbohydrate Counting

The exchange lists are one method used to calculate the amount of total calories, fat, carbohydrates, and protein in your daily intake. Exchange lists are used by diabetics, but also by people who want or need to keep track of fat, protein, or total calories. For example, people attempting to lower their cholesterol through proper diet can use the exchange lists to calculate how much fat is in their diet. People desiring to keep their daily energy intake in the 1,800-calorie range can use the exchanges to calculate total calories.

Carbohydrate counting is another method of diet calculation. Carbohydrate counting is used by people who are focusing primarily on their carbohydrate intake (Gillespie, p. 3). Carbohydrate counting is an effective way for diabetics to control their carbohydrate intake, and so to control their blood sugar. Carbohydrate counting concentrates on foods containing carbohydrates, such as breads, cereals, pasta, rice, grains, potatoes, dairy products, fruit and fruit juice, table sugar, and candy and desserts. Persons using carbohydrate counting for their meal planning are expected to keep their protein and fat intake within acceptable limits, as protein and fat are not counted or calculated (Gill, 2).

Carbohydrate counting has been around since the 1920s. It allows more flexibility in menu planning, as no foods are excluded and only carbohydrates are counted. Persons using carbohydrate counting look at the "total calories" portion of food labels. They can also use printed material from restaurants and food establishments that list nutritional analyses of their menus or purchase books or computer programs that detail carbohydrate information.

Carbohydrate counting operates with the knowledge that the body breaks all carbohydrates into glucose, no matter what the source of the carbohydrate (*Carbohydrate Counting,* 1). One carbohydrate counting exchange equals fifteen grams of carbohydrate and is generally considered to be one serving of starch, fruit, or milk.

Both the Exchange system and Carbohydrate Counting can be used effectively to plan menus. Investigate both so you are informed. You'll be *www.diabeteslife.net* Diabetes Life Network explains carbohydrate counting and explains how to use it for a flexible menu.

www.joslin.harvard.edu Joslin Diabetes Center, located at Harvard University, includes carbohydrate counting for adults and children and includes several approaches to carbohydrate counting.

www.caloriechart.org This site has several free calorie charts listing carbohydrate amounts and also lists related books for sale.

www.childrenwithdiabetes.com This site explains how to plan meals and snack for children, using carbohydrate-counting techniques.

www.diabetesnet.com This site offers carbohydrate-counting cookbooks, kitchen scales, and other related materials.

Figure 4–5 Carbohydrate Counting References

prepared when a customer asks "How many calories is in this barbecued beef sandwich," (easily solved using Exchanges) or "How many carbohydrates are in this angel food cake" (using carbohydrate counting).

Catering Suggestions

Holidays can be frustrating times for diabetics and the people providing meals for them. While current theory has it that no foods need be excluded from diabetic diets (except for severe cases), daily intake must be balanced and be within the person's calorie level. Although an occasional piece of cake might be allowed, holiday meals can have very few options for diabetics.

When designing holiday menus, consider that everyone, including diabetics, can benefit from menu items that are tasty and fun yet lower in fat and concentrated sweets. Rather than having to create separate dishes for diabetics, offer lots of dishes that everyone can enjoy, with perhaps a portion variation for some of the more controlled diabetics.

Many menu items may already fit the bill, especially entrees (serve the sauces on the side). Instead of cranberry sauce, offer stewed apples with almonds, raisins, and cinnamon. Instead of chocolate sauce, offer fruit coulis made with frozen fruit, flavoring extracts and fruit juice concentrate. Whipped cream can be replaced with whipped topping (flavor it with vanilla, almond, or rum extracts, or orange or lemon zest). Tofu makes a creamy base for savory or sweet sauces, requiring little sugar for sweetness (make a creamy dessert sauce with silken tofu, pureed strawberries, and orange zest). Poached or stewed fruit or salsas make low-sugar, low fat accompaniments to roasted meats and seafood. Once you get into this, you will be surprised at how easy it is to convert holiday menus into diabetic-friendly menus.

As a last thought, here's a traditional holiday meal and our thoughts on "diabetic-ing" it:

> Crudite platter with sour-cream based dip (replace the dip with a bean- or low-fat yogurt based dip)

Assorted dinner rolls (no problem)

Roast turkey with giblet gravy (turkey is fine; serve gravy on the side or offer a fresh berry relish)

Cranberry sauce (offer a stewed fruit compote or hot seasoned applesauce)

Mashed potatoes made with milk and margarine (no problem—for a lower-fat version, try using low-fat milk or low-fat chicken stock)

A NUTRI-BAR

Holidays for Everybody

With an eye to individual diabetics' needs, here are some suggestions for festive foods that can fit into a diabetic pattern. For buffets, you might label menu items with the number of exchanges in a serving, so customers can put together a personally balanced meal.

Breakfast

Fresh fruit slices with citrus-honey dip (dip made with two cups nonfat yogurt, one tablespoon orange or lime juice and two tablespoons honey to serve twelve people)

Baked apples seasoned with cinnamon, nutmeg, ginger, and apple juice

Peaches with raspberry sauce (frozen or juice-packed peaches; sauce made with nonfat yogurt, frozen unsweetened raspberries, and orange juice concentrate)

Egg white omelets with fresh chopped herbs and veggies or baked vegetable omelet

Cornbread and zucchini muffins (made with juice concentrate rather than sugar) with raisins and nuts and served with hot fruit compote (stewed apples, pears, peaches and dried fruit)

Baked oatmeal (made with layers of prepared oatmeal, unsweetened canned or frozen fruit, dried fruit and ricotta cheese)

Buffet

Grilled vegetable platter (zucchini, onions, tomatoes, bell peppers sliced, brushed with olive oil, sprinkled with chopped oregano and basil and grilled, served with fresh salsa)

Twice-baked potatoes (stuffed with potatoes mashed with low-fat cottage cheese and unflavored, nonfat yogurt, chopped fresh parsley and onion and garlic powder)

Shrimp and crab stuffed mini-pitas (shrimp and crab chopped with fresh vegetables) or shrimp wrapped with snow peas

Stuffed mushrooms (stuffed with bread stuffing made with water chestnuts, chopped onions, and minced garlic)

Spinach dip (thawed frozen chopped spinach mixed with nonfat yogurt, nonfat ricotta cheese, chopped fresh parsley, and chopped green onions)

(continued)

Crudites with creamy dill dip (dip made with dried dill, low-fat cottage cheese, nonfat yogurt, chopped bell peppers, and black pepper); crudities can be any crunchy veggie, such as jicama, carrots, broccoli, cauliflower, cherry tomatoes, radishes, canned asparagus, canned baby corn, snow peas, or mushrooms.

Desserts

Angel food cake served with a fresh or frozen fruit sauce (puree strawberries with a small amount of orange juice concentrate and vanilla extract)

Chocolate angel food cake (angel food cake made with cocoa powder) served with fresh or frozen berries

Poached pears (poach pears in apple juice flavored with cinnamon and ginger served with ice milk)

Fruit smoothies (made with fresh or frozen fruit, unflavored yogurt and juice concentrate)

Pudding parfaits (made from calorie-controlled pudding mix and low-fat milk, layered with unsweetened granola, chopped dried fruit, and whipped topping)

Fruit tarts (purchase prepared tart shells or make your own meringue shells; fill with calorie-controlled pudding and top with fruit and whipped topping)

Mini-sundaes (made with ice milk or sherbet, topped with chopped nuts, chopped fruit, fruit sauce, and whipped topping)

Ice cream club sandwiches (made with graham crackers, ice milk, chopped fruit and chopped nuts)

Beverages

Flavored coffees served with whipped topping and a sprinkle of marshmallows

Hot herbed tea with citrus slices and mint sprigs

Fruit punch (made with unsweetened juices, sparkling waters, and sherbet)

Fruit smoothies (made with unflavored yogurt or tofu, fresh or frozen fruit, spices)

Canned sweet potatoes with marshmallows and pineapple (have you ever tasted baked fresh sweet potatoes—they put canned to shame; simply bake, cube, and serve with a bit of margarine, or mashed them with a small amount of margarine, nutmeg, and ginger; canned, unsweetened pineapple is fine)

Green beans with almonds (no problem)

Bread stuffing (no problem—a little high in fat, but, hey, it's the holidays!)

1. Prepare a coulis instead of a frosting for baked goods. Puree fresh or thawed frozen berries with a small amount of orange juice concentrate and some liqueur. Pour on plate, place slice of angel food cake on top of coulis and garnish with a fanned strawberry.
2. Purchase fruit packed in juice rather than in syrup.
3. Cut down the sugar and go with some of the "sweet" spices, such as clove, cinnamon, nutmeg, ginger, and allspice, and extracts, such as vanilla, almond, orange, and rum.
4. Offer nuts mixed with dried fruit as snack items, instead of cookies or candy
5. Instead of syrup, used a dried-fruit or fresh-fruit compote, sliced roasted pears, apples, or pineapples.
6. Bake quick breads with less sugar and more applesauce, fruit juice concentrate, and dried fruit.
7. Instead of soda, try sparkling waters mixed with fruit or vegetable juice.
8. Purchase plain yogurt and top with chopped fresh or frozen fruit.
9. Offer unsweetened cereal with chopped nuts, dried or fresh fruit.

Figure 4–6 Reducing that Spoonful of Sugar (How to Reduce Sugar on Menus)

1. Available from the ADA- *www.eatright.org* or 800 366–1655
   a. *Exchanges for All Occasions: Your Guide to Choosing Healthy Foods Anytime Anywhere* (Marion Franz, 1997, ISBN 1-885115-35-0). Based on the Exchange Lists, has menus, recipes and tips for eating out.
   b. *Diabetes Meal Planning Made Easy* (Hope Warshaw, 1996, ISBN 0-945448-61-9) Sample meal patterns and menus show how to incorporate all types of foods into a diabetic menu.
   c. *The New Diabetic Cookbook* (Mabel Cavaiani, 1996, ISBN 0-8092-3164-6). Over 200 recipes easily converted to quantity amounts.
   d. *The Art of Cooking for the Diabetic* (Mary Abbott Hess, 1996, ISBN 0-8092-3393-2) Over 375 recipes which incorporate the Exchanges and nutrient information.
   e. *The American Diabetes Association Guide to Healthy Restaurant Eating* (Hope Warshaw, 1998, ISBN 1-58040-004-3) Analysis of over 2,500 menu items—an insider's view of how food service prepares food appropriate for the diabetic eater.
2. *www.dce.org* is the Web site for the Diabetes Educators practice group of the ADA. Visit the site for ideas on menu planning, recipe development, etc. Available from the Joslin Diabetes Center (for ordering information, 800 344-4501, Eastern Time).
   a. The Joslin Diabetes Gourmet Cookbook—over 500 recipes.
   b . Joslin Diabetes Manual—a reference guide which includes menu planning
   c. *Managing your Diabetes Without Insulin*—a booklet explaining Type II diabetes and how diet fits.

Figure 4–7 Diabetic Resources

Pumpkin pie (a couple of choices here: make a lower-sugar, lower-fat pumpkin custard with canned pumpkin, silken tofu, and apple juice concentrate; this can be baked in a pie shell or in individual dishes)

VEGANS, HONEY, AND SUGAR

A word about **vegans** and sugar. Many vegans avoid honey and sucrose (white or refined sugar). Honey is considered to be an animal byproduct by many vegans so they won't use it. White sugar has no animal properties, as it is processed from cane or from beets. However, many North American sugar processors use filters that contain bone char, made from animal bone. As an alternate to white sugar, vegans may use maple syrup, thawed frozen or canned fruit juice concentrate, date palm sugar, rice or corn syrup, molasses, or dried fruit purees. Be aware of this when designing menus or interacting with vegan customers. Don't be surprised if you are cross-examined about the sweetening content of some menu items.

Remember that in nutrition, you get points for trying. So, if you have to have something sweet and bubbly, skip the soda and have some sparkling water with a shot of syrup, or better yet, mix some sparkling water with fruit juice concentrate. Need cookies to study? Oatmeal and peanut butter raisin have a bit more to them than sugar cookies or cream-filled cookies. When you're cooking, see if you can cut down on some of the sugar and use dried fruit, fruit juice, applesauce, and sweet spices, such as nutmeg, ginger, cardamom, cloves, and anise to replace some of the sugar to do it. Sugar is not all bad, it's just not nutrient dense. A small amount of simple sugar in the diet is okay for healthy people, but it's not necessary. There are lots of other options.

STARCHES AND WHOLE GRAINS

Starches, or complex carbohydrates, are where you should get most of your carbohydrates. The starch group includes fruits; vegetables; unsweetened juices; potatoes; cereals; rice; grains, such as barley, quinoa and spelt; fresh and dried beans and legumes; whole-wheat products; and starchy vegetables, such as winter squash and corn, and lots of other items.

Not too hard to take. So-called "starchy" foods are easy to prepare and easy to enjoy, as well as being on the less expensive end of the cost scale. The more "whole foods" you can add to your menu, the better. In other words, try for whole-wheat bread instead of white, brown rice instead of white rice, whole-wheat or vegetable pasta instead of plain-wheat pasta, real-live fruit or fruit juice instead of green M & M's™, etc.

A word about bread. Like many foods, bread can contain all three types of carbohydrates—simple, complex, and fiber. You can purchase bread that is enriched, fortified and whole grain. Enriched bread and flour products, such as breadsticks, croutons, pasta, and hot and cold cereals have had the B vitamins, thiamin, riboflavin and niacin, and the mineral iron added during processing. Rice and corn products, such as flour or grits, can be used to make bread. Even though many people ignore the bread portion of their sandwich, it offers lots of nutrients.

"Fortified" and **"enriched"** mean that manufacturers have added back nutrients that have been lost during processing or have added nutrients that will enhance consumer health. Sometimes this is done voluntarily, but many times it is done at the direction of the federal government. See the discussion about iodized salt for more details on fortification and enrichment.

Whole grain means that the good stuff, the bran, the germ, and the endosperm, has been left in. Many of the nutrients in whole grains are attached to the bran, including vitamins and minerals and fiber. The germ is the "incubator" for the seed and comes packed with all the vitamins and minerals needed to grow more wheat and to make humans healthier. You've probably seen wheat germ being sold in stores. If you eat whole-grain bread, you can skip buying the wheat germ as a separate product.

FOOD FOR THE MIND

Sources of Low-Fat Complex CHO

Bagels, breadsticks, corn tortillas, English muffins, popcorn, pita, rice, pretzels, whole-grain cold and hot cereal, low-fat cookies and crackers, pizza crusts, fresh fruit and juice, fruit canned in juice or water, unsweetened frozen fruit, dark green leafy vegetables, potatoes, squash, corn

ALCOHOL

What would a chapter on carbohydrates be without a mention of **alcohol?** Anything that ends with–ol is an alcohol. All alcohols are not edible, all do not cause intoxication, and all are not what you would think of as being related to beer or vodka. Methanol, the simplest alcohol, is also called wood alcohol and will cause blindness and death. During the Great Depression, in the 1930s, itinerant people who couldn't afford their daily "fix" would drain the methanol used in car radiators as antifreeze. They would heat the methanol, attempting to skim off the "poison" and drink it. This resulted in fatal internal damage. Today, methanol is used for duplicator fluid, windshield washer fluid, and paint stripper.

Ethanol is the edible alcohol found in beer, wine, and hard spirits. Produced by distilling fruit or grains, ethanol adds flavor and "punch" to alcoholic beverages. Your liver can detoxify a small amount of alcohol every day.

1. Add dried fruit, fresh berries, nuts and seeds to muffins, quick breads (like carrot cake and zucchini bread), and cookies.
2. Use oats and oatmeal wherever you can. Dust the top of muffins and quick breads, use as a thickening ingredient instead of bread crumbs, add to yogurt.
3. Have popcorn, veggie sticks, fresh or dried fruit instead of low-fiber snacks.
4. Use brown rice and vegetable or whole-wheat pasta instead of white-rice and white-flour pasta.
5. Bake potatoes instead of frying or mashing them. Leave the peels on for potato salad.
6. Stop peeling! Where possible, use unpeeled fruit and vegetables.
7. Fruit juice smoothies instead of soda or coffee.
8. Read labels. If it says "high fiber" then choose it.

Figure 4–8 Upping the Fiber on the Menu

A NUTRI-BAR

The Whole Grain and Nothing But the Whole Grain

Grains are great, but they are not all created equal. Direct your passion for pasta and your bounty for bread towards the whole-grain aisle. Refined grains may have had some of their nutrients processed away. Refined grains are more quickly digested and absorbed, causing blood sugar levels to rise too quickly. Whole grains are digested more slowly, allowing for a slow and even rise in blood sugar. Whole grains have soluble and insoluble fiber. The soluble fiber, such as that found in oats, barley, and millet, can help lower cholesterol, and the insoluble fiber, such as that found in wheat berries and bran, can help lower the risk of certain cancer.

Instead of	*Head for the*
white rice, bread and potatoes	brown rice, whole grain breads and sweet potatoes or yams
white rice or pasta in soups or as side dishes	barley, millet, kasha, whole wheat pasta, quinoa
just oats for breakfast	sneak oats into cookies, muffins, stuffings, zucchini bread or carrot cake, veggie burgers

If too much alcohol is taken on a consistent basis, the liver becomes overworked and will eventually begin to scar and break down.

Metabolism

Alcohol is not actually a carbohydrate, fat, or protein, but it seems to be most closely linked to carbohydrate metabolism, with seven calories per gram. Alcohol is metabolized in different ways by different people. Because of their smaller body size, smaller livers and higher body fat, women become intoxicated more quickly than men do. Women's body composition does not allow for as much alcohol metabolism as men do. Many people of Asian descent lack or have inefficient forms of gastric and liver enzymes that assist in alcohol metabolism and so do not handle alcohol well.

Beverage	*Serving Size*	*Calories*
White table wine	4 ounces	80
Red table wine	4 ounces	85
Dessert wine	4 ounces	180
Light beer	12 ounces	80
Beer	12 ounces	135
Bloody Mary	4 ounces	90
Margarita	4 ounces	150
Vodka	1.5 ounces (90 proof)	110
Rum	1.5 ounces (86 proof)	105
Whiskey	1.5 ounces (80 proof)	95

Figure 4–9 Beer Bellies Anonymous

Damage

Nobody can handle large amounts of alcohol for long periods of time. The liver is just not set up to handle the constant detoxifying. The morning after an alcohol session may bring headache, nausea, body aches, and light and noise sensitivity. As the blood alcohol level comes down, the hangover gets worse. When the blood alcohol level hits zero, the hangover peaks and then eventually fades away. Hangovers my happen because alcohol causes dehydration, irritates the digestive tract, and overworks the liver. The liver is so busy detoxifying the blood that is does not have time to help regulate blood-sugar levels. Blood-sugar levels drop, causing fatigue and nausea. If you vomit or have diarrhea caused by alcohol consumption you then create an electrolyte imbalance and more dehydration. Not a pretty picture.

Even less pretty is the damage from long-term use. Years of heavy drinking permanently damage the GI tract. Your stomach hurts, so you don't eat, you just drink. Pretty soon, you develop nutritional deficiencies. You get increased irritation of the mouth, throat, esophagus, and stomach, so you drink to numb pain. You're now at greater risk for cancer and irreversible nerve damage, caused by nutritional deficiencies. Your kidneys are constantly exposed to toxins from alcohol so they begin to break down. Your liver becomes fatty, inefficient, and creates scar tissue from the steady stream of alcoholic toxins; cirrhosis takes only five years to cause fatal liver problems. Alcoholic hepatitis, a chronic inflammation of the liver, can cause death. If it doesn't cause death, the damage it causes is irreversible. Better line up a liver transplant donor. Although the body tries very hard to protect it, the brain eventually suffers irreversible damage from chronic alcohol exposure. Once your brain is affected, it's time to call it quits. It's all physically and mentally downhill from there.

Besides yourself, there are other people that are affected by chronic alcohol use, **Fetal alcohol syndrome** (FAS), which can be caused by as little as an occasional drink during any part of the pregnancy, can result in low birth weight, slow growth rate, and learning impairments. Alcohol use is very, very damaging in the first weeks of pregnancy, when the fetal nervous system is developing. It is very damaging further on in the pregnancy, affecting whatever stage of development the fetus is in. Fetal alcohol syndrome isn't just from chronic use, but could be from one good party.

FAS may not be diagnosed for months after the child is born, but the effects are felt throughout a lifetime. FAS affects how a person learns and relates to others and it has physical consequences that can affect the nervous and circulatory systems.

So is it all or none? Not necessarily. Alcohol has been around since before recorded history. Every civilization seems to have had a method for producing alcohol. In small amounts, two drinks twice a week for men, 1 drink a week for women, according to the USDA, has been thought to have some protective effects. Along with healthy life styles, alcohol is thought to help reduce some forms of heart disease. Just keep in mind that alcohol causes 50 percent more deaths in women than men and causes 60 percent of deaths attributed to liver disease for both men and women. Some people are okay with an occasional drink. Here's who should not even think about it:

1. Anyone under the age of 18.
2. People having alcohol-related illnesses or who are taking medication that will interact with alcohol. Tylenol™ (acetaminophen) and alcohol are thought to be a lethal combination that can cause liver damage.
3. People working with machinery (chefs!) or driving.
4. Pregnant women or women attempting to become pregnant.
5. People with family histories of alcoholism.

FIBER

Fiber has been around as long as there have been plants. And as long as there have been humans eating plants, fiber has been thought to have different health properties.

Fiber is a type of carbohydrate. In plants, fiber gives structure to leaves, stem, fruit and roots. Since fiber can not be digested, it leaves the body pretty much in the same form it entered. Along the way out, fiber grabs fats and takes them along. That is why fiber is said to reduce cholesterol in the blood. Fiber acts like Velcro to sticky fat. Of course, it's all a matter of proportion. If you eat half an apple and a whole pepperoni and sausage pizza, the amount of fiber in the apple is not up to the task of vacuuming out all the fat from the pizza. Once again, moderation is the key.

Soluble Fiber

Soluble and insoluble fiber are the two basic kinds. Soluble fiber, also called pectin, is the white, interior part of an apple or pear, or the juicy part on the inside of an orange. Pectin is what gives apricot nectar its full texture or applesauce its smooth-but-solid texture. Soluble fiber is slightly digestible, but not much.

Soluble fiber helps the body handle glucose. It does this by slowing the rate of absorption of carbohydrates, so not as much sugar is released into the bloodstream. Some soluble fibers, beans and oats, may help to reduce the risk of artery and heart disease (atherosclerosis for the scientists in the audience). Fiber lowers the level of cholesterol in blood and helps the body get rid of cholesterol. Beans, carrots, legumes, citrus, and peas help with this; wheat fiber does not.

Insoluble Fiber

Insoluble fiber, also called cellulose, is the peel of the apple or the membrane around the juicy part of the orange. Insoluble fiber is the transparent cover over beans, the strings in a stalk of celery, or the clear white slipcover on each kernel of corn. Insoluble fiber is what holds plants together, allowing them to hold their shape when you cook them. Insoluble fiber is very indigestible. You can't get appreciable numbers of calories from either soluble or insoluble fiber.

Insoluble fiber is found in peels and skins of fruit and veggies, nuts, and wheat and helps to speed transit time of food. This helps to prevent constipation, diveritculitis, and hemorrhoids. Who wouldn't like to do without those? Insoluble fiber may also help decrease risk of colon cancer.

FOOD FOR THE MIND

Sources of Soluble and Insoluble Fiber

Fresh fruit and vegetable with peels, bananas, berries, beans, seeds, whole grain bread, pasta and cereal, nuts, root vegetables, shredded wheat, bran cereals, lentils, split peas, oatmeal and oat bran, dried fruit

Doctors Kellogg, Graham, and Post

Once people started to get interested in their health, they started to explore the relationship between food and health. Scientific studies and not-so-scientific studies were conducted. Some people published their findings based on beliefs rather than empirical evidence. Fiber became a big issue during and after the Industrial Revolution in the mid-1800s. As people moved away from the country, they ate less "whole" foods, such as unprocessed grains, fruits, and vegetables. Living conditions in the cities weren't very healthy for wealthy or poor people, and the diet was pretty low in nutrients.

Many nutrition theories sprang up during this time, as people looked for ways to stay healthy. A minister, Sylvester Graham (yes, of the cracker of the same name) believed himself quite the healer in the 1830s. His theory was that processed flours, those that had the bran removed during processing, and meat were the root of all disease. He basically believed that eating foods made from white flour, beef, and chicken led to liver disease, cholera, sexual excesses, and bad temper. Graham preached that eating whole-wheat flour and ignoring meat led to good health. Of course, he also believed that cold baths and sleeping by open windows improved health, as well. His high-fiber graham flour was usually eaten as a kind of hot cereal. The story goes that he devised graham crackers as a way to get children to eat enough graham flour, because on its own, graham flour is pretty icky stuff.

Dr. John Kellogg (yes, of the corn flake fame) ran a famous health resort in Battle Creek, Michigan, in the 1870s. Dr. Kellogg must have been quite an inspirational speaker, with one of his favorite mottoes being, "Bran does not irritate, it titillates." Visitors to Kellogg's place were not allowed to eat meat, smoke, drink alcohol, use condiments, or eat anything spicy or pleasurable. They were given large amounts of bran and salad greens, both high in fiber, used for their laxative effect. Kellogg believed that most illness was centered in the digestive tract, and that a clean digestive tract was a healthy one. Fiber earned Dr. Kellogg over a million dollars in his lifetime. If you would like to see a fairly accurate, but racy, account of Kellogg's health resort, rent the movie *The Road to Wellville* or read the book of the same title by C. Boyle Corghessian.

Charles W. Post was a patient of Dr. Kellogg. After being "cured," he decided he could do what Kellogg did, only better. He started his own line of fiber foods, including Post Toasted Cornflakes, Grapenuts (which were broken bits of hard wheat crackers), and Postum, a coffee substitute made from barley and wheat. In 1901, Post made over a million dollars, outearning his own doctor. And there's more fiber intrigue! John Kellogg's brother, William, was so mad at Post that he revved up Kellogg's products, introducing "Kellogg's Toasted Corn Flakes." And the battle continues between these two companies even today.

Fiber research got more legitimate in the 1970s (Fauci, 2) Studies were done that contrasted Western diets with African diets. The African diets were extremely high in fiber. Among people who ate them, there was little to no incidence of diabetes, certain types of heart disease, colon cancer, intestinal disorders, or constipation.

It was found that high-fiber diets decrease the amount of time that food is in the gut. The less time food was in the gut, the less time for toxins to develop. This proved to be the scientific basis for recommending fiber to decrease the incidences of certain diseases.

We briefly mentioned diverticulosis and Crohn's disease (inflammation of the colon) in Chapter Three. Fiber is considered to be an important part of preventing such diseases of the small and large intestine. Populations of people who have high-fiber diets tend to have less incidence of colon cancer

SUGAR SUBSTITUTES

We like to have our cake and eat it too, although we don't want the calories from it. After alchemists gave up trying to change lead into gold, they set their sights on taking the calories out of sugar.

Food scientists have had a reasonable amount of luck with **artificial sweeteners,** also called sugar substitutes or nonnutritive sweeteners. The idea was to find a substance that tasted and behaved like sugar, but lacked sugar's calories. Several government-approved products are currently on the market.

History and Types

Saccharin, a laboratory-produced substance with no links to any natural products, was discovered in the 1880s. Saccharin was considered a prescription pill back then and was found only in pharmacies. It was a boon to diabetics and other people who needed to avoid sugar. Three hundred times sweeter than sucrose, saccharin can be used to sweeten beverages, candy, and drugs (such as vitamins). It cannot be used in the same amounts as sugar, since it is so much sweeter. Therefore, saccharin is not an ingredient to substitute in place of the sugar in cookies, cakes, sauces, or any other products that rely on sugar's bulk. Although it had been around for years, testing was done on saccharin in the 1960s. Because there was found to be a possible link to bladder cancer, the government moved to have saccharin removed from the market. There was a public outcry (not to mention a lot of crying by the companies who produced saccharin or who used it in their products). A compromise was reached. All saccharin and saccharin-containing products carry a warning label. It is up to the consumer to make an informed decision about using it or not.

> FOOD FOR THE MIND
>
> Laboratory animals were given the equivalent of 850 cans of soda per day to assess the risk of using saccharin. To date, there have been no human trials involving saccharin. No documented cases have linked saccharin to cancer in humans.

As a compromise, the USDA set an acceptable daily intake (ADI) for saccharin. The ADI is about 100 times less than the amount that caused bladder tumors in laboratory animals. In order to ingest the ADI for saccharin you would have to drink at least 18 cans of saccharin-sweetened soda per day.

Cyclamates were not so lucky. Saccharin had the playing field, pretty much to itself until the 1950s. Cyclamate had the same shelf life and high temperature tolerance as saccharin, without saccharin's aftertaste.

Unfortunately, more rigorous testing for cancer-causation was in place when cyclamate hit the market. It didn't pass safety standards and was yanked off the market. Cyclamates are allowed in Canada, and there is currently a petition to reallow its use in the United States.

Aspartame was a step forward for sugar substitutes. Made from "natural" products, aspartame is a derivative of protein. Two amino acids (the building blocks of protein), aspartic acid and phenylalanine, are glued together to form aspartame. Protein has four calories per gram, and aspartame is digested as protein. Because it is almost two hundred times sweeter than sugar, very little is used and therefore very few calories are obtained from using aspartame. Aspartame can't be used in cooking, as it falls apart and stops sweetening when subjected to high heat. It can be added to cooked or warm foods. Prove this yourself. Add some aspartame to a steaming hot cup of coffee or tea (be careful!) and let it sit for about 15 minutes. When you go to taste it, you'll find it is not as sweet as it should be.

Aspartame contains phenylalanine, a natural amino acid, found in most protein-containing foods, such as yogurt, poultry, and seafood. Some people are born with a rare metabolic disorder, **phenylketonuria** or PKU. People with PKU must carefully control their **phenylalanine** intake. For this reason, all products containing aspartame must carry a warning on their labels. Check out a can of diet soda and locate the phenylalanine notification.

Acesulfame K is in use in over eighty countries around the world and approved for over one hundred products, including candy, chewing gums, gelatins, pudding and cake mixes, beverage mixes, and nondairy creamers. It stands up very well to heat and can be used in cooking and baking.

Sucralose is an interesting artificial sweetener. It is made from a combination of sucrose and sugar alcohols, such as mannitol. Since there is some sugar in the product, there are some calories. However, sucralose is six hundred times sweeter than sugar, so very little is used. Sugar alcohols are very large molecules and not easily absorbed by the body. For this reason, sucralose is not absorbed very well and contributes little to no calories to food. Sucralose is formulated so that it can be used in the same amounts as sugar. This means it can be used in bakery and dessert recipes.

Uses

So where does this leave us? Artificial sweeteners are very helpful for those people who cannot handle concentrated carbohydrates, like sugar or honey. Artificial sweeteners will not necessarily help with weight loss or decrease the number of dental cavities. A person has to decrease total numbers of calories to lose weight. A double cheeseburger and a diet soda is not the way to lower numbers on the scale. If there are any carbohydrates remaining in the mouth from the bread, then acid-producing bacteria will thrive on them and be much better able to attack your tooth enamel.

Some artificial sweeteners can be used to produce non-sugar-containing items. This does not mean that the products will have no calories, just no sugar. This may be helpful to the chef or baker, depending on the clientele. Remember, you have to decrease total calories from fat and carbohydrates

Cyclamate: 30 times sweeter than sucrose
Cyclamates were banned in the United States in the 1960s, but they are making a comeback. They are stable at high temperatures and have a long shelf-life.

Saccharin (the pink packet) 300 times sweeter (sold as Sweet 'n' Low™)
Saccharin has been around since the 1880s. Because of a possible link to bladder cancer, saccharin-containing products must carry a warning label. Saccharin is stable at high temperatures and has a long shelf life.

Aspartame (the blue packet) 200 times sweeter (sold as Equal™ and Nutrasweet™)
Aspartame is a combination of the amino acids, aspartic acid, and phenlyalanine. Nutrasweet is generally just aspartame, while Equal is aspartame blended with lactose and an anticaking agent.

Aspartame loses its sweetness at high temperatures and has a short shelf life. If added to cooking or baking products, it looses its ability to sweeten.

Acesulfame K (the yellow packet) 200 times sweeter (sold as Sunette™)
Acesulfame K is derived from acetoacetic acid and is relatively new on the scene, having gotten U.S. approval in 1988.

Acesulfame K is stable at high temperatures, has a long shelf-life and is very soluble in liquids.

Sucralose 600 times sweeter (sold as Splenda™)
Sucralose is the new kid on the block, having been approved in the United States in 1995 and in Canada in 1991.

Sucralose is stable at medium temperatures and is processed in such a way that it can be used in the same amounts as sugar in recipes.

Figure 4–10 Sweeter than Sugar

from other sources in a recipe. If you add aspartame to a chocolate chip-macadamia cookie recipe you're back to the cheeseburger and diet cola syndrome. There are so many calories from the fat in a cookie recipe, that the savings from an artificial sweetener are minuscule.

PUTTING IT ALL TOGETHER

Carbohydrates should be major source of daily calories, with intake of carbohydrates being higher than that of fat or protein. Glucose is the main fuel used by muscles and the only fuel used by the brain. Your body derives different amounts of glucose from simple sugars, starch, or fiber. Most carbohydrate-containing foods are naturally low in fat or sodium. Some may be enriched or fortified with additional nutrients. Fruits, vegetables, whole-grain foods, beans and root vegetables are good sources of carbohydrates.

Carbohydrate foods may be of some concern to some people. Diabetics do not have to simply restrict sugar. They need to plan balanced diets using a variety of foods. The Exchange Lists of Meal Planning are a structured way for diabetics to plan meals. Vegans exclude all animal products, including sucrose and honey. Phenylketonurics have to avoid aspartame, an artificial sweetener containing phenylalaine.

Alcohol is a type of carbohydrate that raises many issues. Excess use of alcohol can cause long term physical and mental damage. Alcohol intake during pregnancy can result in FAS.

Simple sugars, starches and fiber add interest, taste and texture to menu items. They are easily prepared, economical and generally enjoyed by a vast audience. Savvy food professionals will use carbohydrates to their advantage.

FYI: A BOWL OF CARBO FUN FOR THE WHOLE FAMILY

In June 2001 General Mills opened the " Cereal Adventure" in the Mall of America, right outside Minneapolis, Minnesota. For those of you unfamiliar with the Mall, it is the largest indoor mall in the world, with its own zip code, post office, and bus station. It is a destination stop for tourists visiting that part of the world.

According to a press release from General Mills, the "Cereal Adventure" is designed to be a "celebration of the long-time breakfast standard, which is growing in popularity at other mealtimes as well." The 16,000-square-foot space has cereal-theme games, shows, and playground equipment situated in entertainment areas with names such as Cheerios Play Park, Lucky Charms' Magical Forest, Trix Fruity Carnival and Cocoa Puffs Chocolate Canyon. The Wheaties Hall of Champions has tributes to sports entertainment.

The Total Nutrition health site and the General Mills Farm Factory educate visitors in the production techniques for cereal manufacturing. Visitors are offered an opportunity to create their own cereal combinations.

And what's a theme park without a nosh? The Cereal Adventure Café offers breakfast and snack foods. Finally, a public place where it's okay to have Cheerios for dinner. And you thought carbohydrates were boring.

FYI: FRUIT PUREES

Cooking and Baking With Fruit Purees

Fruit Is in

Fat is out, but flavor is in for many of your customers. Fat adds texture, creaminess, flavor, moisture, mouthfeel, color, and, in the case of baking, leavening to menu items.

Fruit has many of the properties of fat. Natural fibers can add texture and mouthfeel, juice can add moisture and creaminess, and natural sugars add color and taste. The secret is in selecting the right fruit in the right medium (fresh, frozen or dried) for the item to be prepared.

Commercial and From-Scratch Fruit Purees

Fruit purees are commercially available in frozen and canned forms. Applesauce is probably the fruit puree most familiar in the kitchen. Keep a supply of sweetened and unsweetened applesauce on hand to be used as a fat replacer in baked goods. Fruit purees are also available in a rainbow of flavors, formulated for mixing into drinks. These can be used to replace some of the fat in salad dressings, baked goods, soup, salsa, spreads, and dips. We have seen the following flavors, available from various companies in five- and thirty-pound pails: mango, strawberry, white peach, red raspberry, banana, sweet ginger, prickly pear, Fuji apple, blueberry, pear, pumpkin, red plum, sweet potato, and passion fruit. Commercially prepared fruit baby foods are another way to obtain fruit purees for your kitchen.

Using fruit purees is nothing new. In addition to applesauce, pumpkin is made into a puree before going into a pie or custard, as is sweet potato. Sorbet, that never-had-fat-in-it dessert is a combination of pureed fruit and sweeteners. For years, chefs have created sauces from coulis, which are cooked or fresh seasoned pureed fruit or vegetables. Vinaigrette salad dressings are enhanced by the addition of pureed raspberries, oranges, or strawberries—no additional fat, just flavor!

Take Out the Fat, Put in the Fruit

Fruit purees are going one step further nowadays and are being used to replace some of the fat in recipes, especially sauces and baked items. Instead of butter- or cream-based sauces, chefs are turning to fruit and vegetable reductions as the main ingredient. For example, fresh apples and pears can be peeled and chopped and allowed to reduce (cooked over low heat with a minimum of fluid, such as juice, stock, or wine) until almost caramelized. This reduction can be seasoned with a hint of white or cracked black pepper and chopped raisins and used as a fat-free sauce for ham, pork, or poultry. Orange juice concentrate and fresh, chopped oranges can be reduced, seasoned with ginger and pepper and used as a sauce for fish, seafood, or poultry.

Call It Coulis

Coulis can be used as a dessert sauce or as an ingredient in an entrée sauce. Prepare a berry coulis by blending fresh or frozen strawberries, raspberries, and other seasonal berries until smooth. Add honey and white wine (if desired) and blend to combine. The coulis can be strained if the seeds need to be removed. Serve a berry coulis with angel food cake, banana bread, sorbet, frozen yogurt, or sliced fresh or canned fruit. Coulis adds flavor and color with no fat. Coulis can be made from any fruit which can be blended to yield a sauce-like texture. Bananas can be added to thicken a coulis; melon or fruit juice can be used for thinning. Frozen fruit used for coulis should be unsweetened and should be thawed before using.

Salad dressings and savory sauces can benefit from coulis. Add berry or citrus coulis to vinaigrette or French-style dressings as well as to wine or beef-based hot sauces. For cold sauces, flavor mayonnaise with berry coulis for a fruit salad dressing or with pureed orange and grapefruit, seasoned with rosemary, for fish or poultry dishes. Coulis for this purpose can be frozen, so utilize the over-ripe fruit in your walk-in rather than discarding it.

Morning, Noon, and Night

Breakfast can benefit from fruit purees. Replace half (not all) the fat in pancake and waffle recipes with banana puree or applesauce. Soften margarine, cream cheese or butter, whip with peach or strawberry puree and serve as a topping for muffins, corn bread, or pancakes. This is a sweet and colorful way to eliminate some of the fat!

Fruit purees can be used as accent ingredients in cooking, such as a touch of pineapple-lemon puree in a fragrant rice dish (puree canned, drained pineapple with lemon juice). Use peach or apricot puree with orange juice concentrate as a glaze for vegetables (such as carrots) chicken, duck, pork, or ham. Mix citrus or peach fruit purees into sweet potatoes or poultry stuffings. A touch of mango or pineapple purees can be added to curry sauces and also to salad dressings. Pineapple puree can be added very lightly to tomato salsas to create a sweet yet tangy flavor profile.

Baking with Fruit

Fruit purees are very popular ingredients in baking right now and can be used for part or all of the fat ingredients (butter, oil, eggs, etc.). There are approximately 900 calories or 100 grams of fat saved for every 4 ounces of fruit puree used instead of fat in a baking recipe. Fruit puree staples of baking are applesauce, which has a neutral flavor, and prune puree. Prune puree should be used only in chocolate or hardy baking recipes, as its very sweet flavor and dark color will not show up well in delicate or light-colored items. Applesauce or prune puree can be substituted for equal amounts of fat. So, calculate the total weight or measure for butter, margarine, oil, or egg yolks called for in a recipe and use fruit purees instead.

Fruit concentrates, especially orange and apple, which are neutral in flavor, are being used to replace sugar and some of the egg yolks in baking recipes. As baking recipes are balanced, be sure to try a test run, substituting only one ingredient at a time, to ensure a successful product.

You can prepare your own fruit purees or purchase them. Applesauce (remember, always use an unsweetened applesauce for baking) is probably a ready-to-use product in your kitchen, as are fruit juice concentrates. If you have the time (and it's the right season) try preparing a fresh pear sauce. Stew peeled and sliced pears with cinnamon, sugar and nutmeg until they are a sauce consistency. This can be used as a dessert sauce on its own and can be used as a baking ingredient.

Most dried fruit can be pureed and saved. Date, prunes and raisins are probably the most popular. To make about two pints of dried fruit puree, place 18 ounces of dried, pitted fruit in a blender with 8 ounces of water, 1 teaspoon of lemon zest and 2 tablespoons of vanilla extract. Puree until smooth. Store refrigerated in an airtight container until ready to use. This should last approximately two weeks in the refrigerator.

Fresh fruit can be pureed and used as a fat replacer. Be sure to use ripe, even overripe, fruit and puree as needed. Fresh fruit puree has a very limited shelf-life, but can be frozen for up to three months until needed. Thawed fruit puree will be thinner than fresh (freezing breaks down the natural fibers), so correct for that in the recipe.

Canned fruit purees and fruit baby food are convenient products to have available for fat substituting. If possible, order the unsweetened variety. If unsweetened is not available, than you will have to correct your recipe for sugar content.

Fruit purees can be used with convenience baking mixes. If the mix directions call for oil, substitute an equal amount of applesauce. If the flavor and color is appropriate, you can use prune puree or banana puree. If the batter looks too thin, a small amount of flour and water may be added. If you have the fruit and the time, experiment with freshly pureed mango in pound cake; canned, pureed pineapple in pineapple upside-down cake; pureed pears in zucchini bread; and pureed peaches in a yellow layer-cake. The butter and margarine is going to get pretty lonely on your kitchen shelf!

Nutri-Words

Alcohol: a form of carbohydrate that has seven calories per gram. Alcohol is known to cause mental confusion, dehydration, and liver toxicity.

Artificial sweeteners: chemical or natural substances that have the sweetening ability of sucrose, but lack the calories.

Carbohydrates: a group of compounds which include sugars, starch and fiber. Carbohydrates should be the main source of energy in the diet and are generally thought to contribute four calories per gram eaten.

Carbohydrate counting: a system in which foods are assigned carbohydrate values which a person fits into a daily carbohydrate allotment.

Complex carbohydrates: long chains of simple sugars.

Diabetes: a disorder of the endocrine system that affects carbohydrate metabolism

Exchange Lists for Meal Planning: a system of meal calculation employed by the American Diabetes Association/ American Dietetics Association, that allows the consumer to select appropriate amounts of carbohydrates, fats, and proteins.

Fetal Alcohol Syndrome (FAS): caused by alcohol use during pregnancy. FAS can be manifested in physical and mental retardation.

Fortified and enriched: processes that either return nutrients lost during manufacturing, as in polishing rice, or adding nutrients to foods for consumer benefit, as in adding calcium to orange juice.

Fructose: simple sugar found naturally in fruits and vegetables.

Glucose: a common simple sugar, used by the body for energy and found in the blood. A blood test for "sugar levels" is a blood glucose test.

Insulin-dependent diabetes: the form of diabetes that requires regular injections of insulin in order to have proper carbohydrate metabolism.

Lactase: The enzyme necessary to break down lactose.

Lactose intolerant: people who are lacking the ability to produce the enzyme lactase and are, therefore, unable to digest lactose-containing foods.

Lactose: natural sugar found in dairy products.

Phenylalanine: an amino acid found in the artificial sweetener aspartame.

Phenylketonuria: an inborn error of metabolism (birth defect) in which ingestion of phenylalanine can cause toxicities in the body.

Simple sugars: sugars consisting of only one or two sugar molecules, such as glucose and galactose.

Soluble and insoluble fiber: complex starches that cannot be digested in the human intestinal tract. Soluble fiber dissolves in water; examples would be the pulp of oranges or grape. Insoluble fiber does not dissolve in water; examples would be the apple peel or the "strings" in a celery stalk.

Soy milk: a fluid pressed from soy beans that has the texture and the appearance of dairy milk.

Starch: long chains of glucose molecules. Starch is the main form of stored energy in plant foods, such as potatoes and rice.

Vegan: vegetarians who refrains from eating any form of animal product, including honey.

Whaddaya Think?

1. You've just landed a great job of team chef for a professional football team. The coach wants the menus to be at least 60 percent carbohydrate. Suggest some breakfasts and lunch and dinner entrees that will delight the players and please the coach (we don't want the chef stuffed into a trash can).
2. There is a three-day conference of gluten-intolerant bicyclists from all over the world at your hotel. Design a three-day menu, including a grand buffet, for them.
3. Can you think of at least ten different food items that contain simple sugars, starch, and fiber altogether? (Hint: an apple is an example; the peel has fiber, and the interior has both sugar and starch).
4. Design a Sunday brunch for a lactose-intolerant group. Remember, they still want quiche and omelets and desserts.
5. You're the food-service manager at a residential camp for diabetic children and teenagers. With what are you going to stock the vending machines?
6. Why do diabetics need both diet and exercise?
7. What types of "fancy foods" will you offer your diabetic customers for the holidays?
8. How can you get more whole-grain, high-fiber foods into your daily diet?
9. Point out some of the flaws in Dr. Kellogg's and Dr. Graham's diet theories.
10. How are you going to sweeten vegan desserts and beverages?

Critical Application Exercises

1. Visit a natural foods store. Make a list of all the products you find that would be suitable for a gluten-intolerant customer. Could you prepare some of these products yourself or is it necessary to purchase special products.
2. You're opening the All-Carbo Café. Design a breakfast buffet and a fast-food menu that meets the needs of your carbo-loading customers.
3. Do a web search for lactose free food products and recipes. Report your findings.

4. Analyze the following menu, using the Exchange Lists for Meal Planning:

   5 ounces of skinless turkey breast, sauteed in 2 teaspoons of butter, fresh herbs and garlic, and 2 ounces of sun-dried tomatoes

   4 ounces of baby carrots glazed with 2 ounces of orange juice and fat-free stock

   4 ounces spinach pasta tossed with balsamic vinegar and chopped, fresh basil, and lemon zest

   1 small pear poached and served in 4 ounces of apple juice, cinnamon, ginger, and 2 teaspoons chopped walnut
5. Your customers are asking for desserts without refined sugar (translation: no white sugar or sucrose). Suggest at least ten desserts that can be made with sweeteners other than sucrose.

References

Carbohydrate Counting. Diabetes Life Network, December 20, 2001, *www.diabeteslife.net/living/nutrition/carbo.html*.

Fauci, A. S., Braunwald, E., Isselbacher, K. J. et al (1998). *Harrison's Principles of Internal Medicine.* New York; McGraw-Hill.

Gillespie, S. J., and Kulkarni, K. D. (1998). "Carbohydrate Counting in Diabetes Clinical Practice." *Journal of the American Dietetic Association*, August, 98:8: 897–905.

Magic Chocolate Cake
(Yield: 3 nine-inch-round layer cakes)

Ingredients

10 ounces all purpose flour
5 ounces cocoa powder (unsweetened)
4 ounces cornstarch
1 tablespoon baking powder
1 teaspoon baking soda
7 ounces large eggs (or 6 egg whites and 1 teaspoon oil)
1 pint prune puree
20 ounces apple juice concentrate
3 teaspoons vanilla extract

Method

1. Sift together dry ingredients.
2. In a separate bowl, whip eggs with puree, concentrate, and vanilla.
3. Add dry ingredients to egg mixture and combine until well-mixed.
4. Pour into greased nine-inch layer pans. Bake at 350 degrees (25 degrees less for convection) for 30 minutes or until knife inserted in center comes out clean.
5. Allow to cool. Serve with sliced seasonal fruit or fresh fruit coulis.

Nutritional Analysis: 200 calories per serving, 2 grams protein, 4 grams fat, 15 milligrams cholesterol, 36 grams carbohydrates, 100 milligrams sodium, less than 1 gram dietary fiber.

Glorious Glazed Carrots
(Yield: eight three-ounce servings)

Ingredients

1½ pounds sliced carrots
2 cinnamon sticks
3 ounces peach or pineapple puree
2 teaspoons ground ginger
2 teaspoons chopped fresh parsley

Method

1. Steam carrots with cinnamon stick until carrots are tender.
2. Combine puree, ginger, parsley.
3. Toss cooked carrots with puree and serve hot.

Nutritional Analysis: 112 calories per serving, 0.8 grams protein, 1 gram fat, no cholesterol, 26.2 grams carbohydrates, 14 milligrams sodium, 1.2 grams dietary fiber.

Lose the Fat Oatmeal Raisin Cookies
(Yield: 6 dozen 3/4-ounce cookies)

Ingredients

½ pound margarine
6 ounces prune puree
6 ounces brown sugar
6 ounces white sugar
4 ounces egg whites
1 teaspoon vanilla extract
10 ounces all-purpose flour
2 teaspoons baking soda
1 pound rolled oats (not cooked)
6 ounces raisin puree
6 ounces whole raisins

Method

1. Cream margarine, prune puree and both sugars until well-combined.
2. Add egg whites and vanilla. Mix until well-combined.
3. Add dry ingredients. Mix until well-combined.
4. Add raisin puree and raisins. Mix only to blend.
5. Bake on greased cookie sheets at 375 degrees (25 degrees lower for convection) for approximately 8 minutes or until crisp.

Nutritional Analysis (serving = 2 cookies): 140 calories per serving, 3 grams protein, 4 grams fat, 20 milligrams cholesterol, 22 grams carbohydrates, 80 milligrams sodium, 2.3 grams dietary fiber.

Chapter 5
Fats

Chapter Overview

Objectives

After reading this chapter, the student should be able to:

1. *Identify and explain the breakdown products of dietary fats.*
2. *Explain the difference between the different types of cholesterol and how they affect the body.*
3. *Identify dietary sources of saturated and unsaturated fats.*

4. *Describe how dietary fats are necessary in the body.*
5. *Discuss the various physical problems and diseases that arise from elevated fat intakes.*
6. *Demonstrate how unsaturated fats are hydrogenated and explain how this affects nutritional value.*
7. *Make decisions about selecting and purchasing specialty oils.*
8. *Identify appropriate uses for fat substitutes.*
9. *Discuss the American Heart Association Guidelines as they relate to consumer health and to menu design.*
10. *Design menus that incorporate principles of low fat ingredient selection and low fat cooking techniques while preserving the integrity of the menu.*

Introduction

Fat is a good news, bad news sort of substance. In this chapter, we'll discuss the nutritional and the culinary aspects of dietary fat. Let's see if we can come to a happy agreement between the "melt more butter on my croissant" crowd and the "just say no (to fat)" crowd.

Are all fats created equal? They should be so lucky! Fats differ in chemical structure, appearance, taste, and use. What all fats have in common is 9 calories per gram and the fact that they are very dense in calories. Four ounces of baked or steamed potatoes have about 90 calories, while the same amount of fried potatoes has about 200 calories. A medium-sized fresh apple is about 60 calories, with no fat, while a medium-sized avocado can be as much as 360 calories, all from fat. The Exchange Lists for Meal Planning lists a baked potato as having about 80 calories of starch, 3 cups of popped (not buttered) popcorn is also 80 starchy calories, but one-eighth of an avocado or one slice of bacon is 45 calories, all from fat. A whole egg, which includes the yolk, is about 75 calories, while the same amount of egg whites are only about 40 calories, with no fat. You have to know a little bit about nutrition in order to understand why all of those salads (heaped with grated cheese, bacon bits and salad dressing) are not helping you lose weight.

THE LANGUAGE OF FAT

All fat contains the same amount of calories. However, different types of fat can cause damage and disease to the body while other types of fat can actually contribute to health. You've probably heard people discussing their cholesterol levels or examining a label to find out the saturated and unsaturated fat content of a food. A teaspoon of olive oil and a teaspoon of butter both contain about 45 calories. But that's where the similarity ends.

FOOD FOR THE MIND

All fats contain nine calories per gram. All fats contribute the same amount of energy to the body. How the body uses them makes the difference.

Triglycerides

Just a quick review of the **digestion of fat**. You'll recall from your reading in Chapter 3 that fats are broken down in the small intestine and further processed by the liver, with assistance from the pancreas and the gallbladder. Fat molecules are made of **fatty acids** and glycerols. Your body is looking to separate the fatty acids from the glycerols. The fatty acids, some of them

A NUTRI-BAR

Reduce Fat Does Not Mean Reduced Calories

Fat has nine calories per gram, carbohydrates and proteins have four calories per gram. When selecting foods that are reduced in fat, read past the "Now, with less fat!" part of the label. If fat is taken out, then something must be put back in. For example, reduced fat baking products may have less fat because some of the egg yolks have been eliminated. However, something has to replace the volume, texture, and taste that was lost with the fat. In the case of reduced-fat baking products, egg yolks may be partially replaced with egg whites and soy products. Yes, you are trading nine calories per gram for four calories per gram, but you are still consuming calories. Reduced fat means less calories from fat, but does not mean less calories overall.

essential, are then used for energy, to assist in some reactions, to become parts of body chemicals, such as hormones and many other important body business. Some fatty acids contribute to disease, rather than helping out the body. The glycerols are components of blood and some fat metabolism. We won't be discussing glycerols very much in this text. Just to confuse matters, researchers have assigned different names to different types of fat, depending on their structure.

Triglycerides are a form of fat that may be an indicator of heart disease. Diabetics and people who are obese tend to have higher triglyceride levels and also to have higher rates of heart disease.

The good news is that a lot of triglycerides and that other nuisance fat, cholesterol, can be lowered with the right selection of food, maintaining a desirable weight, stopping smoking, and exercising. As a food-service

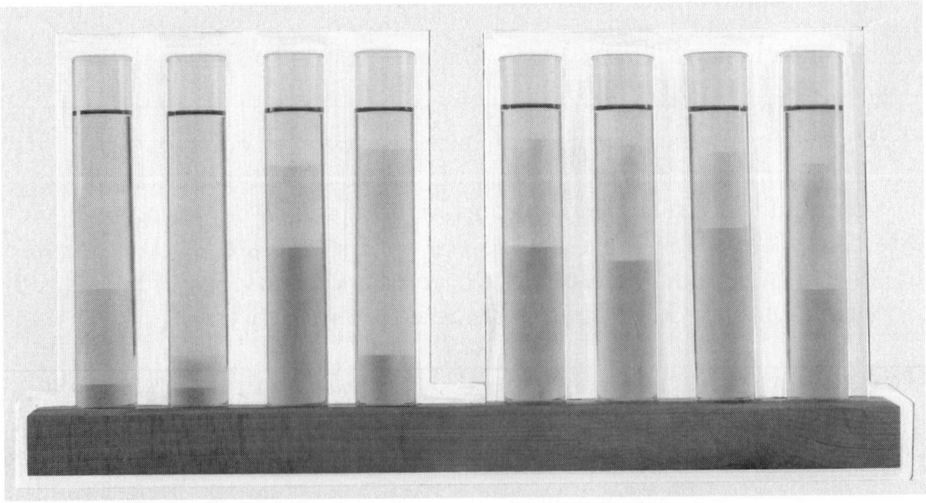

Fats come in all shapes and sizes. Shown here, from left to right are butter, coconut oil, corn oil, olive oil, sunflower oil, safflower oil, canola oil, and peanut oil.

professional, you can offer foods that are moderate in cholesterol for those customers wanting to enjoy dining out while watching their cholesterol. For example, in addition to traditional breakfast offerings, you might add egg white omelets stuffed with seasonal grilled vegetables or mushrooms or baked French toast, made with egg whites. Offer sorbet sundaes along with nonfat milk ice cream for dessert or a chocolate angel food cake served with a raspberry coulis.

Some people may have problems handling high-fat diets. Both the pancreas and the gallbladder contribute enzymes and emulsifiers that help the body to break down and absorb fat. If either organ is not functioning properly, then the body lacks the chemicals necessary to easily digest fats. People who have undergone radiation therapy or who have cystic fibrosis or Crohn's disease (a chronic and debilitating inflammation of the colon) may develop a malabsorption syndrome or inability to tolerate fat in the diet. These customers will appreciate lower-fat menu items, so they can enjoy dining out without feeling ill afterwards.

FOOD FOR THE MIND

Butter versus Margarine: Judging a Book by Its Cover

The cover may look the same, but the book is definitely different!

One tablespoon butter: 100 calories, 11 grams fat, 8 grams saturated fat, 30 milligrams cholesterol, 85 milligrams sodium

One tablespoon margarine: 100 calories, 11 grams fat, 2 grams saturated fat, 7 grams unsaturated fat, 115 milligrams sodium

Saturated Fats

Dietary fats are either **saturated** or **unsaturated.** Saturated fats are very strong substances and are fairly solid at room temperature. Saturation refers to the amount of hydrogen that a molecule of fat is holding onto. If a molecule of fat is holding onto the most hydrogen it can, then it is called saturated.

1. Cholesterol: found in animal products, such as egg yolks, whole-milk products, animal fat, and organ meats. Thought to "clog" the arteries, leading to elevated blood pressure, damaged arteries, and heart disease.
2. Dietary fat: principal form of energy storage in the body, necessary for healthy skin, hormone production, temperature regulation and the metabolism of vitamins A, D, E, and K. A diet too high in fat can lead to many undesirable and dangerous physical conditions.
3. Hydrogenated fat: a method to convert unsaturated, liquid fat to solid, saturated fat, such as corn oil margarine.
4. Lipid: for this text, used interchangeably with dietary fat.
5. Monosaturated fat: found in olive oil, avocados, and some seafood; missing one group of hydrogen atoms, making it easy for the body to break down.
6. Polyunsaturated fat: found in corn oil, cottonseed oil, and some nuts; missing more than one group of hydrogen atoms, making it easy for the body to break down.
7. Saturated fat: found in animal fat and skin, dairy products, coconut, and palm oil; has all the hydrogen groups it can hold, making it a very strong molecule, difficult for the body to break down.
8. Triglycerides: a combination of three fatty acids and a glycerol, triglycerides are the fat found most in food and stored in the body; used as a good source of energy.

Figure 5–1 Fat Vocabulary

Imagine a glass of iced tea. Then imagine adding teaspoon after teaspoon of sugar, until you can't stir the tea. That tea is "saturated" with sugar. When you use a paper towel to wipe up some spilled water, the towel becomes saturated with water, meaning it can't hold any more water. Saturated fat molecules do the same thing with hydrogen, holding onto as much hydrogen as possible.

Saturation makes for a very strong molecule that is difficult to break apart. For this reason, saturated fats give very good texture and mouthfeel to food. Chefs often times prefer to use saturated fats, such as butter or bacon fat, in their cooking. Saturated fats contribute texture and taste to many menu items. For example, butter or hydrogenated vegetable oil (like Crisco™) give the correct texture and taste to cookie dough. Unfortunately, saturated fats are difficult for the body to break down. Excess saturated fats are stored in the walls of veins and arteries, narrowing them and causing a decrease in elasticity and in volume. This ultimately leads to various disease states.

Examples of saturated fats include the marbling in steak, butter, egg yolks, and bacon grease. Most saturated fats are found in animal products, with several exceptions. Palm oil, tropical oils, and coconut products are plant products that contain saturated fat. So you can't feel virtuous if you stop adding whole cream to your coffee and switch to a coffee lightener made from coconut oil. Both cream and coconut oil are saturated fat and will produce the same damage in your body as saturated fats from animal products.

Hydrogenation or Margarine, Bane of the Chef's Existence

Ever wonder how corn oil is miraculously changed into solid oil? It's done through a process called **hydrogenation.** Hydrogen is introduced to vegetable oil molecules to create saturation where there was none. Nature made corn oil to be liquid. Humans fooled around with nature and added some chemical bonds where there weren't any before. When you make mayonnaise and whip lots of air into the oil, you are creating a type of hydrogenation.

> FOOD FOR THE MIND
>
> Examples of unsaturated fats: soy, cottonseed, corn, safflower, canola, olive, walnut, peanut, sesame seed and hazelnut oil, peanut butter, oil found in nuts, seeds, and olives
>
> Examples of saturated fats: fat found in dairy products, egg yolks and meats, coconut, palm, and tropical oils

For years it was thought that hydrogenated vegetable oils, like the type found in margarines or solid vegetable shortenings were healthier than animal fats, such as butter or lard. It's now thought that the bonds made from adding hydrogen to vegetable oil, called trans-fatty acid bonds, may do just as much damage to the veins and arteries as animal fat. Moral to the story: sparing use of any type of fat.

Nowadays you can get light, fat-free, reduced calorie, butter-margarine blends and cholesterol-lowering margarine. The big deal is trans-fatty acids. Trans-fatty acids are formed when naturally unsaturated oils, such as canola or corn, are hydrogenated, as we've said above. If you have to use margarine, select the healthiest one. Read the label. Be sure the margarine is low in saturated fat. Usually, the softer the margarine, the lower the saturation. Be sure it doesn't have trans-fatty acid. Once again, the softer the better; some tub and squeezeable margarines don't have trans-fatty acids at all.

On the other hand, certain manufacturers have created margarines that are almost medicinal. They were formulated with plant sterols. These natural substances, isolated from pinesap or soy, don't allow the body to absorb cholesterol. This type of margarine should not be used for cooking, but rather used in small amounts by people who need to reduce their cholesterol. Other margarines are not as concerned about reducing cholesterol as they are in helping with weight loss. They are reduced in calories. These, too, should not be used in cooking, as they contain too little fat to yield an acceptable product.

Margarine was an invention of need. During World War II, there was a shortage of dairy products. It was discovered if you solidified vegetable oil and added some color, the resulting product could be used like butter. After the war and the discovery of the relationship between animal fat and heart disease, margarine hung around for a long time.

Cholesterol

Saturated fat from plant products is simply called saturated fat. Saturated fat from animal products is called **cholesterol.** It's important to understand the distinction. A manufacturer can produce a sandwich cookie with a filling that contains coconut oil. Coconut oil has a smooth texture and a silky mouthfeel. It's also saturated as all get-out. It will clog up your arteries as fast as a double bacon cheeseburger. However, the cookie manufacturer can put "contains no cholesterol" on the label, since cholesterol is found only in animal products. Knowledgeable consumers will read the ingredient line, see the coconut oil and then make a decision whether the cookie tastes good enough to risk heart disease.

As has been stated above, your body will synthesize the cholesterol you need to create hormones and other body chemicals. Some people inherit a gene that tells their body to create higher levels of cholesterol than is needed. In those cases, people have to be very, very careful about limiting the cholesterol in their diet, as their body already overproduces cholesterol. Even with healthy diets and exercise, cholesterol-lowering medications are sometimes necessary to help keep cholesterol at the proper level.

There are different types of cholesterol. When you go for a blood test, the doctor measures for total cholesterol and then the different types of cholesterol. With all the different types of cholesterol combined, you want a level that measures 200 or below. It is thought that cholesterol readings below 200 decrease the possibility of heart disease and high blood pressure. People with cholesterol over 240 have twice the risk of heart attacks, over 300 have three times the risk, etc.

Fat	*% unsaturated*	*% saturated*
Canola	94	6
Olive	86	14
Corn	87	13
Soy	85	15
Peanut	82	18

Figure 5–2 Cooking Fat Comparison

HDL (high-density lipoprotein) and **LDL** (low-density lipoprotein) are two of the types of cholesterol at which your doctor will look, in addition to total cholesterol. HDL cholesterol is thought to be the less harmful of the two types of cholesterol while LDL cholesterol can do more harm to the arteries. The doctor will look at your overall cholesterol to be sure that it is under 200 and will look at the ratio of your HDL to your LDL to make sure the ratio is in normal limits. The higher your HDL and the lower your LDL, the better for you.

Elevated cholesterol has recently been linked to another medical condition, osteoporosis (Kenney). It's been found that the same type of double-bacon cheeseburger diet that makes your circulatory system resemble the Los Angeles freeway system at rush hour (clogged and ready to blow) can also thin the bones. Low-density lipoproteins not only help to block arteries, but also can invade bone structures and eat away at them, sort of like fatty Pac-men. Yet another reason to keep the saturated fats down to a minimum.

Unsaturated Fats

Unsaturated fats are found only in plant products. A **monounsaturated** fat, such as olive oil, has one area on its molecule that is unsaturated. Put another way, a monounsaturated fat has a hole where one hydrogen used to be. A **polyunsaturated** fat has many areas on it molecule that is unsaturated. Unsaturated fats, such as corn, soy, safflower, canola, sesame, hazelnut, and cottonseed oil are all liquid at room temperature. Unsaturated fats are not holding onto as much hydrogen as they can and are weaker molecules than saturated fat. Think of saturated fats as having a double chain link fence surrounding them and unsaturated fats as having a single fence with lots of holes in it.

Many chefs are working with olive, hazelnut, walnut, avocado, sesame, and other specialty oils to incorporate more unsaturated oils into their recipes and menus. Each oil has its own flavor, color, and cooking properties, leading interest to foods without including saturated fats.

BREAKDOWN AND STORAGE OF DIETARY FATS

Saturated fats are big, unapproachable molecules and require a lot of energy to be broken down. Unsaturated fats are less formidable and require less energy to be taken apart. For this reason, the body will store any saturated fat it does not absolutely need. The storage repository for saturated fat in the body is in fat cells. Dietary fat is stored within each fat cell in a part of the cell called the "vacuole." When you cut down calories to lose weight, the vacuoles in the fat cells empty, but the fat cells are still there. When you begin to eat more calories and have excess calories, the fat cells suck up the excess calories, stored as fat.

If veins and arteries begin to get clogged with cholesterol (since you are an animal, any saturated fat in your body is called "cholesterol"), you can begin to see the start of hypertension (high blood pressure) and heart disease.

Unsaturated fats are more readily broken down by the body. As their "fence" has lots of holes in it, it is easier for the body to break it down. It is obvious if someone is storing a lot of unsaturated fat, as unsaturated fats are carried in the "fatty pads" of the body. You can figure out where those are. Any extra weight you carry around puts a strain on the heart. The heart has to work harder to supply blood to the extra areas you have created. If you were designed to be a 120-pound person, but are a 180-pound person, your heart has 60 more pounds to take care of, day and night, all the time. How long do you think your car's engine would last if you carried four or five heavy sandbags in the trunk all the time? By carrying around extra weight from fat, you are forcing your own "engine," the heart, to overwork on a constant basis. If this happens over a long period of time, your "engine" will start to show signs of wear and tear.

Extra saturated and unsaturated fat can cause damage in your body. Fat is easily deposited but very hard to eliminate from the body. Excess fat adds excess weight or clogs passageways and creates extra work for the heart, lungs, organs, muscles, and joints.

USE OF FAT IN THE BODY

But before we start saying lots of disparaging things about fats, let's talk about fat's good points. Fat is an essential nutrient. Your body can produce some of the fat it needs while some must be gotten from the diet. Even if you don't eat any foods that contain cholesterol, you will still have some cholesterol circulating in your blood because the body produces the cholesterol it needs. Cholesterol is an important part of many natural body compounds, such as certain hormones and also helps the body to absorb vitamins and other nutrients. Vitamin D can be synthesized by your body from dietary cholesterol.

Fat is an efficient source of calories, meaning that it is a good source of energy. Foods that are high in fat are high in energy. During certain times of life, this is very important. For example, an infant needs a lot of energy to grow, but has a very small stomach and not very much ability to store energy. Breast milk and infant formulas have a high fat content that meets infant needs. An infant put on a low fat diet would not grow or develop properly. A person hiking Mount Everest will need an enormous amount of energy, but will not want to carry a lot of heavy food packages. Special hiking foods are very high in unsaturated fats, supplying lots of energy in a small package.

Just a Little Every Day

Fat is a very efficient source of energy and is an essential part of the diet. Because it is so efficient, you require very small amounts of it on a daily basis. About 60 to 70 percent of the energy you need at rest comes from fat calories. Resting energy needs are things like breathing, blinking, swallowing, muscle contractions, etc. Saved or stored energy is in the form of fat, to be used when needed. What are we trying to say? Don't fill up your shopping cart on the fat-free aisle and think you are doing your body a favor. Plan a balanced diet that contains not more than 30 percent of calories from fat every day, and enjoy a vinaigrette here, a little feta cheese there.

Visceral fat is the fat cover around organs. Visceral fat shields the organs from bruising, acting as an insulator and cushion. Don't see the reason for this extra insulation? Just check out someone jogging down the street. All the internal organs are getting bounced around. Without visceral fat, you'd have bruised kidneys every time you ran.

Ever wonder why it sometimes seems that men can lose weight more easily than women? Part of the reason is the way fat is distributed in the body. Fat stored in different parts of the body has different characteristics. Fat stored above the waist is called "yellow fat," and is more metabolically active. Fat stored below the waist is called "brown fat" and is not very metabolically active. This means that when your body needs extra energy and goes into its stores, it will use all the yellow fat before it begins to use brown fat.

Women have more brown fat then men. Mother Nature having a cruel joke. The yellow fat/brown fat ratio is the reason why it's harder for women to change a pants size than a shirt size. The body needs to use up all the yellow fat on top before it will begin to touch the brown fat on the bottom. You might notice, in both men and women, that when people diet to lose weight, you notice the weight loss first in their face. This is the yellow fat/brown fat ratio working again.

American Heart Association Recommendations

The American Heart Association (AHA) is dedicated to improving cardiac health. The AHA issued new guidelines in 2001 (the last update was 1988). After a great deal of research with large, diverse groups of people the AHA has added some new recommendations to their original ones. The 2001 guidelines recommend more fiber and less sugar in the daily diet and reduced the amount of suggested salt, about 30 percent from the original guidelines. Rather than just suggesting that unsaturated fats should be eaten, the 2001 list makes specific recommendations for the intake of monounsaturated fat. There is more emphasis on increasing exercise and reducing weight as being important for heart health. And very importantly, there is an acknowledgment that genes play a role in heart disease. People with family histories of heart disease should be even more vigilant about their diet and lifestyle.

The new AHA guidelines are closer to the USDA Guidelines, creating less confusion for the consumer. Both the AHA and the USDA guidelines encourage consumers to take a holistic approach to health, thinking about their health, their lifestyles, including smoking cessation, exercising and stress reduction, and their diet.

Some heart-healthy topics still need further research, like the effectiveness of anti-oxidants, very-low-fat diets, increased soy protein, and the use of omega-3 fatty acids as tools for reducing heart disease.

HOW FATS CONTRIBUTE TO HEALTH

Fats and carbohydrates are both **protein-sparing** nutrients. This means that the body uses fats and carbohydrates to do the day-to-day tasks and leaves protein for the more important jobs, like building and maintaining muscle and keeping the immune system strong.

1. Be sure to include more physical activity and maintain correct weight, especially if you've had an increase in obesity in the past decade.
2. Genes influence the way people respond to fat, cholesterol, and salt. Tailor your lifestyle (including diet and exercise) to your family history.
3. In agreement with the World Health Organization, people do need some fat in their diet. The current recommendation is at least 15 percent.
4. 10 to 15 percent of total daily calories should come from monounsaturated fat (the 1988 guidelines recommended 10 percent of less from saturated, 10 percent from saturated and remainder from monounsaturated).
5. 25 to 30 grams of daily fiber should come from food, not supplements (this is about 1 ounce of fiber).
6. Choose a diet moderate in sugar, as sugar supplies "empty" calories. Most foods that are high in sugar are low in vitamins, minerals and fiber.
7. Sodium intake should not exceed more than 6 grams of salt per day (about 1 teaspoon of salt).

Figure 5–3 American Heart Association Recommendations, 2001 Modifications (adapted from the American Heart Association Guidelines 2001, *www.aha.org*)

Different parts of the body work more efficiently with different types of fuel. For example, the brain works *only* with glucose while muscle tissue prefers fat. During exercise, the body uses a combination of carbohydrates and fat for energy.

Fats add flavor and texture to foods. The fatty-acid portion of the fat molecule is a carbon chain of varying lengths. The difference in the chain lengths is what causes different flavors in food. Butter and olive oil are both fats, but they have different flavors, colors, and even heating tolerances. This is due to the difference in carbon chain lengths.

Some portions of certain fat molecules may contribute to health. Omega-3 fatty acids, found in fish and some plants, are said to contribute to heart health. Other fatty acids help to regulate blood clotting and blood vessel opening and closing.

American Heart Association
www.Americanheart.org (1-800-AHA-USA1)
National Heart, Lung and Blood Institute
www.nhlbi.nih.org (301-592-8593)
American Red Cross
www.redcross.org (Web site lists local numbers)
American Academy of Family Physicians
www.familydoctor.org (800-274-2237)
American Dietetic Association
www.eatright.org (800-366-1644)

Figure 5–4 Heart Healthy Resource Guide

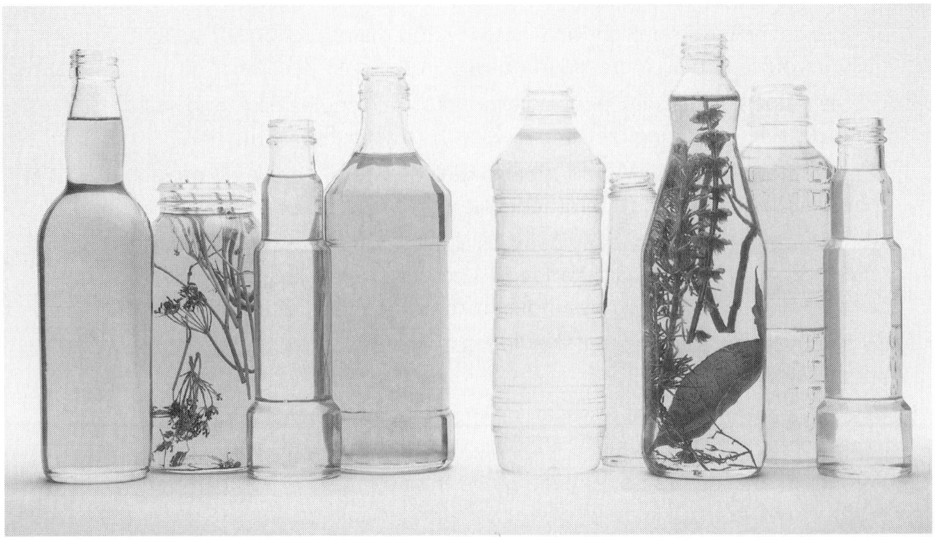

Fats and oils can be incorporated into healthy news.

The Good News

Fat is not all bad, we just tend to get too much of it. As we've said, your body uses fat to insulate organs, regulate temperature and is the preferred source of energy for muscles at rest. All fat from food is not bad. In fact, some has a protective effect for the heart.

Omega-3s

Omega-3 fatty acids, found in fish, soybean and canola oil and walnuts and flaxseed may actually contribute to heart health. Researchers wondered how it was possible that native populations in Alaska, Norway, and Greenland could eat very-high-fat diets and have very, very low incidences of heart disease and high blood pressure. How could this be?

The answer was found in their diet. Specifically, in the type of fat in the diet. All the fat in their diet came from fish, seafood, and fish oil. These foods are naturally high in omega-3 fatty acids. Upon closer examination it was found that omega-3s reduced the amount of hardened material (called **plaques)** that form on artery walls (Bonna, 1).

You've heard the term "hardening of the arteries," more commonly known as arteriosclerosis? Cholesterol and saturated fats tend to attach themselves to the walls of the body's arteries. If this extra fat is not eliminated, calcium attaches itself to the fatty deposits. This creates a calcification, or hardening, of the arteries. If there are a lot of plaques, the arteries lose their elasticity and become narrow. Blood cannot flow normally and the heart must work harder. This can lead to high blood pressure and damage to the heart muscle.

Which leads us back to omega-3s. Populations that have diets high in fish and seafood tend to have less arterial plaque. The conclusion is drawn that a diet high in fish and seafood will reduce the risk of heart disease, since omega-3s found in the fish reduce the possibility of hardened arteries.

There is not currently an RDA for omega-3s, but it is recommended that a healthy diet should include two to three fish meals per week, with small amounts of vegetable oils as well.

Fish oil supplements, in liquid and capsule form, have been available for many years. Perhaps some of you have been chased around the house by an older relative with a big spoon and an even bigger bottle of cod liver oil. The current thinking is that fish oil supplement may not be the way to go. Since nutritional supplements are not regulated by governmental agencies, consumers cannot be sure of the source of the fish oil or how much omega- 3s are actually contained in the supplement. There is the possibility of contamination with impurities during processing. It is possible to take toxic levels of fish oils and that can lead to cerebral strokes (*FDA Consumer*, 2) or liver damage. To keep the whole body healthy, stick to food when trying to get your omega-3s.

In addition to heart health, omega-3 fatty acids have also been linked to decreases in certain types of cancer. Once again, populations that consumed large amounts of fish and seafood tended to have less colon and breast cancer. Omega-3s are an essential nutrient for brain development, growth and function. Maybe that's why some people call fish "brain food." The brain is made largely of lipid (fat), and depends heavily on omega-3 fatty acids to work properly. Pregnant women who include seafood in their diet are ensuring that their child's brain develops properly. As discussed above, pregnant women shouldn't take fish oil supplements.

Olive Oil

There is no such thing as miracle oil, one you can use as much as you want as often as you want. There are no oils that you can pour on foods and use like a medicine to chase heart disease away.

However, between 1985 and 1990 the sales of olive oil doubled (Margen, 5). The Mediterranean diet was popularized (see page 16 for the Mediterranean food guide pyramid), capitalizing on the fact that there was a much lower incidence of heart disease among populations that used olive oil as their main source of fat. It didn't hurt that the promotions stressed the cholesterol-lowering properties of a diet high in olive oil.

Extra virgin olive oil means the olives are hand-picked from the best of the crop and are squeezed at room temperature and cold-pressed. The freshly pressed oil is checked for aroma, taste, and color. The best of the batch is called extra virgin olive oil, and the remainder is virgin olive oil.

The next grade down is pure olive oil, made from Grade-B olives. These olives may have had a solvent added to coax more oil out of the olives and then may be heated (to get rid of solvent). Pure olive oil can be pale and bland. If it is too bland, it may be blended with a bit of extra virgin, to perk it up.

Light olive oil has nothing to do with calories. The "light" in this case has to do with color and flavor, used as a marketing tool. Olive oil is delicate, and

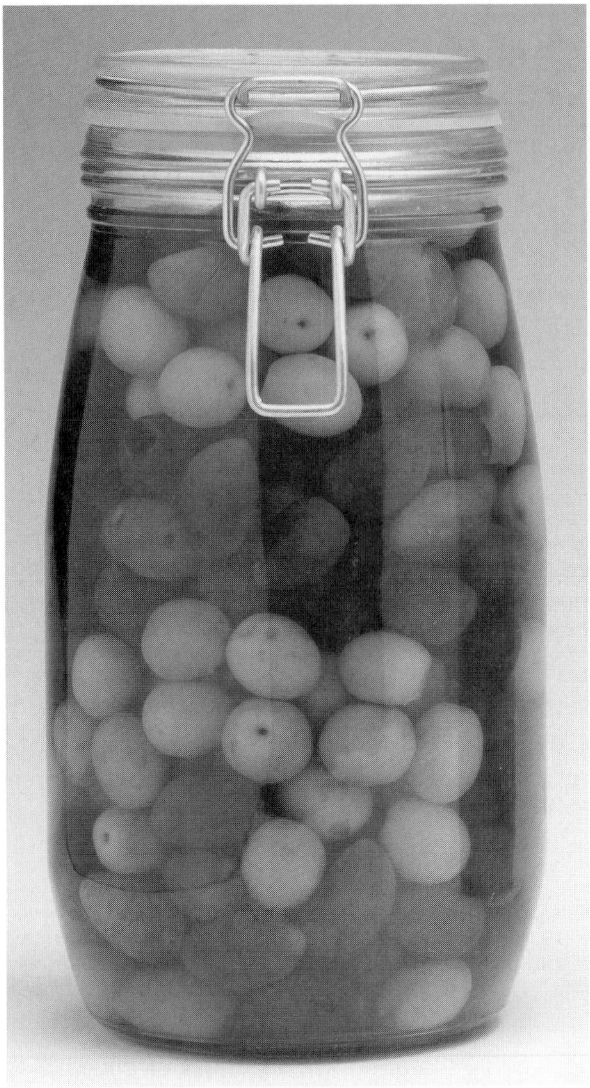

Olives and olive oil come in many varieties.

to be honest, a lot of flavor is lost in heating. Be sure to store it away from heat or light. If you refrigerate olive oil it can get cloudy and thicken.

Olive oil has a wonderful taste and aroma. It is monounsaturated, which many health-care professionals feel may actually help heart health. Olive oil is a great ingredient for the culinary professional. Just beware. Too much olive oil can cause excess weight to amass just as much as its less glamorous polyunsaturated cousins.

The Bad News

As we've been attempting to emphasize, fat is an essential part of everyone's diet. However, on a regular basis, many people consume much more fat than they need. Your body likes to hold onto as much fat as it can, not knowing where it's next meal is coming from. Holding onto extra fat does not give you

Heart attacks have been linked to diet, smoking and obesity and also to several factors over which we have no control. From the annals of the American Medical Association come:

1. Cardiac "events" tend to occur most often between 4 to 6:00 P.M. and on Monday and Friday.
2. Periodontal (gum) disease doubles your heart attack risk. Bacteria may enter the bloodstream and cause blood clots that lead to heart attacks.
3. Body shape seems to influence heart disease. Being overweight is bad. If you have more of that weight in your abdomen (affectionately known as your gut) than your hips, you are more prone to heart disease.
4. A bald spot on the very top of the head has been linked, in men, to a three times higher than average risk for heart attack.

Figure 5–5 Amazing But True

an unlimited amount of energy or lots and lots of fat-soluble vitamins. Unfortunately, that double order of fries can lead to all kinds of nasty conditions, including obesity, diabetes, cancer and heart disease. Read on.

Cardiovascular Diseases

Hypertension (HTN) or high blood pressure can be a contributing factor to heart disease, heart attacks, and strokes. A high-fat diet can be a contributing factor to hypertension. In 2000, over 50 million Americans had HTN (Kenney, 2). HTN causes the heart to work harder than usual and can accelerate **atherosclerosis,** or hardening of the arteries. HTN raises your risk of heart disease by three times and your risk of a stroke by seven times. Think about letting all the hoses in your car's engine get 80 or 90 percent clogged up and still expecting the engine to run consistently at 60 miles per hour. You know that eventually the engine will either wear out from having to run harder just to keep up ordinary performance or will blow a hose. Just about the same thing happens with a heart that is depending on fat-clogged arteries. A heart attack can occur when the heart has just been trying to compensate too long with clogged arteries. A stroke can occur when some of the clog (a combination of dead blood cells and cholesterol called "plaque") breaks off and blocks the blood flow to an artery supplying blood to the brain.

A NUTRI-BAR

Get Your "-emias" in Line

Just some of the diagnoses that come from the double-bacon cheeseburger diet regimen:

Hyperlipidemia: any elevation of fat found in the blood; could be elevated cholesterol, triglycerides or a combination

Hypercholesterolemia: elevated cholesterol levels in the blood

Hypertriglyceridemia: elevated triglyceride levels in the blood

less than 120 and less than 80	Considered optimal; some athletes have blood pressures of 110/60 (very low blood pressures should be monitored).
less than 130 and less than 85	Considered normal. Exercise and weight loss might help in lowering high normal.
130–140 and 85–89	
140–159 and 90–99	Stage One high blood pressure
160–179 and 100–109	Very high blood pressure

Figure 5–6 Various Blood Pressure Levels (information adapted from the American Heart Association)

The most common way to check for hypertension is to have your blood pressure taken. Blood pressure cuffs measure the pressure your heart exerts at different times. The measurement is expressed in millimeters of mercury.

Let's take a **blood pressure** reading of 120/80, which is considered to be normal. The top number, called systolic pressure, is a measurement of the highest pressure within the arteries when the heart beats, in this case at 120 millimeters of mercury. The bottom number, called the diastolic pressure, measures the lowest pressure in the arteries when the heart is resting and filling with blood, getting ready for the next beat.

Blood pressure can be influenced by age, heredity, ethnic background, smoking, state of fitness, and weight status. Almost half of all Americans over the age of sixty are to some degree hypertensive. Hypertension is higher in people with African-American, Hispanic, Native American, Indian, and Pacific Islander backgrounds. People with diabetes are thought to be at higher risk for high blood pressure and heart disease, as diabetes can affect the circulatory system (Kenney, 2). The less fit you are, the harder your heart has to work, kind of like a car that never gets a tune up. And the more weight you have to carry around, the harder your heart has to work, making it work faster with a resultant rise in blood pressure.

Obesity

Obesity has been rising at an alarming rate in the United States in the last ten years. The problem with obesity is not just cosmetic, or that airline seats seem too skimpy. If you load your diet up with excess fat, then you load your body up with excess fat. Your body is still very much running on caveman instinct. It doesn't say, "Oh, he'll never get into that tuxedo on Saturday, let me get rid of this extra fat." Unfortunately, your body's response is, "Oh, good, extra fat; let's store it away for when we'll need it—you just never know when that next meal might get here."

As your body works in this hyper efficient way, your arteries, your organs and your love handles get stuffed with fat. The extra weight associated with fat can be a strain on your back, hips, knees, and ankles as they try to carry the extra baggage around. Extra weight makes your heart pump harder, as it tries to circulate blood to expanded territories.

The extra strain on your circulatory system can sometimes result in Type II diabetes (see Chapter 4 for a discussion on diabetes). With the increased rise in obesity, we are seeing more and more cases of diabetes in the United States. More children are obese and more are becoming diabetic as a result of obesity. The damage done from diabetes, such as vision loss, circulatory system and nervous system damage, and heart disease can be slowed down but cannot be reversed. It's frightening to know that in the year 2000 more children under the age of thirteen were diagnosed with Type II diabetes than in the eight years previous to that. Obesity was at least one of the causes in most of these cases.

Cancers

Groups of people who eat diets high in saturated fat over long periods of time have been found to develop more cancers, especially prostate, breast, and colon cancer. Although we are not absolutely sure of the reason, it is thought that certain fats actually promote tumor growth, some protect cancer cells from destruction and some interfere with the body's ability to produce "fighter" cells that destroy cancer cells. More practically, if a person is very overweight, a doctor may not be able to physically feel an abnormal growth delaying the diagnosis and treatment of cancer.

It is also thought that plant foods, such as fruits, vegetables, and whole grains have a protective effect against many cancers. If you are eating a diet high in fat, it's felt that you are probably not eating a diet high in plant foods. This makes sense since you usually don't follow a double order of nachos and cheese sauce with a fruit salad.

FAT SUBSTITUTES

Fat substitutes have been getting a lot of play in the food technology community for the past thirty or so years. Just imagine, all the potato chips, ice cream, and hollandaise sauce you desire with no calories!

Several obstacles faced the food technologists trying to create fake fats. Fat substitutes have to have the flavor, texture, and mouth feel of vegetable or animal fats and have to be able to stand up to heat. Fat substitutes were not as easy to develop as sugar substitutes, which could be generically "sweet" with no real texture or mouthfeel. Food technologists have tried lots of methods and ingredients over the years. Fat substitutes made from cellulose or oats or egg whites provide only four calories per gram, versus the nine from fat. Working with starch or protein to get them to hold onto more water made them appear creamy. However, the oats and egg whites had to be processed under high heat. This limited what the user could do with them, as they were already cooked. Over the years there have been frozen desserts, pastries and whipped toppings made with lower-calorie fat substitutes, but none were very well-liked by the public.

As we discuss below, chefs have their own way to cut back on the fat on the menu. By using an assortment of cooking techniques and flavoring agents, chefs can cut out the fat without cutting out the flavor. However, the quest for a no-calorie fat continued.

Several companies were able to develop fat-based no calorie products. Fatty acids were manipulated so that the human body was not able to absorb them. This gave the mouthfeel and taste of fat without the calories and these products could withstand the heat, so you could cook with them. These products had no taste, but chefs could work with that.

A more important problem was that several of the fat-based fat replacers caused abdominal cramps and diarrhea and blocked the body's ability to absorb vitamins A,D, E, and K. No calories was one thing. No nutrients was another!

The FDA stepped in and said products containing these fat replacers had to have a warning on the label for consumers. The FDA also limited the fat replacers use to certain salty snacks. The feeling was that snack food did not constitute a large part of people's daily intake and that snack foods were not generally eaten with high-nutrient-containing foods, so little damage would be done. In other words, the FDA was saying that most people only ate a few potato chips every day, and did not eat an apple or steamed broccoli when having the chips, so nutrient interference would be kept at a minimum. The manufacturers added additional vitamins to products containing the fat replacers to compensate for those not absorbed.

THE CULINARY APPROACH TO FAT MODIFICATION

Fat, as a cooking ingredient, is smooth, silky, and satisfying. And yet, as a culinary professional, you are up to the challenge of reducing or eliminating the fat and still keeping the flavor and the texture of menu items.

Who doesn't like the silky luxury of butter, egg yolks, cream, and cheeses? On the enjoyment side, fats provide flavor, mouthfeel, color, moisture, and general wonderfulness to foods. On the cooking side, fats allow the chef to grill and fry food without having it stick; acts as a binding and emulsifying agent for sauces, soups, and baked products; provides creamy textures; and thickens liquids and solids.

A NUTRI-BAR

This Has Nothing to Do With Nutrition

Look at a marbled steak or an untrimmed roast—if the beef fat is pearly white, the animal was probably fed on corn; if slightly yellow, than its been fed on wheat. Corn-fed animals are thought to be more tender, and are probably more expensive. On the other hand, raw chicken can have a yellow, white, and even blueish-black skin. This has to do with the breed of the bird and tells nothing about the fat content or the tenderness (black-skinned chickens are bred in Asia for their supposed medicinal value). Egg yolk color and nutrient level will be influenced by feed. Want an almost orange yolk with lots of beta carotene (vitamin A)? Feed your chickens carrots, sweet potatoes, and marigolds.

Unfortunately, on the health side, too much fat outweighs the health benefits which adequate amounts of fat provide. As we've said, overindulgence in fats, especially saturated fats, can be a causative agent in many diseases, such as diabetes, heart disease, gastrointestinal diseases, and pulmonary diseases.

Ingredient Selection

Remember that, except in extreme cases of illness, a small amount of fat is necessary in the diet. Fat helps transport nutrients through the blood, protects organs from damage and helps build and maintain tissue components. Fat also triggers the brain's satiety center to deliver the message "I've had enough," although we don't always listen. So, we are not looking to eliminate all sources of fat, just limit them a bit. Remember, one ounce of solid fat (as found in butter, avocados, olives, etc.) has approximately 220 calories, so a little goes a long way.

As we've discussed earlier in the chapter, hydrogenation helps solidify unsaturated, liquid fat. Technically speaking, to get a liquid fat to turn into solid fat, you've got to open up some of the bonds holding the liquid fat together and force in some hydrogen. The more hydrogen fat holds, the more solid it becomes. More and more research is showing that manmade solid fats have little to no health benefits, and may actually cause some damage.

As a culinary professional, you've had to be ready to explain your use of small amounts of butter in "healthy" foods. Remind your customers that for years, margarine was thought to be healthier than animal fat. What's now coming to light is that the new bonds formed by playing around with Mother Nature may cause just a much heart disease as the natural bonds in butter. These trans-fatty acids, formed when naturally unsaturated fat is mechanically saturated, may do as much harm, if not more, than animal fats, which are naturally saturated.

1. Use cornstarch and flour slurries instead of **roux** (equal measures of fat and flour) to thicken sauces.
2. Use vegetable, wine, and stock reductions instead of fat-based sauces.
3. Try low-fat fresh or canned milk instead of cream or whole milk.
4. Roast, grill, oven-poach, barbecue, stir-fry, broil, poach, steam, pressure cook, stew, or braise instead of frying foods.
5. Purchase lean cuts of meat and trim excess fat before preparing.
6. Prepare stocks, soups, and meats a day prior to use, refrigerate, and skim off fat.
7. Try low-fat yogurt in place of sour cream in recipes.
8. Use vegetable oil spray or nonstick cookware.

Figure 5–7 Lose the Fat: Culinary Techniques for Keeping the Flavor and Reducing the Fat

The following books take a moderate approach to fat-reduced recipes, offering purchasing and serving guidelines for ingredients and menus

The American Cancer Society Cookbook written by Anne Lindsay, William Morrow and Company, (1988), ISBN 0-688-07484-7

Culinary Nutrition for Foodservice Professionals written by Carol A. Hodges, Van Nostrand Reinhold (1990) ISBN 0-442-22686-1

Healthy and Delicious (400 professional recipes) written by Sandy Kapoor, John Wiley & Sons (1996) ISBN 0-471-13158

Healthful Quantity Baking written by Maureen Egan and Susan Davis Allen, John Wiley & Sons (1988), ISBN 0-471-54022-6

In Good Taste written by Victor Gielisse, Prentice Hall (1999), ISBN 0-13-591595-3

The Professional Chef's *Techniques of Healthy Cooking* by Culinary Institute of America, Van Nostrand Reinhold (1993) ISBN 0-442-01126-1

Figure 5–8 Resources 'R' Us

Decrease the Fat, Increase the Flavor

Fat does indeed add magic to foods, but with a little informed sorcery (and saucery) menu items could appear sinful and creamy without all the fat.

Read the Label

When selecting meats, choose USDA "choice" grade. USDA choice is good for the waistline and the bottom line, as it is less expensive and has less marbling than the higher grades. Be sure to trim external fat and use low-fat cooking methods. In addition to beef, pork and veal have lean cuts that can be utilized on the menu. The saturated fat in most poultry is concentrated in the skin. Contrary to popular belief, the skin can be left on during cooking and removed before serving. This will allow for maximum flavor, juiciness, tenderness, and color with a minimum of fat. Seafood is always a "go" when getting rid of fat. Grill, bake, steam, poach, stew, or barbecue fish fillets, strips, or steaks; add cooked shrimp to green or pasta salads to create a new, low-fat entrée.

You don't have to say good-bye to dairy products when reducing fat—just adjust your inventory. Non- and low-fat yogurt can be used instead of sour cream or heavy cream in some recipes. Canned, evaporated skimmed milk can be used to replace cream in soups and sauces. Some cheeses are available naturally in lower-fat forms, such as part-skim mozzarella or neuchafetel (a low-fat form of cream cheese), and others are available in nonfat versions.

Vegetables and starches can be used as the "creamy" factor in some dishes. Carrots, root vegetables (such as beets, winter squash, turnips), and potatoes can be cooked until soft and pureed to create soups and sauces that appear and taste buttery and creamy. For example, carrots and potatoes cooked together and pureed with fresh or dried thyme, onion powder and white pepper makes a thick, sunburst-colored soup which tastes full of cream but isn't. Pureed potatoes (mashed potatoes thinned with nonfat milk) can be seasoned with garlic and rosemary to create both a "cream" of potato soup or a "creamy" garlic sauce for vegetables.

Here is the technique for making your own soft, low fat cheese

1. Yogurt cheese: this can be used to replace sour cream or whipped cream cheese in recipes.
   Line a china cap or strainer with cheese cloth or coffee filters. Add one gallon of nonfat plain yogurt and allow to drain over night, refrigerated. That's it! One gallon of yogurt should yield about 1½ quarts yogurt cheese.
2. Nonfat fresh cheese: this has the texture of ricotta and will last for two or three days in the refrigerator.
   In a medium saucepan, heat 4 quarts of nonfat milk and 3 quarts of nonfat buttermilk. As curds are created by the heat, remove them and save. Cook until all the milk has transformed into curds.
   The curds can be used as is, formed in a layer pan into a solid, or puree to be used in desserts, sauces, soups, and salad dressings

Figure 5–9 It's the Cheese!

A roux, the chef's thickener, is traditionally made with equal parts of butter and flour. In place of roux, pureed cooked beans, pureed cooked vegetables, rice, or potatoes can be used instead. Allow enough cooking time to have thickening occur and to incorporate flavors. By the way, pureeing is a method that gives the allusion of creaminess. Puree some of a vegetable or bean soup and add back to the remaining soup-it will appear that you have cooked with cream or butter.

Flavor Enhancers

The culinary rule is that if you take something out, you have to replace it with something. So, if you take out the fat, think about what you will put back. Nobody will appreciate a fat-free chicken breast if it is colorless and tasteless.

If you are using stocks or broths instead of fat, be sure they are flavorful. You can reduce them (allow them to cook over low heat to evaporate some of the water and concentrate the flavors) to intensify the flavor. Lemon or lime juice, white or black pepper or wines heighten flavor without fat.

Fresh and dried herbs have no calories or fat and enhance the taste and color of menu items. Paprika, cumin, red pepper flakes add color, as do curry powders and turmeric (the "yellow" in mustard).

Pureed vegetables make colorful, fat-free sauces. Puree green, yellow, and red peppers and create a tri-colored base for chicken and fish. Spinach can be pureed, mixed with low-fat milk and seasoned with pepper and nutmeg or mixed with garlic and onions to be used as a sauce for fish or poultry or as a base for "creamy" spinach soup.

Think Convenience

Desserts are a special part of the meal. If you don't have the time to create special low-fat treats, think convenience items. Frozen, ready-to-use angel food cake can be thawed and served over a pool of fresh pureed strawberries or sliced fresh fruit. Graham crackers can be layered with canned or fresh sliced fruit and frozen yogurt or sorbet to create a dessert "club

Here is a partial list of all the different cooking methods that do not require the addition of fat

Bake and roast: place meats on racks to allow fat to drip away. Roll meat in cracked pepper, coarse salt, or dried herbs to seal in the moisture. Wrap potatoes, beets, yams, and whole, peeled onions in foil and roast until tender.

Barbecue and grill: marinate lean meat cuts before cooking to maximize moisture and tenderness. Rather than sauté or fry, barbecue or grill vegetables and potatoes.

Sauté: you don't need fat to sauté; try vegetable stock or broth, vegetable juice, tomato puree, or non-stick pans.

Steam: sprinkle meat or veggie with fresh or dried herbs and citrus juices to enhance flavor without fat.

Poach: poaching doesn't mean waterlogged chicken or fish. Create a court bouillion with chopped carrots, celery, onions, white wine and herbs, use de-fatted chicken or vegetable stock or broth or vegetable and fruit juice.

Smoke: you can "smoke" meats, fish, and vegetables on the stovetop. Using disposable pans, fill the bottom pan with wood chips, perforate the top pan and fill with seasoned product, cover and allow to "smoke" over medium heat (be sure your ventilation system is in good shape before you do this).

Braise and stew: trim meats of excessive fat and cook with fresh or frozen veggies, potatoes, grains, and fresh or dried herbs. If liquid is required, use vegetable juice or puree, tomato puree, or de-fatted vegetable stock.

Figure 5–10 Just a Reminder

sandwich." Frozen ice milk or sherbet can be made into a low-fat sundae, topped with frozen or canned fruit, dessert syrups, chopped raisins, and vanilla wafers. Pudding mixes can be made with low-fat milk, combined with a low-fat whipped topping for a fast "mousse;" serve this with sliced bananas and canned mandarin oranges.

If you have time, create a fruit tart with a graham cracker crust, low-fat pudding, and canned or frozen fruit. Bake apples or pears with cinnamon and ginger and serve with low fat ice cream or yogurt. Canned pumpkin can be mixed with egg whites, evaporated canned skimmed milk, nutmeg, cinnamon and lemon zest and baked in a pie shell or as custard.

EGG SUBSTITUTES

Puffy French omelets, savory Italian frittatas, spicy Chinese egg foo yung, airy Spanish tortillas—all feature Mother Nature's almost perfect creation, the egg. Without it, where would quiche, strata, soufflé, or egg salad be? There's just one minor health detail that might concern your customers.

In the ongoing battle of cholesterol versus man, the humble egg yolk is constantly under attack. The yolk is Mother Nature's cruel joke, as it is packed with health-giving fat-soluble vitamins and artery-clogging saturated fat, the infamous cholesterol.

The jury is still out on the importance of limiting dietary cholesterol versus lowering total fat intake. Some authorities feel that the key to heart health is to lower all fat in the diet while others feel that the accent need only be on the lowering of saturated fats.

Be that as it may, Americans still tend to overdo it on saturated fats but are trying to change. According to the USDA, egg products (such as egg substitutes) account for over 25 percent of all egg use in the country.

Ersatz Eggs

Egg substitutes have several roles to play in order to give a successful performance. They must lend the same moisture, mouth feel, texture, and color as egg yolks do, while leaving the saturated fat by the way side. This is accomplished in various ways.

Commercial egg substitutes are generally made from pasteurized egg whites, with vegetable oil, cellulose gums, beta-carotene, nonfat milk, salt and emulsifiers, and stabilizers added for texture and color.

"Egg whites are thin after pasteurization," explains Trudy Cravens, RD, Worthington Foods, a manufacturer of egg substitutes. "They pour like water, lacking the texture, mouthfeel, and appearance needed. By adding dairy notes, beta carotene (for color) and stabilizers we can put back the vitamins, flavors, colors, and baking properties."

The upside of commercial egg substitutes include the convenience of an almost whole egg-like product and pasteurization. Pasteurization eliminates some of the danger from salmonella contamination (although mishandling brings the danger right back) and extends shelf life. Most commercial egg substitutes are shipped frozen. Kept properly frozen, egg substitutes can last up to a year. Egg substitutes can be easily poured, more convenient than cracking and separating eggs. The downside is that egg substitutes are more egg-spensive than shell eggs and are not as quickly available, as they must be thawed. They usually fairly high in sodium, used as a preservative.

Vegan Eggs

Most commercial egg substitutes are egg and dairy based. There is at least one product on the market that is plant-based, especially suitable for vegan vegetarians and for people with an allergy to eggs or dairy. A dry product called Egg Replacer, produced by Ener-G Foods (800-331-5222 or *www.ener-g.com*) is the gold standard for plant-based egg substitutes. It comes packed in one-pound boxes, which translates into the equivalent of approximately 80 large eggs. Egg Replacer's ingredients include potato starch, tapioca flour, carbohydrate gum (for body), citric acid, and calcium carbonate (for leavening). One and one half teaspoons of Egg Replacer mixed with two tablespoons of water replaces one large egg. Once reconstituted, Egg Replacer must be handled with the same Hazard Analysis Critical Control Points (HACCP) care as fresh eggs. Egg Replacer can be used to replace whole eggs in baking recipes or when eggs are used as a moistening ingredient in casseroles. Egg Replacer does not have the texture or flavor to be used in

Here are some tried-and-true formulas for replacing eggs (each formula is the equivalent of one large egg)

1. One tablespoon nonfat dry milk powder, 2 large egg whites, 3 drops of egg shade: sprinkle milk powder over egg whites, beat until smooth; add egg shade and beat until blended.
2. Two ounces soft tofu, 2 drops egg shade—mash or blend and use in stir-fries, as "scrambled eggs" or in baking.
3. One tablespoon flour, 2 teaspoons water, one teaspoon vegetable oil, 2 drops egg shade: blend all ingredients until well-combined and use as egg sub in baking and sauces.
4. One-quarter cup of mashed bananas or applesauce or pureed beans or mashed potatoes or pureed fruit can be substituted for one egg, depending on the use (for example, banana or fruit can be subbed for eggs in baking, potatoes or beans in soups or casseroles, etc).
5. Two egg whites per whole egg.

Figure 5–11 One Up on Mother Nature

recipes where eggs are the stars, such as in omelets, sauces, scrambled eggs or quiche. Egg Replacer must be used like a whole egg, so meringues, which require only egg whites, or Hollandaise sauce, which requires only egg yolks, are out. At this time, Egg Replacer is the only commericially available vegan egg substitute. You can experiment on your own with various ingredients, such as tofu, nut flours, or fruit purees to devise your own vegan egg substitute.

Other non-animal ingredients to replace eggs are soft tofu, mashed beans, mashed potatoes, and fruit purees. You will have to match the substitute with the menu item. For example, tofu can be scrambled with chopped vegetables and herbs to create a dish close to scrambled eggs—use it as an entrée or as a filling for breakfast burritos. Fruit purees, such as banana and apple, can be used to replace some of the egg in baking recipes and pureed or mashed beans can be used as a thickener, instead of eggs, in soups and dips.

Grow Your Own

If purchasing egg substitutes is not in your budget, you can create your own. Purchase frozen egg whites or separate white from shell eggs. Egg shade, a food coloring that specifically mimics the buttery golden color of egg yolks, can be used to color the whites.

When creating your own egg substitutes, you will have to tailor your creation to the use. For example, if you are making egg-white omelets, you need only use egg whites colored with egg shade—you might add a bit of milk for texture. If you are going to use your own egg-sub creation for a binding agent, as in casseroles, sauces, and soups, you will have to add a bit of fat, such as vegetable oil or melted margarine. If you are working with baking recipes, then you will have to experiment with a combination of egg whites, oil and milk to balance the baking formula. Rule of thumb is generally two egg whites and one teaspoon each of water and oil to replace each large egg. Tofu, which is high in unsaturated fat and low in saturated fat, can also be used in baking recipes.

There are some things that egg substitutes just don't do all that well. Hollandaise sauce, having the main ingredients of butter and egg yolks, comes to mind. No matter how it's done, margarine and egg substitute does not make an acceptable Hollandaise. The same can be said for flans and custards and some baking recipes that rely heavily on the fat in the egg yolk for flavor and texture. For these items, it would be better to offer alternates, such as wine reduction sauces, meringues, and mousses.

Take Out the Eggs

Some menu items will never miss the whole egg. For example, cheese strata (a multilayered, baked-cheese sandwich over which a savory custard sauce is poured) can be transformed into a lower-fat, whole egg-less product. Alternate layers of thinly sliced bread with thinly sliced tomatoes, mushrooms, onions and low-fat cheese (such as skim milk mozzarella). Create a sauce with heated non- or low-fat milk, beaten egg substitute, white pepper, crushed garlic and a hint of nutmeg. Pour the sauce over the strata and bake until bubbly. Sweet or savory quiche fillings can be made from a base of heated low-fat milk (soymilk can be used for a vegan option) and egg substitute. Beat the two ingredients together and add sweet ingredients (chopped dried, fresh, or canned fruit, sugar or syrup, orange or lemon zest, cinnamon, ginger, etc.) or savory ingredients (diced onions, peppers, garlic, tomatoes, mushrooms, low-fat sausage, ground pepper, basil, thyme, oregano, etc.), pour into an unbaked shell and bake until golden brown.

Yolk-less Baking

Egg yolk-less baking presents more of a challenge, as most baking formulas are a balance of fat and fluid. Quick bread, muffins and sponge cakes respond well to the loss of yolks, as they have other sources of moisture and leavening. Try banana bread or zucchini bread using egg whites, mashed banana or zucchini and thawed orange juice concentrate to replace the whole eggs. Lemon-pie filling (made with sugar, lemon juice, lemon zest and egg substitute) tastes and look rich without the fat from the yolk.

Many breakfast items can go yolk-less. Baked or griddled French toast can be made with egg substitutes rather than whole eggs. Add some chopped dried fruit, such as raisins or dates to replace some of the texture lost with the yolk. Offer three egg omelets "your way," which can be any combination of one or two egg whites with one whole egg, three egg yolks, etc. Add chopped veggies for color and texture. The same mixture can be used to create a morning scramble or as a filling for breakfast burritos. Layer this mixture with cooked hash browns and bake until crispy for a morning casserole. As an alternate to egg substitutes, soft tofu may be used instead.

FYI: NUTS TO NUTRITION

Okay, so you've studied the Food Guide Pyramid, you've read the news, and you're ready to cut back on the saturated fat and cholesterol. So what are you going to do about your brain's satiety center screaming, "give me some fat!"

Well, nuts to you and your satiety center. The American Heart Association wants you to limit the saturated fat and to replace it with unsaturated fat. Unsaturated fat can be found in some vegetables (avocados and olives come to mind), seafood and . . . nuts!

Yes, nuts have lots of calories from fat. You still need to calculate so your diet is 30 percent or fewer calories from fat. With your fat allowance you can choose from pecans, pine nuts, walnuts, almonds, pistachios, hazelnuts, peanuts, chestnuts—you get the idea.

Nuts are not just fat calories. Most varieties contain protein, fiber, folic acid, and some other vitamins and minerals. The fat that the nuts have is polyunsaturated and monounsaturated, the "heart healthy" kind. If you feel the need for some luscious and creamy, nuts are the way to go.

Lots of research bears out the benefits of nuts. Several studies show that people who include five or more servings of nuts per week had fewer heart attacks than people who didn't (La Bell, 3). Walnuts has been seen to lower blood cholesterol in some people, almonds have shown some signs of helping to prevent colon cancer and pecans seemed to assisted some people in lowering the LDL (low density) cholesterol in their systems.

A very interesting weight-control fact came out of this nutty research. Several studies compared weight loss among dieters eating a low-fat menu versus dieters eating a moderate-fat diet, with the fat coming mainly from nuts. Dieters on both types of diets lost the same amount of weight. The low-fat dieters tended to gain back small amounts of weight while the nut-eaters kept their weight stable.

So forget the butter moo and step up to the pate de peanut butter.

Nutri-Words

Atherosclerosis: a form of heart disease, characterized by high blood pressure and elevated blood cholesterol levels. Depending on the extent of the disease, surgery may be necessary, after which diet and exercise play an important role in preventing reoccurrence.

Blood pressure: the amount of pressure exerted by the heart during various phases. Norms have been established for blood pressure at rest and during exercise.

Cholesterol: cholesterol is the name given to saturated fats from animal sources. Humans are able to synthesize their own cholesterol, in addition to storing cholesterol gotten from the diet. There are several types of cholesterol in the body with the ability to do different levels of damage. A blood test can determine a person's cholesterol level.

Digestion of fat: fat is broken down to fatty acids and glycerol by the action of the digestive organs, enzymes and other chemicals produced by the body.

Egg substitutes: low-fat products that have some of the characteristics of eggs, without the saturated fat of eggs.

Fat substitutes: chemical compounds that have some of the characteristics of fats, without the calories or damaging effects (such as found in cholesterol).

Fatty acids: end products of fat digestion. Some of the fatty acids are essential, necessary for the smooth functioning of the body.

Flaxseed oil: pressed from flax seeds, thought to have some health benefits, such as antioxidation of damaging substances and reduction of cholesterol in the body, when combined with a healthy lifestyle.

High-Density Lipoproteins (HDL): are the form of cholesterol thought to do the least damage to the body.

Hydrogenation: a method to convert unsaturated, liquid fat to solid, saturated fat, such as liquid corn oil to margarine.

Hypertension: elevated or high blood pressure. Usually an indication of a disruption or disease-state in the body.

Low-Density Lipoproteins (LDL): are the form of cholesterol thought to do the most damage to the body.

Mono- and poly-unsaturated fats: the degree of unsaturation tells the consumer how easily the body can break down and absorb the fats they have selected. Olive oil is a popularly used monounsaturated fat. Corn oil or canola oil are polyunsaturated fats.

Obesity: elevated body weight, beginning at ten per cent above ideal body weight. Obesity may be a causative factor for poor health, including hypertension, heart disease and diabetes.

Omega-3 fatty acids: found largely in fish oils, thought to have a protective effect against certain types of heart disease when combined with a healthy lifestyle.

Plaque: a solid mass of fats, especially cholesterol and saturated fats, fiber and muscle tissue that collects on artery walls. Eventually, calcium adheres to the plaques, causing the loss of elasticity and narrowing in the artery. Excessive plaques on artery walls can lead to high blood pressure and heart disease.

Protein-sparing: nutrients, usually carbohydrates or fat, that take the place of protein in some body reactions. This allows protein to be used efficiently where it is needed.

Roux: a mixture of equal parts fat and flour, used to thicken sauces, soups, and stews.

Saturated fats: are generally from animal sources, such as the fat found in egg yolks, bacon and whole fat cheeses.

Triglycerides: are a combination of three fatty acids and a glycerol and are the fat found most in food and in the body and used as a good source of energy.

Unsaturated fats: fats generally found only from plant sources, such as walnuts, corn oil, olives and avocados.

Whaddaya think?

1. How do fats from plants and animal differ?
2. What's the big health deal about saturated fats?
3. Take a road trip to a large grocery store and then a natural foods market. What kind of specialty low-fat or fat-reducing kinds of products did you see? Would you use any of them?
4. Suggest a decadent dinner menu that has only unsaturated fats for the fat calories.
5. Give us some good news about fat.
6. What are you doing to avoid atherosclerosis?
7. Why does being overweight or obese open you up to more diseases?
8. What types of fats and oils would you choose for customers trying to reduce their cholesterol?
9. Have you tried products that contain fat substitutes? Cruise the snack aisle to scope some of them out.
10. What's the relationship between meat grades and amount of fat?

Critical Application Exercises

1. Compile some good news about dietary fat:
   a. Prepare an explanation for your customers how you can use some fat in meal preparation and still serve healthy meals.
   b. Explain to the professional running team you are preparing meals for what types and amounts of fats they need in their diet.
2. Make a list of the kinds and amounts of saturated fats you have eaten in the last three days. What would the American Heart Association say? Do you need to make any changes in your intake?
3. Review information on olive oil:
   a. If your restaurant serves salad, seafood sauteed in olive oil and serves olive oil to customers instead of butter, suggest the different types of olive oil you would recommend for purchase (and which types would be used for which foods).
   b. Explain to your customers why olive oil is considered to be so healthy.
4. Eggs have gotten a bad rap. Some of your customers are requesting yolk-less meals:
   a. Suggest five breakfast entrees that do not need egg yolks.
   b. Suggest five dessert items that minimize the use of egg yolks.
   c. Explain to your customers the good news about egg yolks, when used in moderation.

References

Bonna, K. H., (1992). "Habitual Fish Consumption, Plasma Phospholipid Fatty Acids, and Serum Lipids," *Archives of Internal Medicine*, January, 55:1, 1126–1134.

"Fish Oil Supplements" (1990). *FDA Consumer,* October, p. 30.

Kenney, J. (2000). "Cholesterol and Osteoporosis," *Communicating Food for Health*, May, 10:5, p. 60.

Kenney, J. (2001). "Coffee and Heart Disease," *Communicating Food for Health*, February, 10:2, p. 24.

LaBell, F. (2001). "Nuts about Nutrition," *Prepared Foods*, March 20: 3, pp. 69–70.

Margen, S., and Ogar, D. (2000). "Olive Oil: It's' Good But Not Miraculous." *Los Angeles Times*, December 11, p. S5.

Margen, S., & Ogar, D. (2001). "The Skinny on Fats, Both Good and Bad," *Los Angeles Times*, January 15, p. S3

"Obesity and Diabetes Increasing at Alarming Rates" (2001). *Patient Care*, April 15, 25:4. p. 9.

(No One Will Believe It's Low Fat) Custard Pie
(Yield: 2 nine-inch pies or 12 individual tarts)

Ingredients

1 quart low fat milk
6 ounces egg whites with egg shade or egg substitute
8 ounces sugar
2 teaspoons vanilla
½ teaspoon lemon zest
½ teaspoon nutmeg
2 teaspoons applesauce
2 nine-inch baked pie crusts or 12 individual baked tart shells

Method

1. Scald milk over double-boiler or in a small steam-jacketed kettle.
2. Mix all dry ingredients (except zest) together and stir slowly into milk.
3. Constantly stirring, add remaining ingredients. When all ingredients are added, stir and heat for 2 minutes.
4. Remove from heat and pour into baked tart shells or graham cracker crusts.
5. Refrigerate until firm, approximately 2 hours.
6. Garnish with fresh, frozen or canned fruit slices, such as strawberries or peaches, or with burnt sugar.

Nutritional analysis: 216 calories per serving, 10 grams protein, 2 grams fat, 5 milligrams cholesterol, 43 grams carbohydrates, 140 milligrams sodium, no dietary fiber.

Lemon without the Yolk Pie Filling
(Yield: filling for 1 nine-inch pie shell)

Ingredients

8 ounces egg whites with egg shade or egg substitute
8 ounces sugar
12 ounces hot water
3 ounces lemon juice
2 tablespoons fresh lemon zest
1 nine-inch pie shell, baked and cooled

Method

1. Combine egg substitute and sugar in double-boiler; stir until completely blended.
2. Add water, juice and zest and stir continually until mixture is thick and smooth.
3. Pour into pie shell.
4. Refrigerate to set, at least 2 hours.
5. Garnish with grilled pineapple slices

Nutritional analysis: 189 calories per serving, 8 grams protein, 2 grams fat, 2 milligrams cholesterol, 40 grams carbohydrates, 236 milligrams calcium, 110 milligrams sodium, no dietary fiber.

Chapter 6

Protein

Chapter Overview

Nitrogen in Protein
The Burger or the Sprouts
Body's Need for Protein
Uses of Protein in the Body
Amino Acids
Protein Digestion
Protein Myths
Populations With Special Protein Needs
Seniors
Cystic Fibrosis
Gluten Intolerance
Vegetarians
Different Types of Vegetarians
How to Design Menus
Calculating Protein Needs
Consequences of Too Much/Too Little Protein
Selecting High-Quality Protein
High-Protein, High-Fat, Low-Carbohydrate Diets
Putting it all Together
FYI: Vegetarian and Beyond

Chapter Objectives

After reading this chapter, the student should be able to:

1. *List some historical health claims made about protein.*
2. *Calculate personal daily protein needs.*
3. *Explain protein's role in the body.*
4. *Detail the consequences of too little or too much protein in the diet.*
5. *Suggest how to design menus that contain high-quality protein.*
6. *Define the various types of vegetarians, including how protein adequacy is met.*
7. *Convert an omnivore menu to a vegetarian menu.*
8. *Explain the need for amino acids and how to obtain them from the diet.*
9. *Discuss the rationale given for low-carbohydrate, high-protein diets.*
10. *List reasons to avoid protein supplements.*

Introduction

Protein *is that mysterious nutrient that people claim will provide rippling biceps, beautiful hair, strong fingernails, and smooth skin. Protein is added to shampoos, hand lotions, sports drinks, and snack foods. Whatever the claim, protein is one of nature's prime inventions.*

In this chapter, we will explore what protein is made of and how this make-up affects the way your skin looks and feels, why you do or don't get frequent colds and how you are doing in the muscle-tone area.

We'll look at normal protein needs and compare them to the needs of athletes and to those people who choose a weight reduction diet that is very high in protein. We'll examine the new trend toward less animal protein and the

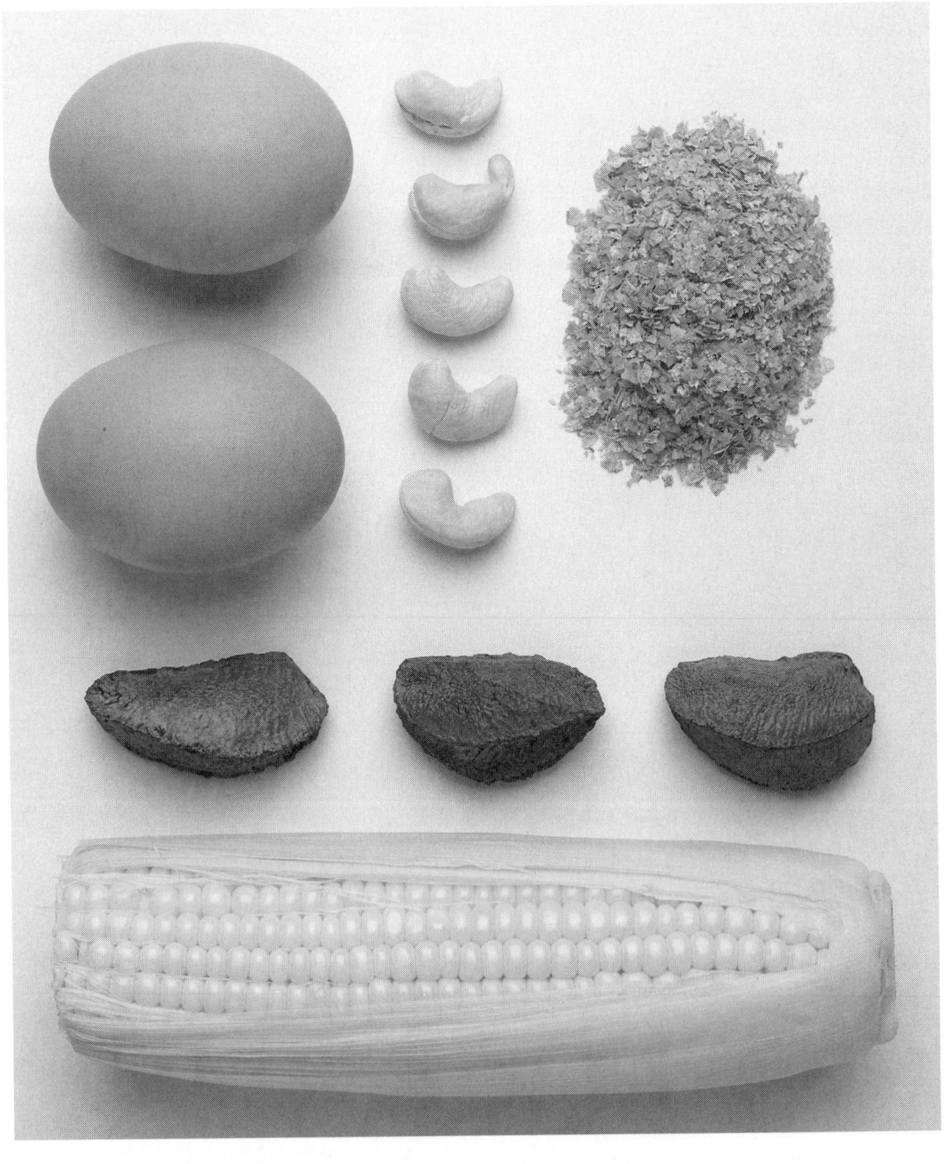

Protein comes in all shapes and sizes.

increasing popularity of vegetarian menus. This chapter will prepare you to enter the world of protein nutrition and to make informed decisions about your health, your diet and menu design.

NITROGEN IN PROTEIN

Protein differs from fats and carbohydrates in that it is the only calorie-containing nutrient with **nitrogen.** Whether from animals or plants, all proteins have four calories per gram and should be about 10 to 15 percent of your daily calories.

The Burger or the Sprouts

At any one time there are usually several best-selling diet plans that promise weight loss. Although they promise the same thing, these diet plans usually are very different. Just recently there were two top diet plans, both designed by MDs and both promising lots of weight loss. One was a strictly **vegan,** very-low-fat, low-protein, high-carbohydrate diet. The other was a high-protein (with ensuing high fat), no-carbohydrate diet. People lost weight on both plans.

So, which would you choose? The steamed veggie and brown rice platter or the all-you-can-eat cheeseburger (sans buns). Not too hard to figure out what the majority of people selected. However, it's not the immediate weight loss that should be questioned, but the ability to maintain weight loss. A good question to ask would be what types of health problems might result from following either of these diet plans.

We hope that you are wondering how someone can eat all the steaks, chops, cheese, eggs, and burgers they want and not suffer any health consequences. Good question!

Food and Amount	*Grams of Protein*
Grilled pork chop, 2 ounces	35
Grated parmesan cheese, 1 tablespoon	3
Cooked garbanzo or black beans, ¼ cup	4
Cooked pasta, 1 cup	7
Milk or yogurt, 1 cup	8
Egg, 1 large	6
Baked chicken, 2 ounces	30
Tofu, 3 ounces	7
Cheddar cheese, 1½ oz	11
Brown rice, 1 cup	5
Peanut butter, 2 tablespoons	8

Figure 6–1 Protein Content of Selected Foods

BODY'S NEED FOR PROTEIN

This brings us to this chapter's topic: protein. Protein is essential for sustaining life and keeping body systems in good repair. Too little protein can result in poor growth and healing, immune function problems, breathing difficulty, and even heart problems, such as dangerously low blood pressure or irregular heart rhythms. On the other hand, too much protein, eaten over long periods of time, can result in kidney disease, poor liver function and vitamin deficiencies and may play a role in some forms of heart disease and cancer. What's the answer? Balance!

USES OF PROTEIN IN THE BODY

Your body produces and uses thousands of proteins, each with its own job. Proteins are found in the internal organs, the muscles, and the skin, in the blood, and are part of the **immune system.**

Without protein, your body doesn't do very well as it lacks the building material necessary to keep you functioning correctly. Too much protein causes problems, too, as excess protein puts a strain on the liver and kidneys and may produce more toxic byproducts than the body can efficiently get rid of.

Let's do some protein science and then we can get back to our cheeseburger-orgy question.

Protein comes from the Greek word *protos,* meaning "of the utmost importance." Both animal and plant proteins are made mainly of protein and water. Protein provides the structure and carbohydrates and fats provide the energy. If the body doesn't get enough protein from the diet, than it starts to cannibalize itself, breaking down muscles and internal organs to obtain the protein it needs. The only organ ever spared is the brain. Survivors of long-term starvation have been found to have vital organs that have shrunk by one-quarter to one-third of their size. Even the heart was affected. The brain, however was always its full size. Smart instincts, preserving the body's control center.

AMINO ACIDS

Whole proteins are not exactly what the body is looking for. It's the **amino acids** that make up the protein chains that the body can use. Proteins are chains made from the twenty different amino acids contained in plant and animal protein.

Nine of the amino acids are **essential amino acids.** In nutrition, "essential" means the body's got to have it but is not capable of making it. Essential nutrients must be obtained from the diet. You can get essential amino acids two different ways: animal products or combining a couple of plant products. Animal proteins, such as meat, dairy, seafood, or eggs, contain all the essential amino acids. Plant proteins have some amino acids. Beans, legumes, nuts, and soy have one group of essential amino acids. Wheat, rice, and other grains have another group of essential amino acids. When you eat

Essential Tryptophan Valine Threonine Phenylalanine Lysine Leucine Methionine Isoleucine Histidine *Nonessential* (*denotes conditionally essential- research is still being done) Glutamine* Glycine Tyrosine* Serine Proline Glutamic Acid Cysteine* Aspartic Acid Arginine* Asparagine Alanine

Figure 6–2 Essential and Nonessential Amino Acids

one food from each group, such as rice and beans or peanut butter and bread, you get all the necessary essential amino acids from a combination of foods. We'll discuss the issue of combining plant foods to obtain protein a little later in the chapter when we discuss vegetarian eating patterns.

PROTEIN DIGESTION

A quick review of protein digestion. Protein digestion begins in the stomach. Hydrochloric acid and protein-specific enzymes are produced by the stomach with the aim to unravel protein strands and get at the amino acids. The protein strands are mostly unraveled in the stomach and completely unraveled in the small intestine. Remember active transport from Chapter 2? Active transport is how individual amino acids get across the walls of the small intestine and into the blood stream, where they can travel to where they are needed.

Protein is a very busy nutrient. Like a nice shape? **Collagen,** one type of protein, gives skin, hair, and bones their shape. Collagen is the most prevalent protein in our bodies, as we have lots of items that need to stay in the correct shape.

Keratin, a very tough, fibrous protein, is the protein that makes up a large portion of the hair and nails.

Less glamorous proteins take energy and turn it into physical work. Not energy, like what you get from carbohydrates and fats, but actually flexing and gripping and contractions that involve muscle action. Every time you type on a computer keyboard, climb stairs, lift weights, blink, or breathe, you need protein to fire the right muscle contractions.

Enzymes are made of proteins. Enzymes help to start reactions, such as jump-starting digestion, breaking down toxins or absorbing vitamins.

A NUTRI-BAR

Just in Case You Needed to Know

The next time you need some scintillating cocktail conversation, you can enthrall your audience by reciting the essential amino acids: histidine, isoleucine, leucine, lysine, methionine, phenylalaine, threonine, tryptophan, and valine.

Web Site	*Comment*
www.talksoy.com	United Soybean Board, information on soy products, health and nutrition research
www.cdrf.com	California Dairy Research Foundation has information on the use and health value of dairy products
www.aeb.org	American Egg Board has information on egg protein nutrition and use
www.calpoly.edu/~dptc	California Polytechnic State University's Dairy Products Technology Center
www.ag.uiuc.edu/~stratsoy/new/wecom.html	University of Illinois, Urbana-Champaign's soybean center
www.porkcouncil.com	National Pork Council
www.beefcommission.org	National Beef Commission

Figure 6–3 Express Protein

Hormones are also made of protein. Hormones are your internal busybodies, sending and delivering messages as needed to ensure the smooth running of your fuel-efficient system. For example, insulin is a hormone that tells the body how to handle glucose in the blood, as we've discussed in Chapter 4. Thyroxin is the hormone that tells the thyroid how to handle your metabolism. Hormones tell children how much to grow and adults how many hours to sleep or how much to eat.

If you're not eating enough protein, then you're not doing your immune system any favors. Antibodies are specific proteins found in the blood that attack and neutralize viruses, fungi and bacteria and anything else that doesn't belong in your system. Your white blood cells, lymph fluid, and antibodies are all necessary for a well-functioning immune system and rely on protein as their building material.

Protein tells your circulatory system how much fluid to keep and how much to discard. In this way, your body has the correct fluid balance, which means your tissues get nourished correctly and your heart can pump at a normal rate. If there is too little protein in the diet, then the body cannot maintain correct fluid levels. If fluid levels are incorrect, fluid tends to flow out of the veins and arteries and into the surrounding tissue, causing **edema.** Edema is uncomfortable, resulting in swelling and pressure. Edema can cause blood pressure to rise and can cause damage to joints and muscles.

Another aspect of correct fluid balance is the maintenance of correct acid levels in the body. Protein also assists in this. At any time, you have a balance of acid and alkaline in your body fluids, your lungs, and your muscles. If there is the right amount of fluid, then the amount of acid in the blood and other body fluids are diluted correctly and everything works as it should. If the blood becomes too acidic, it can affect the entire body. Incorrect acid levels can lead to coma, shock or death.

Protein is a real workhorse. It seems like it has its own muscles to help out. Proteins carry lipids, vitamins and minerals around the body in the blood. If you don't have enough protein, then the body doesn't get nourished correctly, as there are no delivery people around to bring what's needed to where it's needed. Protein also helps to transport toxins from used-up nutrients away from the muscles and organs. If there is a protein deficiency, then you can have a build up of toxins.

Your body much prefers carbohydrates and fat for energy, but will use protein in a pinch. Converting protein to energy is a clunky, inefficient mechanism. It's not a pretty process. The body can start to break down it owns muscles for energy if there are no other sources of energy available. This happens in cases of extreme starvation.

PROTEIN MYTHS

For as long as people have been eating protein-containing foods, there have been myths about its "magical" qualities. Here is some information about some of the more popular protein legends:

1. Protein-enhanced shampoos and lotions will help to strengthen my hair and fingernails.

No way: The portion of your hair and nails that you can see are already past saving. They are basically dead tissue, waiting to be discarded. The portion of your hair and nails you can't see, the stuff that starts right below the skin, is what needs nourishing. That comes from a balanced diet and lots of fluids. Soak and condition to your heart's content. If you don't have a good diet, your hair and nails will never look healthy.

2. If I want to "bulk up" my muscles, I need protein or amino acid powders.

Have you been listening? All proteins are made from amino acids. Most people eat too much protein. One cheeseburger gives you about 30 percent of your protein needs for the day. Throw in some grilled chicken, a cheese pizza, tuna salad, or a beef burrito, and you've got all the protein your body can handle for the day. Not only are they expensive, protein powders can cause liver and kidney overload. Have a peanut butter sandwich and save your money.

3. Lots of people are having collagen injections to give them plumper, more kissable lips. That collagen is from an inert plant source, right?

Wrong! Collagen is a type of animal protein that helps to keep muscles in shape. Most plastic surgeries involve animal (usually pork or beef) collagen that has been pasteurized to prevent cross contamination. Collagen injections don't last, as the collagen is slowly absorbed into your system just like any other kind of protein.

4. Some people take insulin by mouth and others have to inject it.

Insulin is a hormone, made of protein. Medical-grade insulin is recovered from human cadavers and from pork. If you actually ingested (swallowed) insulin, your body would digest it, just like any other kind of protein. You'd get no medical benefit from it, as your body would treat it just like egg or meat protein. Insulin is injected to bypass digestion so it can be directly absorbed into the blood stream and used by the cells to metabolize glucose. As described in Chapter 4, some people take a medication that can jump-start their pancreas. This medication is sometimes mistaken for insulin, which it is not.

As we've previously mentioned, protein digestion is centered in the stomach. Enzymes (which are protein!) and gastric acid work to break protein down into amino acids. To illustrate this mechanism for yourself, make some gelatin, any flavor and let it gel. Now place a piece of fresh pineapple (canned won't work because the heating inactivates the acid and enzymes) on one portion of the gelatin and some fresh papaya on another portion. Watch the gelatin slowly get digested. This is the same thing that happens to meat, cheese, beans, and eggs in your stomach, although there's a little more churning and activity in your stomach.

POPULATIONS WITH SPECIAL PROTEIN NEEDS

Some people have difficulty with protein digestion. As you get older, you secrete less of the acid and enzymes needed to break down proteins. Antacids also affect how you digest protein, since the job of an antacid is to suppress the amount of acid the stomach secretes.

Seniors

Some older people get into a real Catch-twenty-two. If they eat a meal with a lot of protein, they get a stomachache because they lack some of the chemicals to digest the protein. They take an antacid to relieve the stomachache and wind up being able to digest even less protein as their hydrochloric acid production is suppressed. The answer to this conundrum? Eat several small meals with a small amount of protein rather than one big meal with lots of protein.

Cystic Fibrosis

People with cystic fibrosis lack some of the enzymes needed to digest protein. This is a dilemma, as cystic fibrosis patients have an increased energy need. Cystic fibrosis patients often have to plan high-carbohydrate, high-fat, low-protein menus.

Gluten Intolerance

In Chapter 4, we mentioned **gluten intolerance.** Gluten is the protein found in wheat and wheat products, like bread, baked goods, and pasta. If someone with gluten intolerance eats wheat protein, they can be chronically fatigued, have intestinal damage and malabsorption syndrome. **Seitan** is a popular vegetarian ingredient made from wheat gluten. Seitan has a chewy texture and can be grilled like beef as "steaks" or slices of "roast." Seitan is commercially sold in smoked, barbecued, and herb flavors. Some people assume that seitan is made from soy, just like tofu. Being even more detective like, tempeh, another chewy, entrée-like vegetarian ingredient is made from soy but can have flour or wheat added to it for flavoring. Reading food labels is going to become one of your new hobbies.

Vegetarians

When you talk about protein, you usually include a discussion about vegetarians, since vegetarians exclude some or all types of animal products. Many non-vegetarians can't imagine how one can get sufficient amounts of protein without animal products. Nowadays, more and more people are becoming vegetarian, semi-vegetarian, or just attempting to cut back on animal protein consumption. You better bone up on your vegetarian knowledge.

What really is acceptable to various types of vegetarians? It's always helpful to know the players if you're the one responsible for the scorecard. The following is an introduction to some of the philosophies to which some of your vegetarian customers may subscribe. Vegans and vegetarians are the major categories you'll probably find.

Different Types of Vegetarians

Consider the word "vegetarian." It has several meanings. "Vegetarian" can be the umbrella term for all people who exclude some or all animal products from their diet (as in vegans, fruitarians, etc.). It is also the term used by people who used to be categorized as "lacto-ovo" vegetarians.

Let's clarify that. "Lacto-" means dairy and "ovo-" means eggs. **Lacto-ovo vegetarians** exclude animals from their diet, but include animal products, such as cheese, sour cream, and yogurt made from cow, goat, or any other kind of animal milk. Lacto-ovo vegetarians will accept animal products that they perceive do not harm or make an animal suffer. For many years, people, when asked what type of vegetarian they were, would respond "lacto-ovo."

In the past several years, the "lacto-ovo" has been dropped and vegetarians—formerly known as lacto-ovo—are now known simply as "vegetarians."

To reiterate, then, a "vegetarian" can be a lacto-ovo vegetarian or can be one of any type of vegetarian. Depending on the situation, it is important to clarify. When asked to write a "vegetarian menu," for a group of people with whom you are unfamiliar, you need to ask, "Will we be including or excluding dairy?" Their answer will tell you how to proceed.

What is this word vegan, anyway? It was coined by a British vegetarian group, who pronounces it "vee-gan" (rhymes with "can"). Vegans are understood to exclude meat, fish, poultry, eggs, dairy and honey from their diets and fur, wool, leather and animal-tested products from their life.

Why do vegans not include dairy or eggs in their diet? After all, the animals are not killed to obtain them, you say. Many vegans will tell you that just because an animal is not killed doesn't mean it doesn't suffer. Most vegans are dedicated to animal rights, which would include forcing animals to produce food and be "shackled" in miserable conditions. Vegans may also point out that not only do food-producing animals suffer, thus harming them, but the genetic engineering, hormones, chemicals, and diseases of animals raised in close quarters could also harm you. And that's as politically vegan as we're going to get.

When people speak about "vegan nutrition issues," they are usually speaking about the amount of protein found in a vegan diet. Up until several years ago, protein planning or protein combining was thought to be essential. The two-minute explanation of this is as follows: essential amino acids, found in proteins, are necessary for growth and repair of tissues and muscles, for the formation and maintenance of a healthy immune system, etc. Animal proteins contain all the essential amino acids while plant proteins each contain some of them. It was thought that you conscientiously had to combine plant foods, such as rice and beans or lentils and pasta, in order to guarantee the intake of complete proteins. We now know that as long as you eat lots of different foods each day, by hook or by crook, you'll have the proper protein intake. Just as omnivores (people who include every type of food product in their diet) can follow the Food Guide Pyramid without eating specifically calculated foods, so can vegans, as long as they are eating a varied, well-balanced nutritious diet. So, vegans shouldn't live just on apples and broccoli—throw in some soymilk, humus, or a bean burrito, too. By the way, soy is an almost-complete protein food. Soymilk, edamame (fresh soybeans), tofu, or soy burgers can add a lot of fast protein to the diet.

Any type of vegetarian will choose the vegetarian lifestyle for any number of reasons. We have heard for health reasons, religious reasons, ethical reasons, environmental reasons, "it's the way I was brought up, and I'm used to it" reasons, and economic reasons, to name a few. Some people remain vegetarian their entire life, some are vegetarian for long periods of time, returning after brief "omnivore" sojourns and some people are "semi-vegetarian," coming and going on the vegetarian lifestyle.

Please remember that there are all different levels of each type of vegetarian. Some lacto-ovo vegetarians may eat dairy and eggs, but not wear leather or use animal-tested products. Some lacto-ovo vegetarians may only eat dairy, some may only eat eggs. Some vegetarians may exclude leather or animal testing from their lives but attend a horse race. Everyone does what he or she thinks is right.

You should be ready to do a lot of label reading if you are going to offer vegetarian menus. You will have to decide if you will offer only vegetarian (lacto-ovo), only vegan or combinations.

Processed foods contain animal protein in many forms. Whether cutting back on animal protein for health reasons or vegetarian reasons, you have to become a junior scientist when it comes to label reading. For example, **rennet,** also called "enzymes" on many labels, is what takes milk and turns it into the solid curd known as "cheese." Vegetarians are okay with eating milk but do not want to ingest animal rennet. Animal rennet is a natural enzyme found in animal stomachs. So, to get animal rennet, the animal must be killed. There are synthetic enzymes that are fine for vegetarians and vegans. You have to read the label and do some investigation, because some manufacturers merely list "enzymes." Unless you ask, you have no way of knowing the source of the enzymes.

How about the stuff that makes things gel? Gelatin and aspic are animal-derived, but agar and carrageenan, derived from sea vegetables, are plant-derived. They all form a gel, and are used as thickener, so you have to read the labels to see exactly what was used.

How to Design Menus

When it comes to designing menus, the easiest and simplest way to go is to start with vegan and then add non-vegan ingredients, rather than having to prepare four or five versions of the same thing. For example, you can prepare a Greek salad made with fresh greens, tomato wedges, sliced red onions, black olives, diced green bell pepper and herbed croutons with a rosemary vinaigrette. It's vegan and everyone can have it. You can offer Feta cheese on the side for vegetarians, and anchovies for omnivores (people who eat everything). This way you've prepared only one dish to which ingredients can be easily added, rather than preparing two or three different dishes. Apply the same principle to lasagna (layers of pasta, sliced zucchini, tomatoes, mushrooms, red onions, eggplant, and spinach with tomato sauce) or to burritos (black-bean and brown-rice filling). Menus are easily adaptable for lacto-ovo. Four-cheese lasagna, ravioli, or tortellini; pastas with cream or cheese sauces; pizzas with cheese and other toppings; macaroni and cheese; cream soups; quiche; frittatas; omelets and egg salads; baked potatoes topped with sour cream; and vegetables with hollandaise sauce are all examples of vegetarian items. Commercially prepared mayonnaise and salad dressings, which may contain eggs or cheese, can be used. A breakfast menu could be a sautéed vegetable omelet with a bagel and cream cheese, lunch could be a vegetable quiche and a cream of broccoli soup and dinner could be baked eggplant with a yogurt and tomato sauce. Desserts could include puddings, ice cream, custards, and baked items topped with whipped cream or butter cream icing.

To adapt the same recipes for vegan, you'll have to look at your budget and do some product tasting to use soy- or grain-based cheese, cream cheese, and sour cream. Tofu can be used in place of eggs in some dishes, but you'll have to experiment to perfect this technique.

CALCULATING PROTEIN NEEDS

Vegetarian or omnivore, what's the correct amount of protein? In calories, 10 to 15 percent of your daily intake should come from protein. If you want to work out exact amounts, healthy adults need about 0.8 grams of protein per kilogram of body weight. Use this formula:

1. Convert pounds of weight to kilograms (pounds ÷ 2.2)
2. Multiply kilograms by 0.8 This equals the protein RDA (in grams) for a healthy adult. If you'd like to convert this to ounces, there are 28 grams in 1 ounce.

What's the buzz? Although still high in fat (unless you select a low fat soymilk or tofu), soy products are very low in saturated fats. Soy's proteins and isoflavones (natural plant estrogens) are thought to reduce cholesterol, reduce the risk of heart disease and ease symptoms of menopause. Conveniently, The United States is one of the world's largest growers of soybeans (although close to 75% of the crop is exported or used for animal feed).

Tofu is probably the most familiar soy product. Nothing more than coagulated soymilk (think: cheese making), tofu is available in different firmness and flavors. Silken tofu is custard-like and can be the "cream" in pies, soups, custards and sauces. Soft tofu blends well and can be used instead of dairy in smoothies, salad dressings and dips. Firm and extra firm tofu are toughies and can be marinated, chopped, diced sautéed, baked. You get the idea.

Tofu has a neutral flavor so it will take on whatever personality you give it. Marinate tofu in fresh or dried herbs, salad dressings, vinegars, barbecue sauce, chili sauce, etc. If you need a really firm tofu, such as for grilling or roasting, you can drain blocks of tofu. Place tofu between weights, like several china dinner plates, and allow to drain for several hours. This will condense and compress the tofu and works well for tofu "steaks," fajita strips and barbecued tofu sandwiches.

There are commercially available flavored tofus, both sweet and savory. Try almond-flavored tofu for dessert items, and barbecue, Southwestern, Mediterranean and Asian flavored for entrees.

Freezing is okay for tofu and makes it chewier in texture. Drain tofu and slice before freezing. To use frozen tofu, let it thaw in the frig, squeeze out excess fluid and marinate or cook.

Soymilk is available in several flavors and fat levels. Soymilk is naturally high in protein but low in calcium, Vitamins A, D, and B_{12}. If nutrition is a concern, look for fortified brands. Look in the store for vanilla, almond, mocha and chocolate soymilk.

There is life beyond tofu. Tempeh is a firm cake of pressed, fermented soybeans, sometimes mixed with grains, such as rice or wheat. Tempeh's mild, smoky flavor and chewy texture works well in chili, casseroles, stir frys and hot sandwiches. Tempeh is sold in blocks and is usually available in various flavors. Soy nuts are roasted soybeans and have a nutty, peanut flavor. Use them in Thai dishes, as salad toppings and as an ingredient in baking and trial mixes. Soy cheese and yogurt can be used just like their dairy cousins. Soy cheese is available in various types, such as mozzarella and cheddar. Soy yogurt is generally available as a sweetened, fruit flavored product. Use it as is, in sauces or freeze it for a fast dessert. Frozen soy milk (also rice milk) is the soy equivalent of ice cream and is available in many flavors and forms (sandwiches, popsicles, etc). Meat analogs, such as tofu dogs, burgers, crumbles, breakfast strips, "fake" sandwich meat are generally made from soy protein and are designed to mimic their animal counterparts. Experiment with different brands to find the type that have the flavor and texture acceptable for your customers. For example, several brands of soy burgers must be fried to be palatable, which may defeat the purpose of your healthy offering.

Figure 6–4 Soy 101

Although not a soy product, seitan is a popular vegetarian meat substitute. Originally processed by Buddhist monks, seitan is in wide nationally and international production. Seitan is compressed, fermented gluten (wheat protein). It is available in blocks, strips and crumbles and can be frozen until ready to use. Seitan has a very firm texture and will hold up to poaching, roasting, grilling and baking. Serve it as a "steak" (marinated in lemon or limejuice, garlic and onions) or add it where you would use beef or chicken strips. There are commercially available meat analogs made with seitan, some in the shape of roasts, which can be flavored and served just like roast beef.

Soy products have been around for the last two thousand years or so—definitely not a fad! Incorporate them into your menus for health and interest.

SOY INSTEAD

Instead of:	*Soy Sub:*
8 ounces ricotta cheese	8 ounces mashed firm tofu or 5 ounces okara
8 ounces milk	8 ounces soy or rice milk
8 ounces yogurt	8 ounces blended silken tofu or soy yogurt
1 large egg	2 Tablespoons blended firm tofu
1 ounce baking chocolate (has dairy)	3 ounces unsweetened cocoa powder and 1 Tablespoon soy oil
1 pound ground beef (for burritos, meat sauce, etc)	1 pound diced firm tofu, 12 ounces crumbled seitan or tempeh (marinate for extra flavor before cooking)

SOY SUGGESTIONS

Tempeh: marinate in Italian dressing or barbecue sauce and grill or dice and mix into soups or chilies, slice and grill and serve as a "tempeh" dip sandwich

Soy Milk: use in place of regular milk in puddings, custards and sauces, make hot chocolate or coffee beverages, use in soups

Soy Crumbles: sauté, bake or grill with fresh or dry herbs and use as pizza toppings, in chili, in "beef" and mac casseroles or "meat" sauces, in tacos, with tofu as a "morning scramble."

Soft Tofu: use instead of ricotta cheese in stuffed shells and lasagna, make fruit smoothies, use in salad dressings, scramble instead of eggs (remember to season with pepper, hot sauce sautéed veggies, etc.)

Silken Tofu: use instead of mayo or sour cream in recipes, use to make pudding, pie fillings or custard, smooth out sauces (tofu Alfredo or primavera) or soups and make a frosting by blending a small amount of tofu with instant pudding mix

Firm Tofu: add to brochettes instead of meat, use in stir frys, cut in cubes to make an egg-less or chicken-less salad (toss with celery, onions, pickles, regular or vegetarian mayo), grill, roast (use the same seasonings as you do for meat) or bake with bread stuffing

Figure 6–4 Soy 101 *(cont.)*

Here are some fast (but not thorough) definitions for quick reference:

Vegans: do not eat meat, fish, poultry, dairy products, eggs, or any foods that contain these ingredients. They do no use leather products, fur, wool, honey, or any products which have been animal-tested.

Vegetarians: do not eat meat, fish, or poultry, but do eat dairy products and eggs. Vegetarians may vary on their stance about leather, honey, etc.

Fruitarians: vegans who also exclude the eating of any product which would kill off the plant (such as a carrot, which is the whole plant).

Raw Foodists: vegans who do not allow their foods to be heated over 118°F (feeling that the nutritive components of food are inactivated at higher temperatures).

Pescans: vegetarians who include fish and seafood in their diet (not very common).

Figure 6–5 Veggie Fast Guide

Protein needs can increase when you are growing during childhood, are building during pregnancy or weight training or when you are repairing, during an illness or recuperation from an injury.

You want to eat the correct amount of protein every day. As we've said before, both too much and too little protein can cause problems. Too little protein can lead to permanent learning impairment in children. It can damage the heart, brain, and other organs in adults, as seen in starvation or anorexia.

Veggie Appetizers: use the following suggestions to create an elegant statement with passed hors d'oeurves or as a light dinner buffet

COLD: cold tortellini or mini- ravioli stuffed with mushroom, herbed cheeses, grilled vegetables, and spicy tomatoes served with tomato-basil or harissa (Moroccan pepper sauce) dipping sauces. Mini-bruschetta topped with sautéed mushrooms, onions, and tomatoes, garnished with fresh basil.

Stuffed mushrooms or cherry tomatoes (stuffings to include herbed rice or grilled vegetables) with a lemon-dill vinaigrette. Deviled eggs. Assorted crudities and breadsticks with flavored hummus, tapenade (chopped olive dip) and yogurt- and sour cream–based dips. Caponata (marinated eggplant combined with tomato puree, olives, and celery). Assorted marinated vegetables and olives.

HOT: Potato skins stuffed with chopped, seasonal vegetables, flavored mashed potatoes (try rosemary, horseradish, and garlic) and topped with yogurt-cucumber dressing. Grilled fruit and vegetable skewers (use various flavored marinades). Mini spring rolls (steamed rice paper wrappers) steamed and fried won ton and egg rolls stuffed with shredded fresh vegetables and herbs. Fried, breaded ravioli, and steamed gnocchi with tomato and cream-based dipping sauces. Vegetable (sweet potato, green bean, carrot, etc.) tempura with dipping sauces.

Figure 6–6 Vegetarian Catering Ideas

Many people eat too much protein. Over the long haul, you can cause kidney or liver damage by eating too much protein. Some vitamin needs are tied to the amount of protein you eat. This has to do with the items proteins need to be absorbed and used by the body. If you eat too much protein, you can be leading yourself into vitamin deficiencies.

> FOOD FOR THE MIND
> How Much Protein Is Enough?
> One method of measurement is the RDA, depending on your health status:
> The RDA for women (aged 19 to 24) is 46 grams of protein; for men the RDA is 58.

CONSEQUENCES OF TOO MUCH/TOO LITTLE PROTEIN

Too much protein puts a strain on the kidneys, as they have to get rid of all the end products of protein digestion. High protein intakes tell the body to get rid of minerals. The more protein you eat, the more bone calcium you lose, and no, you can't solve it by putting cheese on your burger. Animal protein is more acidic than plant protein and tends to make it easier for the body to dissolve and get rid of bone calcium.

Over the short haul, if you eat more protein than your body needs, you'll get fat. Excess calories from carbohydrates or protein are turned into fat by the body since fat is a more convenient form of storage. Excess protein will not result in larger muscles, stronger fingernails or thicker skin. It will result in more blubber where you don't want it.

So, you don't want to eat too much protein, but you do want to eat good quality protein. Lean beef, pork, poultry and seafood are good sources of protein, as are eggs, beans, nuts pasta, non- and low-fat dairy and soy products, such as soymilk, tofu or tempeh.

Some desserts can be simple, yet elegant, and some can be all-out!

Fresh berries with orange liqueur and mints—assorted fresh berries can be marinated in an orange, cassis, or honeydew liqueur and garnished with chopped fresh mint (or serve this over an orange or champagne sorbet, garnished with a cookie)

Sliced oranges with dates and nuts—peel and slice oranges or tangerines, plate and garnish with halved dates and chopped nuts

Grapes, grapefruit, and orange juice concentrate—marinate grapes and pink grapefruit in orange juice concentrate. Plate and serve with a selection of cookies or biscotti

Poached pears—pears can be poached in dessert wine, cinnamon, and clove-spiked apple cider or simple syrup and served with chocolate sauce or strawberry puree

Baked apples—flavor with ginger, cloves, mace, cinnamon, and nutmeg and serve alone or "a la mode"—create an apple-cinnamon or pumpkin pie sorbet

Lemon sorbet with biscotti

Soy or rice ice cream—serve with fruit syrups, fruit preserves or chopped berries and nuts

Fruit pies—make the crust without lard or butter and top with flavored nondairy topping

Figure 6–7 Desserts Without Dairy or Eggs

Carnivore	*Instead of*	*Try*
Sweet potatoes	butter, cream, marshmallows	margarine, silken tofu, chopped fruit and nuts
Mashed potatoes	butter, milk	margarine, soy milk, vegetable stock
Cooked veggies	butter	margarine, flavored oils, vegetable stocks, herbs
Stuffing	meat and meat stock	chopped veggies and nuts, veggie stock, fruit juices, corn, dried fruit, chopped nuts
Pie crust	lard or butter	margarine, vegetable shortening or oil
Salad dressing	cheese, mayo	oil- and vinegar-based dressings
Gravy	meat and meat stock	vegetable stock or broth to create onion and mushroom gravy, cranberry and dried fruit sauce

Figure 6–8 From Carnivore to All-I-vore with Vegetarian Holiday Menus

SELECTING HIGH-QUALITY PROTEINS

So, why do you have to eat more plant foods to get lots of protein? You've probably noticed that a portion of grilled chicken is about three ounces of meat, whereas a bowl of beans and rice can be about twelve or fourteen ounces. Four ounces of broiled beef has about forty-seven grams of protein, four ounces of tofu has ten grams, four ounces of cooked beans (like lentils or kidney beans) have nine grams, two Tablespoons of peanut butter have eight and, four ounces of pasta has five grams. You get the idea. Plant protein is less

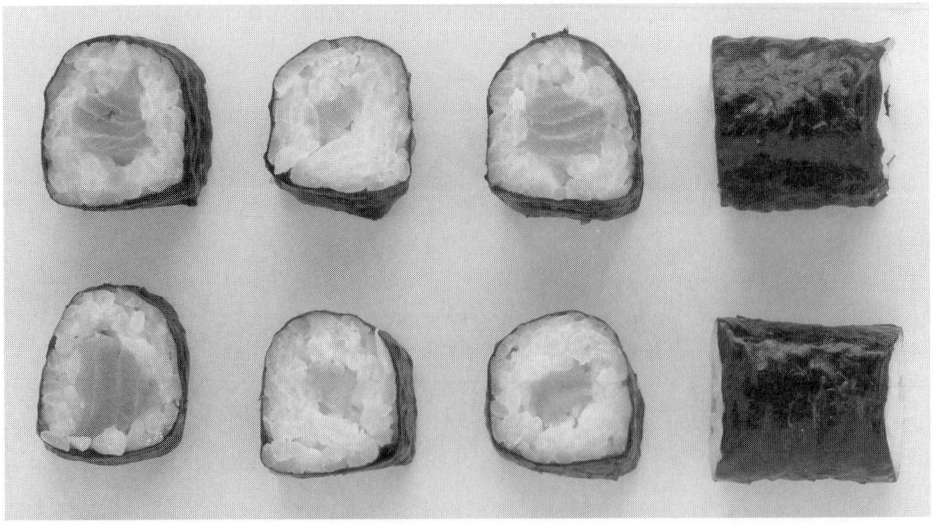

High-quality protein can come in a variety of packages.

High-quality protein can come in a variety of packages.

concentrated than animal protein. There is less concern about eating too much plant protein, as the plant foods that contain protein are generally low in fat and sodium and high in fiber. And, we might note, are usually less costly, which could be an important consideration. Animal protein can be attached to a lot of fat, as in steaks, burgers and sausage. As you know, excess calories from animal fat and protein can lead to obesity, hypertension, and some forms of heart disease and may increase the chances of developing some types of cancer.

HIGH-PROTEIN, HIGH-FAT, LOW-CARBOHYDRATE DIETS

We hope you have been intrigued by the burger diet question that we introduced at the beginning of the chapter. People who advocate low-carbohydrate, high-protein diets claim that carbohydrates raise blood sugar levels to unacceptable heights and create insulin "insensitivity." If body cells become insensitive to insulin, they cannot process glucose the way it should be. The belief is that if the body cannot process glucose, then it will store it as excess energy. Excess energy translates into excess fat. It's claimed that although carbohydrates cause blood sugars to rise, animal fat and protein do not. You are supposed to make the assumption that eating animal fat and protein will not cause the body to store fat, but carbohydrates will. Therefore, a diet high in meat and cheese will keep you lean, while a diet of pasta and fruit

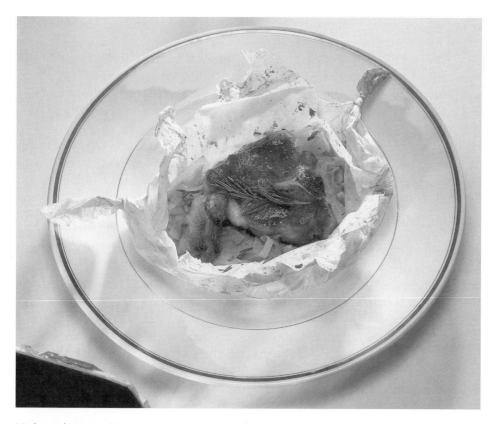

will make you store excess fat. Or, at least, that's the premise of the no-carbs, lots of meat and cheese advocates.

A kernel of truth is sometimes a dangerous thing. While it is true that excess carbohydrates are translated into fat by the body, so are excess protein and fat calories. It is harder for the body to derive energy from protein and fat. If you deprive the body of carbohydrates, it will have to work harder to get its energy from protein and fat.

There are problems with forcing the body to use inefficient fuel. Depending on your health and genetic propensities, you could develop an extremely high cholesterol level in your blood, which could lead to high blood pressure and heart disease. Your kidneys could become overtaxed and damaged. Some people do not do well without carbohydrates. As their bodies burn protein and fat instead of carbohydrates, toxins start to amass in body tissues and blood sugar levels become unstable. This is called "ketoacidosis" and is a condition that occurs with poorly controlled diabetics. It can lead to organ failure over time. You've read discussions of the health problems associated with diets high in fat and protein. These problems don't go away because you're cutting out carbohydrates.

Another point is that all carbohydrates don't act the same. Whole grains, such as oats, barley, brown rice, beans, legumes, and starchy vegetables, such as sweet potatoes, yams, and corn cause blood sugar to rise very, very slowly. These types of carbohydrates contain lots of vitamins, minerals, and fiber, an important part of the diet. If a diet is full of these kinds of foods, there is little risk of insulin "sensitivity," as the carbohydrates are released so slowly into the system.

What's the answer? We will discuss high-protein, low-carbohydrate diets in more detail in Chapter 8. The best answer for a healthy diet is moderation and variety. Too much or too little of any nutrient is never a good idea.

So, after all this discussion, what type of protein should you include in your day-to-day menus? You'll have to determine the calorie amount according to the number of calories you are eating. For example, if you're eating about 1,800 calories per day, and protein calories are supposed to be about 10 to 15 percent of your intake, then you should figure about 180 to 200 calories of protein.

Here's some more help with protein selection. One ounce of skinless chicken breast is 35 calories, one ounce of a turkey drumstick is 55 calories, one large egg is about 75 calories and 1 ounce of link sausage is 100 calories. These are all protein foods. They differ in the amount of fat they have. So, for 200 calories of protein, you can have about 5 ounces of chicken breast, 3.5 ounces of turkey leg, about 2 eggs or 2 link sausage. Remember, you're also getting fat with your protein.

Lean sources of protein foods are nonfat dairy products, like skim milk and cheeses made from skim milk, such as skim-milk mozzarella. Beans and legumes are low fat and high protein. Very lean cuts or beef, pork, veal, and venison contain little fat. That's good for your body, but not so hot for your palate.

Fat contributes juiciness and tenderness to meat, so adapt cooking styles to compensate for the lack of fat. You can marinate meats in wine, vegetable juice, or chopped vegetables to restore some moisture.

Soy products, such as soymilk, tofu, and tempeh are healthy and high in protein, but can be high in fat. Select low- or no-fat versions of these products. Seafood, fish, and skinless poultry are also lean sources of protein.

Does this mean you or your customers must suffer with dry tasteless meals? No, just learn to cook! Cooked beans can be mashed, mixed with chopped peppers, chilies, tomatoes and onions and rolled in a tortilla for a breakfast burrito. Need more filling? Scramble seasoned egg whites or tofu for more protein or add roasted, chopped potatoes or herb steamed rice to take up space.

Pizza doesn't have to be high fat. Just adapt your taste a bit. Instead of extra cheese, use either low-fat mozzarella (you'll never taste the difference) or use less cheese. Pile the pizza high with sliced bell peppers and onions, chilies, mushrooms, and sliced tomatoes; give the pepperoni the night off.

If you're a real meat eater, see if you can cut down on the size of your portion. Select the leaner cuts of steak and skin poultry. See if a meaty type of fish, like swordfish, shark, or salmon, meets your taste needs, so you switch off from meat. Want to really go out on a limb? Grill a portobello mushroom or some marinated extra firm tofu instead of some meat. You'll be delighted with the texture and the taste (if you use your culinary skills to season them).

"Power" smoothies don't have to have a raw egg (blecch!) or protein powder. If you're drinking your breakfast, use nonfat milk or yogurt or tofu for

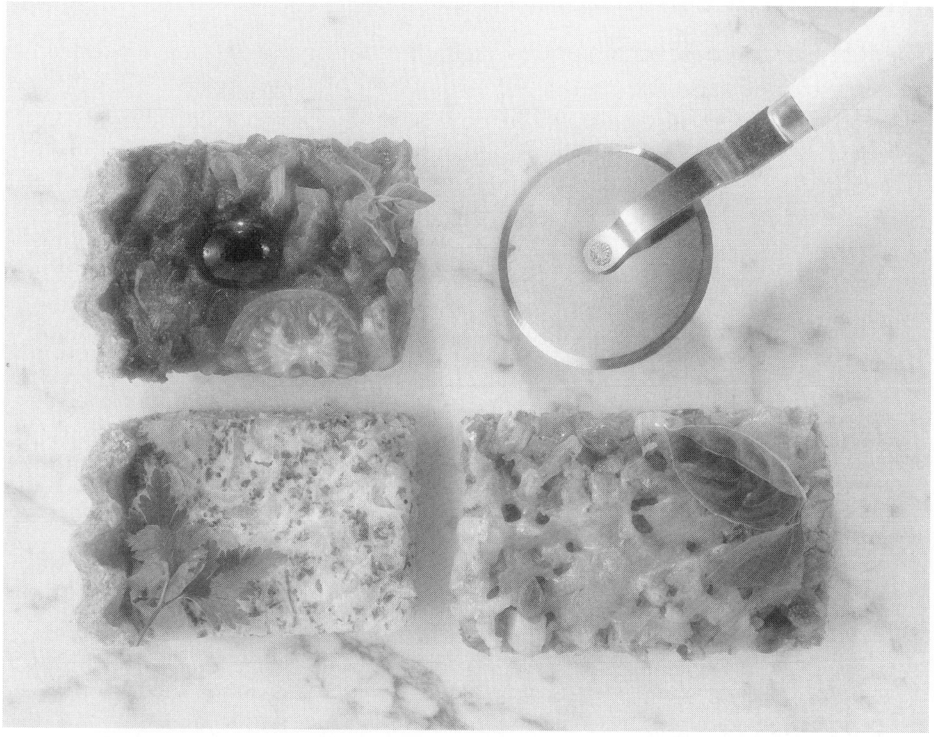

Flan nicoise, creamy onion flan, and scone pizza.

the protein portion of a fruit smoothie. Add bananas, strawberries, orange juice, fresh or frozen berries or peaches to create a filling grab and go meal.

What about the infamous double-bacon cheeseburger? Well, there's not a solution for everything. Have the burger in all its glory, knowing that it should be a once-a-month indulgence (yeah, right). Or convince yourself that a single cheeseburger will suffice. Reducing the number of calories from saturated fat is helpful in any amount. Veggie burgers and soy cheese may or may not be a viable option. Many veggie burgers are high in fat or have to be fried for an acceptable texture. Exchanging one set of calories for another is not a solution. See if you can handle the burger without the cheese or the bacon. Replace the flavor and the crunch with lots of lettuce, tomatoes, onions, sliced cucumbers, shredded carrots and fresh chilies. See what kind of creative solutions you can come up with.

PUTTING IT ALL TOGETHER

Protein is an essential part of life. High-quality protein can be obtained from animal or plant sources. Eating too much protein can result in damage to internal organs and vitamin deficiencies. Not eating enough protein can result in a depressed immune system, poor growth, and an inability to heal. Protein has many roles in the body that cannot be done by any other nutrient. Plant proteins can provide all the essential amino acids required, as long as thought is put into the menu. Lean proteins are low in fat, meaning that the food-service operator will have to use some culinary magic.

FYI: VEGETARIAN AND BEYOND

The Ritz Carlton hotel chain prides itself on meeting every guest's need. This certainly extends to their menu. According to corporate policy, if it's not on the menu, the food-service staff will do what they can to accommodate your

A NUTRI-BAR

Food Service Enters the "Zone"

Dr. Barry Sears's "Zone" diet is a high-protein, low-carbohydrate diet. At the peak of its popularity, there were Zone restaurants, Zone spas, and Zone grocery items.

Profits are important to employers. Healthy employees help to bring in the profits. Dr. Sears convinced several large manufacturers that offering free, healthy meals to employees at medical risk would improve their health and productivity more than just paying for their healthcare.

Diabetic, pre-diabetic, obese, and hypertensive employees were identified at three manufacturing plants. They were offered two "Zone" meals per workday and received nutritional counseling to assist in planning their home meals. Over a six-week period, many of the diabetics lost up to ten pounds. Lab values improved for many of the participants. Productivity among the participants improved an average 13 percent during their "Zone" period.

request. For example, if you want a lower-fat version of the fried chicken salad, they'll grill the chicken. If you prefer your salad vegetarian style, the chef will top it with grilled vegetables.

Many food-service operations are jumping on the vegetarian bandwagon. Vegetarian is not so difficult for appetizers, soups, accompaniment dishes, breads, or desserts. Upscale or restaurant-level entrees can sometime offer more of a challenge. Culinarians all over the country are rising to the occasion. Here are just some of their veggie entrée offerings (note that these are really daring, all being vegan without support of cheese or eggs):

Seeger's (Atlanta): Twenty-five different roasted vegetables with black truffle oil

Daniel (New York): Ivy Award winning chef Daniel Boulud offers a nine-herb ravioli with black trumpet mushrooms, chanterelles, and black truffles

Babb (New York): Carrot flan with pea vines and agnolotti pasta

Mary Elaine's at the Phoenician Resort (Scottsdale, Arizona): Terrine of Victory Farms petit vegetables with yellow tomato coulis and eggplant caviar

The Ryland Inn (Whitehall, NJ): Portobello "steak" au poivre with tempura green beans

KassBah Restaurant and Bar (West Hollywood, CA): Nobile mushroom fettuccine with chanterelle, porcini and morel mushrooms tossed in fennel and mushroom sauce

Naha (Chicago): Chilled white and green asparagus with salad of mache and charred tomato vinaigrette

In the year 2000, the American Culinary Federation's Culinary Team USA competed at the Caterplan World Culinary Grand Prix in Glasgow, Scotland. The team won four gold medals for international culinary excellence. Part of their award-winning three-course hot-food entry was a vegetarian platter of soy nut crusted seitan, sea vegetable, and six-grain sausage, stuffed onions with wheatberry pilaf, kale-wrapped smoked tofu, tofu cakes, and vegetables with carrot and orange jus.

It sounds as if you had better get ready to offer vegetarian entrees on the menu. Here are some ideas, tips, and pointers. Be sure you have a test run before serving any new items in a food-service operation or even for a holiday dinner at home. Most food professionals will tell you "three's a charm" when testing recipes. Try a new recipe three times, preferably on three different groups of people before adding it to your repertoire.

Vegetarian entrees are easily prepared from the ingredients that many food operations keep on hand. Pasta, rice, barley, couscous, beans and legumes, and potatoes can all form the base of vegetarian entrees. Nontraditional ingredients are available, such as tofu or seitan; you decide if you have the time to train your staff and educate your customers about them.

You can decide on the amount of time and money you have for your vegetarian effort. The easiest way (but probably the most costly) is to use convenience products. Veggie burgers are available frozen in a variety of flavors and are easy to prepare. Just substitute a veggie burger for a hamburger patty in patty melts or hamburger platters. Pile high the raw vegetables (sliced tomato, lettuce, onion, bell pepper, shredded carrot, etc.), and you have a quick entrée. A veggie burger can be substituted for a slice of meatloaf, Salisbury steak, Swiss steak, or country-fried steak. Taking it a step further, veggie burgers can be cooked and crumbled into tomato sauces (to make a vegetarian "meat" sauce), used as a filling for tacos, burritos, and omelets, used as a vegetarian pizza topping or used in casseroles (such as tamale, chili, or shepherd's pie) to replace ground meat.

Tofu dogs can be offered instead of regular hot dogs and can be grilled or steamed. Slice tofu dogs into casseroles or soups where you would normally use ham or other smoked meats. One hospital we visited was making a bagel-tofu dog for their pediatric patients. A bagel was toasted on the grill, the tofu dog was sliced length-wise and grilled and then cut to fit the bagel. The bagel was then wrapped in foil and heated in the oven for about 5 minutes. Served with relish, ketchup and mustard, it was a big hit. Vegetarians or those customers watching their cholesterol don't have to be left out of Oktoberfest. Purchase vegetarian sausage and steam with braised red cabbage flavored with caraway, sliced apples, cider vinegar and juniper berries. Soy chorizo is almost indistinguishable from the spicy beef or pork version in flavor and texture, although it is almost fat-free. Use soy chorizo in traditional Spanish, Portuguese, and Central American dishes.

Pasta is an easy way to go for vegetarian entrees. To make a pasta dish acceptable to both vegetarians and vegans (you don't want to have to prepare too many versions of the same dish), select pasta which does not contain eggs. Prepare a marinara sauce (flavorful tomato sauce with vegetables), add sautéed or steamed mushrooms, minced garlic and extra tomatoes, and serve over cooked pasta for a fast entrée. Or toss pasta with sauce, place in steam table pan, top with chopped tomatoes, bell peppers, and onions, cover and bake until hot for a quick vegetarian casserole. Additions to the tomato sauce can include chopped seasonal vegetables (such as summer squash, carrots and different varieties of mushrooms), cooked lentils or white beans, roasted garlic and fresh chopped herbs (try basil or oregano). For a color and flavor difference, use pesto sauce (basil or spinach pureed with pine nuts, olive oil, and garlic).

Beans and legumes are easy to prepare (use canned or dried) and versatile. Make a hearty four-bean soup (try kidney, navy, garbanzo, and black-eye peas), pair it with a baked potato (topped with chopped veggies and margarine), steamed rice or pasta salad and you have a fast vegetarian entrée. Or season red or black beans with onion, cumin, and pepper and serve on a steaming bed of white or brown rice. Cooked beans can be pureed and seasoned and used as a protein-rich sauce to top pasta, rice, or other cooked grains. Toss cooked beans into a rice pilaf for another fast entrée.

Baked potatoes can be topped with chopped fresh and cooked vegetables, cooked beans, salsa and butter, margarine, and dairy or soy cheeses. If you have the space, create a baked potato bar and let your customers create

Tofu's not just for stir fry anymore. Check out the Asian-influenced salads served at Asian-fusian restaurants in the Los Angeles area:

Mishima Restaurant: Tofu salad with chopped lettuce, tomatoes, seaweed, daikon sprouts and dried bonito with a dressing made of mayonnaise, seaweed paste, bonito broth, soy sauce, and rice vinegar.

Tai Yo Restaurant: Tofu on a bed of broccoli sprouts, baby greens, cucumbers, baby radish and green onions with a dressing of miso, ginger, soy sauce, garlic, and peanut oil.

Hirozen Restaurant: Layered tofu salad of julienned cucumbers, daikon radish. sliced tomatoes, shiitake mushrooms, radish sprouts and edible flowers with a dressing made of soy sauce, miso, sesame seeds, and hot peppers.

Zen Grill: Mixed baby greens and soft tofu are tossed with balsamic vinegar, soy sauce and citrus juice, sprinkled with dried seaweed, and a thick garlic-peanut sauce.

Kakemoto: Tofu with asparagus and tatsoi (water spinach) with a dressing made of ginger, miso, sweet rice wine, and slices of tofu drizzled with miso.

Figure 6–9 Do You Tofu?

Glutamine: never heard of it, you say? Ever heard of **MSG** or **monosodium glutamate**? MSG is a form of fermented soy, used as a flavor enhancer

Tryptophan: can't sleep? There's a method to Grandma's madness of warm milk before bedtime. Tryptophan is an amino acid found in dairy and poultry products. It is said to be a "natural soother." Maybe that's why everyone gets so sleepy after Thanksgiving dinner. Some people cut out the middle-man and purchase tryptophan supplements. This can be a dangerous practice, depending on the way the tryptophan is processed. Very little tryptophan is needed to produce the desired effect, so sticking with foods that contain this amino acid is probably the best bet.

Phenylalanine and aspartic acid: not expecting an amino acid with that diet soda? Ever heard of Equal™ or Nutrasweet™? Aspartame is an artificial sweetener used in diet sodas, pudding and gelatin mixes, sugar free candy and bakery items and frozen desserts. Unfortunately, there is a birth defect called "phenylketonuria" or PKU. People born with PKU must avoid the amino acid **phenylalanine,** as they lack the ability to digest it. Eating phenylalanine can cause mental retardation in children, along with kidney and liver damage in adults. Before aspartame, life was easy for PKU sufferers. They simply avoided protein-containing foods. Nowadays, they must read labels on anything that might have aspartame added as a flavoring agent. Don't believe us? Look at a can of diet soda. If it is sweetened with aspartame, then it has a warning on the label for PKU sufferers.

Figure 6–10 Amino Acids in the News

their own hot potato specialties. The same can be done with a pasta bar. Have several types of unsauced cooked pasta, several sauces (all without meat and at least one without dairy), and chopped fresh and cooked vegetables. Customers can then build their own entrees.

If you have the time to create vegetarian dishes, you may want to make your own veggie burgers with combinations of beans and grains. The same recipe can be used to form cutlets and loaves. Prepare this ahead of time, cook off and freeze to be used as needed. Tofu (pressed soy beans) is getting more popular on the market today. A fully cooked item, tofu is bland and takes on the flavor of the ingredients around it. For using in cooked entrees, select firm or extra-firm textures. Tofu is perishable and must be kept refrigerated (where it has a seven-day shelf life).

Tofu can be scrambled, just like eggs and used as an ingredient in stir-fries, casseroles, and in fillings for hot sandwiches. Just remember, tofu must be seasoned or it will come across as bland and boring. Tofu can be marinated and used as a substitute for eggs or meat. A school we visited was making a "turkeyless" tetrazini, using cubed tofu (which they had marinated in poultry seasoning) to replace the meat.

Incorporating vegetarian items into your menu is easy. Get familiar with vegetarian ingredients and start experimenting.

Nutri-Words

Amino acid: building block of protein.
Collagen: connective tissue.
Complementary proteins: combining of two plant foods, such as beans and rice, to form a protein that contains all the essential amino acids.
Edema: accumulation of fluid in the hands and feet or around body joints.
Essential amino acid: an amino acid that is mandatory for proper body functioning. Proteins containing all the essential amino acids can be found complete in animal-containing foods, such as meat or eggs. No one plant food contains all the amino acids.
Gluten intolerance: an inability to metabolize gluten, a wheat protein.
Immune system: the body system responsible for suppressing illness.
Lacto-ovo vegetarian: a vegetarian including animal products, such as dairy and eggs, in the diet.
Monosodium glutamate (MSG): a fermented soy product that contains the amino acid glutamate. Used as a flavor enhancer.
Nitrogen: an essential component found in protein.
Phenylalanine: an essential amino acid, found in some artificial sweetener. Some people are born with phenylketonuria, an inability to metabolize phenylalanine.
Protein: an energy-giving nutrient containing four calories per gram, used in the formation of muscle, skin, blood, tissue, hormones, enzymes, and immune system components.
Rennet: an enzyme used in cheese processing. May be isolated from animal stomachs or can be chemically synthesized.

Seitan: a protein food made from gluten.

Vegan: a vegetarian excluding animal and animal products from the diet.

Whaddaya think?

1. So, how's your daily diet—too much or too little protein?
2. What are the consequences of a long-term diet with too little protein? Too much protein?
3. How do you get your essential amino acids?
4. How does your vegan professor get essential amino acids?
5. What do you need to look for in an amino acid?
6. What has protein done for you lately?
7. What won't protein do for you?
8. Can you calculate exactly how much protein you need every day?
9. Modify this to be (a) lean (b) vegan: double-bacon cheeseburger with mayo and avocado, chili fries, and a chocolate milkshake.
10. Design a luxurious vegan banquet for a holiday get-together.

Critical Application Exercises

1. Play both sides: defend both low-protein diets and low-carbohydrate diets. In your defense, include chef suggestions for menu offerings.
2. The vegans are coming! Design a five-day vegan menu for the summer camp your hotel is hosting:
   a. You'll need breakfast and lunch for five days for fifty vegan teenagers.
   b. Be sure each meal includes complete proteins (has all the essential amino acids).
   c. Remember taste, flavor, and appearance.
3. Explain to the football player for whom you are private-chefing why taking protein supplements are unnecessary. In your explanation, include the types of foods that supply adequate protein and the result of overdoing protein.
4. Design a "meat-eaters" dinner menu that is deceptively healthy. Go small to moderate with protein portions, but include lots of window dressing. To really show your expertise, analyze the menu with the Exchange Lists for Meal Planning.

Flightless Tetrazini
(Yield: serves 10)

Ingredients

Vegetable oil spray as needed
1 pound mushrooms, sliced
6 ounces onions, chopped

4 ounces bell pepper, chopped
1 pound firm tofu, cubed
3 pounds pasta, cooked
1½ quarts prepared white sauce
6 ounces green peas, cooked
6 ounces carrots, diced, cooked

Method

1. In sauté pan, heat oil spray. Sauté mushrooms, onions and peppers until soft.
2. In a steam table pan, combine mushrooms, onions, peppers, tofu and pasta.
3. Toss with sauce, garnish with peas and carrots.
4. Bake at 325 degrees for 30 minutes or until golden brown and bubbly.

Notes: A vegan sauce can be made by using soymilk and margarine to replace cow's milk and butter. For extra garnish, use chopped red, green and yellow bell peppers.

Nutritional Analysis: 932 calories per serving, 12 grams protein, 24 grams fat, 0 milligrams cholesterol, 169 grams carbohydrates, 368 milligrams sodium, 8 grams dietary fiber.

Pumpkin Tofu Pie
(Yield: 2 nine-inch pies)

Ingredients

2 pounds silken tofu, drained
2 pounds canned pumpkin puree
3 ounces vegetable oil
2 teaspoons nutmeg
3 teaspoons cinnamon
1 teaspoon ground ginger
½ teaspoon ground cloves
½ teaspoon orange zest
2 nine-inch unbaked pie shells

Method

1. Combine all ingredients, except pie shells, in a blender and process until well combined.
2. Pour pumpkin mixture into pie shells and bake for one hour at 375 degrees (25 degrees lower for convection) or until knife inserted in center comes out clean.
3. Allow to cool on racks before cutting.

Serving Ideas

1. Make individual pies by using unbaked 3-inch tart shells. Garnish with candied orange peel or crystallized ginger, pineapple sauce, or soy or rice ice cream.

2. Create pumpkin custard by baking without the crust in individual serving dishes. Top custard with butterscotch or caramel sauce, thawed frozen berries, nondairy whipped topping flavored with vanilla and cinnamon or lemon or orange sorbet.
3. Bake these pies ahead of time—they will hold in the refrigerator for up to three days. Freezing, however, will yield a watery pie with a tough crust.
4. Make a pumpkin sorbet—prepare pie filling as listed above, but rather than baking, freeze in individual dishes.

Nutritional Analysis: 238 calories per serving, 8 grams protein, 17 grams fat, 0 grams cholesterol, 119 milligram calcium, 104 milligrams sodium, 2 grams fiber.

Chapter 7

Vitamins, Minerals and Water

Chapter Overview

Chapter Objectives

After reading this chapter, the student should be able to:

1. *Make informed decisions about including vitamins and minerals in the diet.*
2. *Define vitamin toxicity and explain how to avoid it.*
3. *Explain the difference between the properties of fat- and water-soluble vitamins.*
4. *List dietary sources for major and trace minerals.*
5. *Prepare an argument for obtaining vitamins via the diet versus through supplementation.*
6. *Suggest how to prepare food in a manner which retains maximum amounts of nutrients.*
7. *Define herb and botanical standardization and explain how it relates to the consumption of herbal preparations.*
8. *List dietary sources of water and explain how to avoid dehydration.*
9. *Explain how caffeine and alcohol may interfere with nutrient retention.*

Introduction

So, how many of you think a complete breakfast is a Flintstone™ and a cup of coffee? Or do you prefer to slurp your vitamins, stopping at your favorite smoothie stand for a cranberry–apricot–apple–bee pollen shake?

Over six billion dollars are spent in the United States every year on vitamins. Do we need them? Do we need to take them or can we just eat them. The answer is "yes and/or no," depending on the foods you choose.

OBTAINING VITAMINS AND MINERALS FROM FOOD

Dietitians and nutrition professionals will tell you that you can obtain all the vitamins and minerals you need from your diet. Certainly food contains all the vitamins and minerals that a person could need. The question is, are you up to the challenge? You know that if you try, you can eat five or more servings of fruits and vegetable per day, lots of whole grains and fiber-containing foods and a variety of protein foods, such as seafood, poultry, red meat, beans, legumes, and soy foods.

Lots of Things in One Package

Most foods have several vitamins and minerals, so you don't have to eat forty different foods every day. Milk, for example, contains calcium, magnesium, phosphorus, vitamin A, and vitamin D, among other nutrients. So that cup of yogurt you snagged on the run has a lot of things going for it.

Combine that yogurt with an orange, you've got some vitamin C, zinc, and phosphorus. Add some whole-wheat toast and you've got most of the B vitamins, such as folic acid, niacin, thiamin, and riboflavin and the mineral iron. See, getting your As and Bs isn't as hard as it looks.

Everything but Energy

Vitamins do not directly give energy, as they do not contain carbohydrates, proteins, or fats, which are the only sources of energy. Even though you can't get energy, or calories, directly from vitamins, vitamins help the body to use

A NUTRI-BAR

Multiple Multivitamins

Hopefully, your idea of a healthy breakfast is not a fruit-filled doughnut and a multivitamin. You know that most people can get all the vitamins and nutrients they need from the food they eat. "But," you say, "I don't have the time!" Consider this:

1. Most water-soluble vitamins produce only very expensive urine. Your body doesn't store water-soluble vitamins well, so excess just gets washed out.
2. If you take a calcium pill instead of a cup of yogurt, you miss out on the magnesium, phosphorus and vitamins A and D, not to mention the fluid. If you take vitamin C instead of an orange, you miss out on beta-carotene, calcium, fiber, and fluid. We're really not sure if the whole package of an orange helps you use vitamin C more efficiently, but we're pretty sure it works a lot better than just a pill with a single substance.
3. If you insist, do some research on maximum doses. Even water-soluble vitamins can cause problems. Fat-soluble vitamins can become toxic.
4. This is when you might have permission to use vitamin supplements, but only after discussing their use with a health-care professional:
   a. Iron-deficiency anemia—*only* with the doctor's okay. Too much iron can result in hemochromatosis (iron overload) which can cause heart arrhythmias.
   b. Pregnant or breast-feeding women are sometimes prescribed vitamin supplements because of their increased nutrient needs.
   c. If you might be prone to osteoporosis, because of family history, the use of certain medications or chronic disease.
   d. Some tentative research shows that people with family histories of colon cancer, heart disease, and prostate cancer may benefit from some vitamin E.
   e. Strict vegans who don't vary their diets or have small daily intakes.
   f. People who are chronic dieters (under 1,200 calories per day).
   g. People undergoing cancer therapy

energy. Properties in vitamins guide the way for the body to use energy in an effective way. If you are vitamin-deficient, you may not be able to utilize the energy you take in.

GENERAL PROPERTIES OF VITAMINS

Vitamins do help with lots of different activities in the body. Without vitamins, you could not grow, metabolize nutrients, utilize energy or maintain health. At press time, the RDAs have been established for 14 vitamins. This is changing all the time, as new functions for vitamins are discovered.

Vitamins are divided into water-soluble and fat-soluble categories. Today there are eight **water-soluble** B vitamins, Vitamin C and four **fat-soluble** vitamins A, D, E, and K that have been isolated and their properties scientifically tested (Rubin, 5).

People have always known that food was essential for life. They just didn't know what particular substances in foods made them important. There have been many food and nutrition theories over the centuries. Until the 1800s, most societies thought that eating raw foods was unhealthy or could kill you. Forget salads or sushi. Real risk-takers might eat a fresh apple or pear, but would peel the fruit and discard the peel. In fact, if fruit was ever eaten uncooked, it was always peeled. "Peel me a grape" takes on a whole new meaning.

Certain foods were never eaten by some people, relished by others. In the 1700s, tomatoes and eggplant were considered poisonous by the French while their Spanish and Portuguese neighbors included them as a staple.

HISTORY OF VITAMIN DISCOVERY

Vitamin C was discovered in the early 1700s, but no one knew it. The British navy at that time was very powerful and very large. British sailing ships were constantly setting out to discover new lands that could be sources of wealth. Although ships could carry fresh food stores for no more than 10 or 15 days, voyages often lasted for months. After the fresh food ran out, sailors lived on salted meat (you know it as beef jerky), hard tack, a very dry biscuit that had the texture of a three-month-old bagel, rum, water, and any fish or birds they could catch. What's missing? Although high enough in protein and carbohydrates, in other words, energy, this diet was totally devoid of vitamin C.

After several months without vitamin C, the sailors would develop a "sea sickness" or **scurvy.** Since no one knew anything about vitamins, this "sea disease" was attributed to the idea that man was not meant to live on the water, away from dry land for long periods of time. Scurvy was considered incurable. Symptoms included bleeding gums, wounds that never healed, bruising, loss of teeth (caused by gum disease), muscle soreness and, ultimately, dementia. During one especially long voyage to the West Indies, a group of scurvy sailors was put ashore with several officers. The ship was to return in several weeks. If anyone were still alive, they'd be picked up and brought home. The group was not issued any stores, as stores could not be wasted on "hopeless cases."

The group was able to scrounge food on the tropical island, including fresh fruit. The small citrus fruit they ate were probably oranges, but, being unfamiliar with most citrus, they called them limes. Miraculously, after several days of eating the citrus fruit, the symptoms of scurvy disappeared! The group was picked up and returned to England, being sure to take a large stash of "limes" with them. From that time on, limes were added to all British sailors' rations. Perhaps you've heard the slang term for a British sailor, that is, "limey."

WATER-SOLUBLE VITAMINS

So, vitamin C was discovered, but not identified or isolated for at least 150 years. Thiamin was the first vitamin isolated in 1911. To make matters more interesting, vitamins do not exist in just one chemical form. Many vitamins exist as a group of similar compounds. For example, **folic acid** is also known as folacin and folate because it can exist as an acid, a protein and a carbohydrate. For all intents and purposes all the different forms do the same thing in the body.

B Is for . . .

The B vitamins, which include **thiamin, riboflavin, niacin, B_{12},** B_6, and folic acid take care of a large number of functions in the body, including muscle control, nerve function, healthy skin and eyes and the manufacturing of red blood cells. Folic acid has been found to prevent certain kinds of birth defects and B_{12} may prevent certain kinds of anemia. B_{12} is best absorbed from animal sources, so vegans may need to think about special B_{12} supplementation.

Vitamin C helps create a healthy immune system, helps build collagen (the "glue" that helps joints to function correctly), and helps in healing. Don't do too much of a good thing, though, as too much vitamin C can cause gastric upset, diarrhea, and kidney stones. Once again, if you are eating a reasonable diet, you will get an adequate amount of vitamins without worrying about getting too much (Neergaard).

FAT-SOLUBLE VITAMINS

Fat-soluble vitamins are stored in the fatty tissues of the body, so you do have some leftover from day to day. This is not to give you permission to eat healthy one day and live on chips and ice cream the next. You just have a bit of an insurance policy with vitamins A, D, E, and K. There is a possibility of toxicity with fat-soluble vitamins, since you can store them. Vitamin **toxicities** come from **megadoses.** This is almost impossible from food, unless you are juicing 30 pounds of carrots a day. If you eat a varied diet, you can obtain an adequate amount of fat-soluble vitamins without worrying about an overdose. Most vitamin toxicities come from taking too many **vitamin supplements** over long periods of time (Squires, 6).

Water-soluble vitamins are not stored, so there is very little chance of toxicity. But because you can't store water-soluble vitamins, you need to keep up on your levels on a daily basis. So, you need daily dietary sources of all the B vitamins and vitamin C and at least every-other day sources of vitamins A, D, E, and K. Watch it if you are taking vitamin supplements with large amounts of fat-soluble vitamins, as too much of a good thing can result in toxicity.

WHERE TO FIND THE VITAMINS YOU NEED

All the vitamins you need can be found in animal and plant sources. All dairy milk, and some soy milks are enriched with vitamins A and D. If you eat that ever-famous balanced diet, you will get enough E and K. Vitamins E and K are

1. If you take supplements containing the fat-soluble vitamins (A, D, E, K), take them with a fat-containing meal. We're not talking a double order of French fries here, just a swallow of low-fat milk or a "schmear" of butter or margarine on some toast.
2. Always take vitamin and mineral supplements with food. You'll absorb more of them and your stomach won't rebel.
3. If you want to get the most for your money, don't take calcium with supplements that contain zinc or iron. Calcium binds zinc and iron, so your body won't be able to use them. So, if you want to take calcium and a multivitamin that contains zinc and iron, take the calcium in the morning and the multivitamin in the afternoon.
4. Use the KISS (keep it simple, silly) method for supplementation. Choose the least expensive variety with the least amount of bells and whistles. Time-released, food-grade, natural, organic, or chemical-free on the label is not a guarantee of a better or more effective product. When it comes down to it, an orange is still a better vitamin source than the most expensive vitamin C in the world.
5. Repeat after me: no megadoses. Megadoses of vitamins and minerals will not vastly improve your health, may harm you and can interact with other medications you are taking, rendering them ineffective.
6. Forget Tahiti. Exotic-sounding herbals preparations that promise to cure everything from bad relationships to athlete's foot probably will not live up to their claims. If you're lucky, they won't do any harm. If you're not lucky, they can cause harm.

Figure 7–1 A Reasonable Guideline for Safe Vitamin and Mineral Supplements

needed in small amounts and are conveniently found in small amounts in lots of foods, such as green veggies, nuts, plant oils, beans, whole grains, and some meat and seafood. Once again, remember that fat-soluble vitamins are stored and can create a toxic state in your liver, so don't overdo it on the supplementation. Enriched grains and cereals supply you with many of the B vitamins, and salsa, sliced kiwi, and strawberries join oranges to give you lots of vitamin C.

Whole Foods Versus Supplementation

Some people know that they eat a healthy diet all the time and don't worry about supplementing their diet with vitamin and mineral pills. Some people know that they eat healthy some of the time and worry about the times when they don't have time to eat well. And other people think that the tomato sauce and onions on their pizza constitute a healthy serving of vegetables. These people may consider using vitamin supplements occasionally to make up what they're missing.

There's no real substitute for the real thing. A glass of orange juice is more beneficial to the body than a vitamin C pill. It is more enjoyable and healthy to get your calcium from some stir-fried tofu or some strawberry yogurt than from a calcium tablet. It is thought that whole foods have more health-promoting properties than supplements. Eating whole foods delivers the nutrients to you in the original package. That orange you're eating isn't just a packet of vitamin C, but a whole carton of vitamins, minerals, fiber, water, and other natural substances meant to function together. Sometimes it's just not possible to grab those five daily servings of fruits and vegetables. If you decide you need some help from a bottle in the vitamin and mineral department, you should start by consulting a health-care professional. They can give your body and your blood a once over to ascertain what you need.

Food Not Pills

It can't be emphasized enough that **vitamin supplements** are just that—supplements. They are not meant to replace a good diet. Something else to remember, before you purchase that thousand-count bottle of 500 percent of your RDAs vitamins, is that your body only needs 100 percent of any given nutrient. In regards to water-soluble vitamins, the Bs and C, that means that your body will keep what it needs up to 100 percent and wash away the rest. With fat-soluble vitamins, A, D, E, and K, the body will attempt to store what it can't use right away. This can lead to toxicities and ultimately can lead to organ failure. Minerals are water-soluble; so your body uses only what it requires and discards the rest.

If the gasoline tank of your car holds 15 gallons of gas, you don't try to force 20 gallons into it. You know that it runs most efficiently when it is almost full. You also know that trying to add extra fuel will not help its performance. The same is true with your body and vitamins and minerals. Your body absolutely needs 100 percent of the **RDAs** for vitamins and minerals. More than

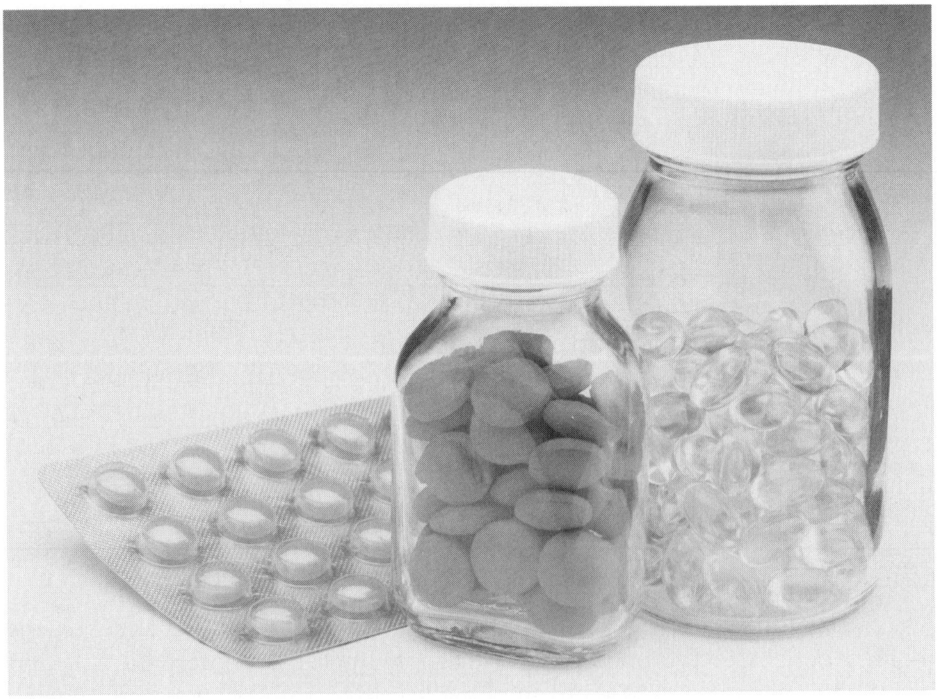

Food or pills? Choose wisely.

that will not help you and could possibly harm you. It's a waste of money and could do damage to take megadoses of vitamins and minerals.

Even the Brownies

Remember that almost all the food you eat contains some vitamins and minerals. For example, that piece of toast you grab on the way out in the morning is probably made from flour enriched with B vitamins and iron. So, now you don't need 100 percent of your Bs and iron, you need a little less. That cup of yogurt you scarf down on the way to class has some calcium, magnesium, phosphorus, and vitamins A and D. So, now you don't need a pill that supplies 100 percent of those nutrients. Unless you eat a diet totally devoid of real ingredients, you are getting at least some nutrients. Check out the label on a bag of cheese puffs or corn chips. Along with the outrageously high fat and sodium content, you'll probably find some real vitamins and minerals contained in the package. The point is that people who take vitamin supplements and eat a reasonable diet are getting far more than 100 percent of their daily needs. When you add megadoses of vitamins and minerals, you go way off the scale of what is required. If you're not careful, your heart and liver could go on strike to protest having to handle such a heavy load.

VITAMINS AND DIGESTION AND ABSORPTION

If you do use vitamin and mineral supplements, remember that they need to go through digestion before they can be absorbed. Taking vitamins with food, even a slice of toast or a slurp of milk will help you get everything from them. If you take vitamins on an empty stomach, you probably won't absorb 100 percent of the vitamins. In addition, some vitamins may stimulate your stomach to secrete digestive acids, which can result in stomach upset.

No-Name Is Not Bad

When it comes to vitamins, you don't have to go for the most expensive brands. Vitamin C is vitamin C. It doesn't make any difference to your body if the vitamin C was extracted from citrus or synthesized in a test tube. Once it's in pill form, vitamin C is just another beneficial chemical. Do select vitamins that come in opaque glass or plastic. Light can break down vitamins, so you don't want them in glass or see-through plastic. Heat can also break down vitamins, so store them in cool places and not over the stove or in the bathroom. Vitamins have expiration dates, so buy 'em and use 'em. Discard them after they've expired, as they won't be doing anything for you. And do keep all vitamins away from children. An excess of fat-soluble vitamins can build up in the liver to toxic levels, causing damage.

CULINARY SELECTION OF NUTRITIOUS FOODS

Chefs and food-service professionals should feel good about being able to please their customers' palates and nourish them as well. Since many adults eat up to 50 percent of their meals away from home, they're relying on eating establishments to serve interesting, tasty, safe, and nutritious foods. Vitamins

Web Site	Comments
www.nal.usda.gov/fnic/etext/000015.html	USDA Food and Nutrition Information Center
www.consumerlab.com	Provides independent testing, results and information on the evaluation of dietary supplements
www.nnfa.org	Nutritional Foods Association represents manufacturers and suppliers of dietary supplements
www.americanutra.com	American Nutraceutical Association. Nutraceuticals are natural substances found in food ingredients thought to promote health
www.herbs.org	The Herb Research Foundation has data on herbs and links to other resources
www.herbclips.com	The American Botanical Council, a research organization for the botanical industry
www.botanical.com	Information on over 800 varieties of medicinal and culinary herbs
www.healthy.net/herbalists	The American Herbalists Guild, a governing board for herbalists

Figure 7–2 Express Info for Vitamin and Nutritional Supplements

fall apart easily when exposed to too much heat, light, or air. Minerals and vitamins can be leached out into cooking water if there is too much used or if they are left to soak. Here are some ideas for keeping the vitamins where they belong, in the food, not in the air or in the cooking liquid.

Fresh Is Best

When you can, use fresh or frozen fruit and vegetables. Canned vegetables have been cooked, so they have lost some of their vitamins. If you need to use packaged fruits or vegetables, use **aseptic packaging** or ultrahigh pasteurized (UHT) fruit and vegetables. These newer processes don't leach out as much of the nutrients as the more traditional canning methods. If you are using canned or processed foods, try to heat them as minimally as possible to save the nutrients that remain. These newer procedures expose food to heat for shorter periods of time. This makes their color and texture more appealing and saves some of the nutrients.

Plan Ahead

Order only enough fresh produce for several days use. As fresh produce "sits," it loses nutrients. Don't cut or peel produce until you are ready to use it, as the exposure to air will destroy some of the vitamins. Don't soak produce to wash it. Water will rid produce of water-soluble vitamins and minerals. Frozen vegetables should not be thawed or rinsed before cooking. Thawing and rinsing makes the texture and the taste less desirable and removes many of the nutrients.

TECHNIQUES OF NUTRITIOUS FOOD PREPARATION

Cooking techniques are as important as preparation techniques for the preservation of produce nutrients. The idea is to get them in and get them out. Exposure to heat and liquid destroys all the good stuff in food. So steam or pressure-cook rather than boil, stir-fry or grill rather than roast; and microwave rather than bake. If possible, reuse cooking liquid. This used to be a typical kitchen technique. It conserved water and added nutrients to one product that had been leached from another. For example, water drained from the pasta was used to cook the beans. Water that vegetables had been cooked in was used to make the stock or a sauce. We are not encouraging cross-contamination here. Use good judgment when reusing cooking water.

Even red meats contain some vitamins, such as thiamin, so select cooking methods for maximum nutrient retention. Cook to doneness, but don't hold the roast on the steam table for a long period of time. You will have to incorporate good nutrition techniques with food safety standards. Whole grains have lots of vitamins and minerals so offer whole grain pasta, breads, cereals and brown rice when you can on the menu. If it fits into your budget, purchase fortified foods, such as orange juice with calcium, soymilk with A and D, and cold cereals with vitamins and minerals.

Free the Radicals

No one has a sure cure for aging or the prevention of all illnesses. The fountain of youth or a cure for cancer has yet to be discovered. We have found, however, that eating the right foods can help to prevent heart disease and some types of cancers. Dietary fiber and certain vitamins, found in fruits and vegetables, seem to have a protective effect against some forms of cancer.

Some vitamins act as **antioxidants.** When your body turns food and air into nourishment, it produces by-products that are toxic. For example, you take in air, extract the oxygen for use by the body and produce carbon dioxide, a toxin, as a by-product. These toxic by-products are called **free radicals** and are thought to cause damage to the cells that may result in cancers and other diseases. Free radicals are rendered inactive by antioxidants. Water-soluble vitamin C and fat-soluble vitamin E are antioxidants. Some studies have shown that people who have diets high in vitamin C or E tend to have lower incidences of heart disease. Does this mean you should start taking massive doses of these vitamins?

No, it means eating lots of highly nutritious foods over a lifetime with an occasional vitamin supplement when your diet isn't what it should be.

FOOD FOR THE MIND

Vitamin A is measured in several different ways. You may see one or all of them on food and supplement labels. **Retinol Equivalents (RE):** are a unit of measurement of the vitamin A content of food, based on the substance retinol. **International Units (IU)** were the first, and considered outdated, measurements of vitamin A. IUs were based on the vitamin activity seen in foods.

MAJOR AND TRACE MINERALS

Minerals make up only about 5 percent of our body weight, but they are essential for life. You can find minerals occurring naturally in foods, in the environment, such as soil and water, and in our bodies.

Vitamin A: Vitamin A is found in the form of retinol in foods of animal origin and in the form of beta-carotene in plant foods.
Great Sources: cooked carrots, sweet potatoes, beef and chicken liver
Very Good Sources: cooked and raw spinach, fresh mango, cantaloupe, romaine lettuce, fortified oatmeal, broccoli and watermelon
Good Sources: Dried prunes and apricots, Corn flake cereal, fresh peaches, black-eyed peas, fortified milk
Vitamin D: Very few foods are naturally high in Vitamin D. Sunlight is a good source of vitamin D, but you have to be careful about getting too much of a good thing.
Good Sources: canned fish, such as sardines and salmon (with bones), fortified milk, fortified cereals
Vitamin E: Vitamin E deficiency is rare, as so many popular foods contain adequate amounts of vitamin E and the body's needs are so small. Vitamin E is actually a group of compounds, called "tocopherols."
Great Sources: Total™ and Product 19™ cold cereals, sunflower seeds, almonds, cottonseed and soybean oil and margarine, strawberries
Good Sources: Commercial salad dressing, corn oil and margarine, peanuts, tomato juice
Vitamin K: Vitamin K is found more in plant foods, especially green vegetables, than in animal foods.
Great Sources: raw cauliflower, raw cabbage, raw spinach, cooked broccoli, whole eggs, cooked green beans, raw tomatoes
Good Sources: corn oil, milk

THE B VITAMINS
Thiamin: Many foods have a small amount of the B vitamin thiamin. Most people get thiamin from foods that have been enriched with thiamin. Thiamin deficiency is seen in alcoholics, as alcohol interferes with the body's ability to absorb thiamin.
Great Sources: wheat germ, fortified oatmeal, soy milk, corn flakes, enriched rice, sunflower seeds, dark meat of turkey
Good Sources: enriched pasta, orange juice, cooked carrots, enriched bread, pecans, lentils, cooked and canned black beans

Figure 7–3 Water Soluble and Fat Soluble Vitamins and Their Sources

There are two classifications of minerals, the **major** and the **trace minerals.** Major minerals are found in greater amounts in the body and are needed in larger amounts in the diet. Among the major minerals are calcium, potassium, chloride, sulfur, magnesium and **sodium.** Trace minerals are needed in smaller amounts and include **iron,** iodine, **zinc, fluoride,** and cobalt. If you eat a balanced diet, then you should be able to get all the minerals you need from the food you eat and the beverages, such as water, dairy beverages and juice that you drink (Rubin, 4).

Taking high doses of single mineral supplements can be dangerous, unless a physician has diagnosed a need. Too much of a good thing, such as iron or calcium, can be toxic. So don't self-prescribe or swallow all the advertising

Riboflavin: Riboflavin was originally called B_2 in Britain and Vitamin G in the United States. To avoid confusion, "riboflavin," meaning "yellow" was agreed upon as this anti-beriberi vitamin's new name.
Great Sources: Cooked beef and chicken liver, yogurt, milk, fortified oatmeal, corn flakes
Good Sources: pork, eggs, cooked mushrooms, almonds, beef, soy milk
Niacin: Niacin can actually be produced in your body from the amino acid tryptophan, as well as being obtained from food.
Great Sources: canned tuna, cooked beef liver, fortified oatmeal, cooked salmon and halibut, corn flakes, peanut butter
Good Sources: cooked mushrooms, canned salmon (with bones), ham, enriched pasta, enriched rice
Folic Acid: Folic acid, also known as folacin and folate, helps the body to synthesize DNA and to form red blood cells. It is available from a diversity of foods.
Great Sources: beef and chicken liver, raw spinach, cooked black and pinto beans, romaine lettuce, artichokes, enriched pasta, soy beans
Good Sources: cooked collards, enriched rice, sunflower seeds, cooked broccoli, oranges and orange juice, cooked crab
B_{12}: Vitamin B_{12} is found naturally only in foods of animal origin. It is important for many processes in the body, including the prevention of pernicious anemia. Vegans need to include specially-fortified products in their diet to ensure adequate B_{12} intake.
Great Sources: beef and chicken liver, cooked clams and oysters, crab, lobster, beef, yogurt
Good Sources: milk, cottage cheese, pork
Vitamin C: Vitamin C is found mostly in vegetables and fruit. Vitamin C, also known as ascorbic acid, helps the body to absorb iron and to maintain immune function.
Great Sources: oranges and orange juice, kiwi, cantaloupe, broccoli, watermelon, strawberries, sweet potato, soy beans, romaine lettuce, fresh pineapple, tomatoes
Good Sources: spinach, okra, winter squash, asparagus, green beans

(*Source: www.nal.usda.gov/fnic/foodcomp*—the USDA Nutrient Database for Standard Reference, Release 13)

Figure 7–3 Water Soluble and Fat Soluble Vitamins and Their Sources *(cont.)*

you see and hear. If you think you have a need for more minerals or vitamins, check with a doctor. Let's look at the popularity of one mineral, following some of the marketing tools and educational information about it.

Calcium 101

Orange juice fortified with calcium, soymilk with extra calcium, fruit-flavored calcium supplements. You can't escape the calcium explosion. Why the sudden interest in this super-white mineral that gives pearls their luster?

Well, pearls, those opaque gems of calcium, are nice to wear around your neck, but its even nicer to be able to stand up straight and smile. Without calcium, you'd have very few pearly whites in your smile, and you'd

MAJOR MINERALS

Potassium: Potassium works with sodium to regulate muscle contractions and nerve impulse transmissions. The major sources of potassium are vegetables and fruit.

Good Sources: bananas, oranges and juice, cantaloupe, baked beans, winter squash, fresh apricots, baked potatoes, yogurt, milk

Calcium: Calcium is very important in the formation of bones, and is also important for healthy nerve function, blood clotting and muscle contraction.

Great Sources: tofu processed with calcium, yogurt, milk, cheeses

Good Sources: molasses, soybeans, spinach, greens, canned salmon (with bones)

Phosphorus: Phosphorus is stored in the bones, and is important for skeletal health and for the processing of energy.

Great Sources: liver, yogurt, sunflower seeds, milk, dark meat of chicken

Good Sources: white meat of chicken, lentils, calcium-processed tofu, soy milk, peanut butter

Magnesium: Magnesium is a factor in more than 250 enzymes and is crucial for cardiac health and nerve function.

Great Sources: cooked lima and black beans, peanut butter, cashews, almonds, sesame seeds

Good Sources: calcium-processed tofu, black-eyed peas, banana, molasses

TRACE MINERALS

Iron: It is important to obtain iron in adequate amounts, but excess amounts can result in toxicity. Iron is an important part of hemoglobin, helping to transport oxygen around the body.

Great Sources: calcium-processed tofu, beef liver, corn flakes, clams and oysters

Good Sources: lentils, spinach, enriched pasta and bread, sunflower seeds, dark meat of turkey, shrimp

Figure 7–4 Minerals and Their Sources

have a decided slouch from a telltale gray bone structure. We have known for years that calcium is very important in the growth and maintenance of bones and teeth. Calcium is also a big factor for a healthy nervous system. We're finding out that calcium may play a role in helping to prevent certain kinds of cancers and even to reduce some of the symptoms of PMS. Calcium has always been important for health. Every day we seem to be finding out even more reasons to maintain adequate calcium stores in the body.

The majority of calcium in your body is in your skeleton and your teeth. A small, but important amount of calcium is found in the blood and is important for correct nerve conduction. Calcium is found in the membrane of every cell in your body, helping with muscle contractions, and is also essential in the absorption of vitamin B_{12}. Among its many jobs, vitamin B_{12} assists the body in utilizing iron, thus helping to prevent certain anemias. Insufficient calcium, insufficient B_{12} absorption. Insufficient B_{12} absorption, lack of energy and many other complications caused by anemia.

Zinc: Zinc is important for immune function and for normal growth and development. Many sources of zinc are from animal products.
Great Sources: beef liver, dark meat of turkey, steak and ground beef, crab, bran flakes
Good Sources: wheat germ, lobster, yogurt, ham, dark meat of chicken, canned beans
Iodine: The thyroid gland requires iodine to function correctly. Except for foods from the ocean and some grains, very few products are naturally high in iodine.
Great Sources: shrimp and lobster, cod and halibut, seaweed, milk, liver, baked potato, iodized salt
Good Sources: whole egg, fortified oatmeal
Manganese: Manganese helps the functioning of several key enzymes in the body. Most people consume enough manganese to avoid deficiency.
Great Sources: wheat germ, fresh pineapple, oatmeal, spinach, cantaloupe, coffee, tea, baked beans, sweet potatoes
Good Sources: cooked greens, beets, broccoli, cocoa
Fluoride: Ninety-nine percent of all the fluoride in the body is found in the bones and teeth. Fluoride is obtained from water from municipal sources, as most cities fluoridate their water. Sources of fluoride include infant formula, mouthwash, toothpaste, and fluoridated water.
Chromium: The importance of chromium has only recently been discovered. It has been shown to help the body to use insulin properly and to properly metabolize carbohydrates and fats.
Great Sources: mushrooms, dark chocolate, prunes, almonds, and asparagus
Good Sources: beer, whole-grain bread and pasta, brewer's yeast.

Figure 7–4 Minerals and Their Sources *(cont.)*

Positive and Negative

Your skeleton functions like the "savings account" for calcium in your body. Your bones are in a constant state of thinning and repair, because of the day-to-day demands of exercise, stress, and normal functioning. Bone is built up all the time, if you give your body the building materials, such as calcium, vitamin D, and sufficient fluid. Some researchers are suggesting that the trace mineral boron may help the body to absorb calcium, as well.

Your body's alternator, if you will, knows how to keep correct calcium balance. Your brain, your kidneys, and your liver communicate with blood, muscles, and internal organs to assess calcium needs. Your personal set of checks-and-balances changes the amount of calcium you absorb from food and how much you lose in urinary output.

Your body knows it needs calcium and will actually change its ability to absorb calcium from food, depending on needs and menu selections. For example, say you recently broke a bone in your foot, but don't change your diet, which is minimally adequate in calcium. Your body will attempt to absorb every milligram of calcium it can from the food and water you take in. Of course, there has to be some calcium in your diet, as your body cannot perform alchemy and create calcium where there isn't any.

Health care professionals speak about **positive** and **negative calcium balance.** Positive calcium balance occurs when you have an excess of calcium in your system caused by need and diet. Negative calcium balance occurs when you have more need for calcium than your body can supply.

You can be in positive or negative calcium balance depending on your needs, your lifestyle and your selection of food and fluids. Positive calcium balance is necessary when you're growing, as in childhood, or when you are building, as in pregnancy, or when you are repairing, as in recovering from a broken ankle or resting up after running a marathon. There is an interesting natural phenomenon related to calcium balance. People who need the most calcium seem to absorb the most. Children absorb almost 75 percent of all calcium they ingest, while thirty-year-olds seem to go down to 20 to 40 percent. So, Mother Nature does seem to have a conspiracy going when it comes to calcium absorption. Your needs don't decrease proportionately as your ability to absorb decreases. So adults need to carefully select foods that are high in calcium so they don't go into negative calcium balance.

If you go into negative calcium balance, then your body has to dip into the "savings account" of your skeleton to get the calcium it needs for muscle contraction, healthy blood formation and other necessary functions. If this continues for any length of time without sufficient replacement of calcium, your bones begin to thin. This is the mechanism that causes **osteoporosis.** It's a vicious circle. If you don't ingest enough calcium, your body removes it from the bones. If you still don't ingest enough calcium, the body continues to withdraw from the skeleton. Pretty soon, your calcium savings account is overdrawn, and you have thinned-out bones that break easily and repair very slowly.

When you hit your mid-thirties, nature tells you, unfortunately, to go into negative calcium balance. How can you meet this challenge? You can eat a calcium-rich diet, you can stay well-hydrated, and you can exercise. In addition to diet, it's been found that weight-bearing exercises, such as walking, running, tennis, weight-lifting, and aerobics, help increase the density of bone. So grab a cup of yogurt or a soymilk smoothie and walk during your work break!

Helps and Hurts

Who is most at risk for osteoporosis? Just about everybody. Both men and women can develop osteoporosis.

"Ten to fifteen percent of men over fifty may have osteoporosis," says Robert M. Zeit, MD, of Healthview Imaging Center in Newport Beach, California, and "osteoporosis can develop in men or women, depending on genetics and lifestyle. Excess caffeine and alcohol and smoking leech calcium from the bones on a daily basis."

What helps? Vitamin D helps your body to absorb calcium; it's no accident that many foods naturally have both calcium and vitamin D. Manufacturers have gotten nutrition-savvy and enriche products with both calcium and vitamin D. Read the label on yogurt, low-fat cheeses, soy and rice milk, and cold cereals, and you'll find both these nutrients. Boron, found in many fruits, veggies, nuts, and beans, helps in calcium absorption as well.

It's thought that the hormone estrogen helps the body maintain calcium levels. After menopause, when estrogen levels decrease, many women opt for estrogen replacement therapy, taking daily doses of estrogen combined with other hormones to prevent the onset of osteoporosis. Others may opt to find estrogen from plant sources. Soy is high in phytoestrogens, or plant estrogens. Populations of women having diets high in soy, such as found in traditional Japanese diets, do not display bone-thinning or other symptoms of menopause. Neither synthetic estrogen or plant estrogen is recommended for women with a history of breast, cervical, or ovarian cancers. It is thought that estrogen may stimulate these types of cancer cells to grow in people with a propensity for them.

Of course, lots of calcium-rich foods is the first line of defense. Exercise is very important in helping the body to build bone, but it has to have something with which to build! There are lots of dairy and nondairy foods that offer good calcium supplies. We'll talk about dietary selection a little later.

What harms? Too much protein or salt, alcohol, caffeine, smoking, and lack of exercise. Lack of exercise will guarantee tissue-thin bones later in life. Protein, salt, alcohol, and caffeine send an incorrect message to your blood and kidneys to vacuum calcium out of the blood. This calcium is lost from the body in the urine. In developing countries, although you see many nutrition deficiencies, you don't see many bone fractions or osteoporosis. This is because the population performs lots of weight-bearing work, walks, doesn't get very much protein, and has less access to tobacco, alcohol, and caffeine.

Believe it or not, some foods are not your friends when it comes to building up calcium. Some foods have lots of calcium, but also contain oxalates, natural substances that inhibit the absorption of calcium. Spinach, which is a great source of iron, has some calcium. But its oxalate content doesn't let you get at it. So have your spinach salad at one meal and your frozen yogurt at another meal. Beans, legumes, and other green vegetables contain oxalates. This doesn't mean exclude them from your diet, as they have other important nutrients. You just need to plan your meals accordingly. Bean burrito at one meal, macaroni and cheese at another meal.

There Will Be a Test

How are calcium levels in your body assessed? This is still a fairly new science, with a lot of disagreement between health-care professionals. Bone scans or bone-density tests can estimate calcium levels. The issue with bone scans is that they measure total bone, which has other minerals. At this point, though, bone scans are the gold standard for assessing bone, or calcium, health. Blood tests are not helpful, because the body tends to keep blood calcium at a constant level. Your blood calcium could be within a normal range, and your bone calcium could be in a negative range.

So how much calcium does everyone need on a daily basis? Just as it is difficult to assess calcium stores in the body, it is difficult to give an exact amount for calcium needs. At this time, health-care professionals will tell you to check your RDA for calcium and attempt to derive as much as possible from the foods you eat. The current theory is that postmenopausal women and men who might need it should get 1,200 milligrams of calcium per day.

One a Day

How about supplements? Some people may feel unable to include enough calcium in their diet. Remember, supplements are not meant to take the place of balanced meals. Calcium supplements may be of some use, but don't take too much. It is possible to have too much calcium from supplements. Excess calcium, taken over extended times will begin to bind zinc and then zinc can't do everything it's supposed to do in the body. If you do decide to take calcium supplements, find some with added vitamin D and boron, which will help calcium absorption.

Calcium Without the Moo

Some people don't like dairy products, some people don't digest them well and some people just can't include enough dairy products in their daily diet to get the calcium they need. There is calcium without the moo.

So, what's your new calcium plan? Include nonfat dairy products, such as yogurt, cheeses, milk, cottage cheese, ricotta cheese, and food made with these ingredients, greens, such as kale, collards, mustard, romaine lettuce and Swiss chard, soy milk enriched with calcium, tofu made with calcium, lots of beans and legumes and nuts and seeds in your daily diet. Purchase calcium-enriched foods, such as cereal, pasta, and juices, cut back or get rid of caf-

A NUTRI-BAR

Nondairy Calcium

Reference: 4 ounces milk = 150 milligrams

Food	*Amount*	*Calcium (in milligrams)*
Fresh orange	1 medium	56
Calcium-fortified Orange juice	4 ounces	up to 160 (read the label)
Tofu	4 ounces	120–300 (read the label)
Broccoli	8 ounces	178
Collard greens	8 ounces	148
Mustard greens	8 ounces	110
Kale	8 ounces	94
Green cabbage	8 ounces	158
Roasted almonds	2 ounces	160
Sesame seeds	2 tablespoons	175
Hummus	4 ounces	80
Cooked beans	4 ounces	60
Blackstrap molasses	1 tablespoon	135

feine, alcohol, and tobacco. Cut back on protein portions. The average healthy adult only needs about four to five ounces of protein per day; think about getting it from calcium-rich foods. Think ethnic foods, such as Japanese, Chinese, Thai, and Middle Eastern. These cuisines tend to include lots of veggies and whole grains that are calcium containing without excess levels of protein.

Many More Minerals

Zinc helps in wound healing, in immune response and is part of many hormones and enzymes. Humans tend to absorb zinc more easily from animal rather than plant sources. Red meat, whole eggs, mollusks (such as oysters), poultry, dairy products, and dried beans are good sources of zinc.

When you purchase toothpaste, you may select a brand that has fluoride. Fluoride is important for the health of bone and teeth and helps prevent cavity formation. Many municipal water supplies have fluoride added for this purpose. Believe it or not, fluoridated water was a really hot topic in the 1950s. The use of fluoride to help dental health was discovered in the early 1950s. It was also the time of the Cold War in America. Many citizens thought that fluoridation of city water was a Communist plot, and that the government was trying to control people's minds by adding chemicals to the water. It took many years before most municipalities in the United States

A NUTRI-BAR

Get More Calcium on the Menu

1. Instead of purchasing salad dressing, blend nonfat yogurt or calcium-enriched tofu with chopped onions, cucumbers, fresh parsley, and garlic. Yogurt or tofu can also be used instead of mayo to add a bit more calcium.
2. Cut back on the iceberg and add chopped Romaine or shredded cabbage, Chinese cabbage, or collard greens to salads.
3. Cultivate kale—it's easy to cook, just steam it or blanch with chicken or vegetable stock and serve as a bed for other veggies or grains.
4. Use calcium-fortified orange juice as an ingredient for baking, sauces and salad dressing.
5. Make a calcium smoothie (see recipes below).
6. Use blackstrap molasses when baking carrot cake, gingerbread or zucchini bread, bran muffins or peanut butter cookies. Use instead of maple syrup on pancakes or waffles.
7. Go ethnic—lots of stir frys, hummus, falafel (chick pea fritters), Indian and Thai vegetable curries, etc.
8. Add more to the soup—think lentils, black-eyed peas, chick peas, shredded greens, etc.
9. Garnish! Chopped nuts and sesame seeds brighten up rolls, muffins, cereals, soups, pasta and salads.
10. Cut back on the coffee. One or two cups a day are okay. Try out decaffeinated teas and coffees, herbal teas, and grain beverages.

A NUTRI-BAR

Calcium With and Without the Moo

With Moo

4 servings
8 ounces nonfat vanilla yogurt
8 ounces lemon sorbet or sherbet
4 ounces canned pineapple tidbits, drained
4 ounces calcium fortified orange juice
1 teaspoon orange zest

Place all ingredient in a blender and process until smooth. Serve chill, garnished with a pineapple or orange wedge

Nutritional Analysis: 184 calories per serving, 4 grams protein, 2 grams fat, 20 milligrams cholesterol, 34 grams carbohydrates, 55 milligrams sodium, 2 grams dietary fiber, 80 milligrams calcium.

Without Moo

4 servings
8 ounces calcium-processed silken tofu
8 ounces calcium-enriched orange juice
4 ounces sliced bananas
4 ounces canned peaches, drained and chopped
2 ounces fresh or frozen (thawed) strawberries
4 ounces chopped ice
1 teaspoon soy powder (optional)

Place all ingredients in a blender and process until smooth. Serve chilled, garnished with a whole strawberry of an orange wedge

Nutritional Analysis: 198 calories per serving, 8 grams protein, 4 grams fat, 34 grams carbohydrates, 20 milligrams sodium, 2 grams fiber, 60 milligrams calcium.

voted to allow fluoride to be added to their water. Nutrition has always been so controversial!

Your thyroid gland is the "alternator" of your body, controlling metabolism rates and iodine is the fuel that the thyroid needs. Iodine can be found in iodized salt, sea products, such as ocean fish, nori, sea vegetables that are popular in Asian cuisine, and some dairy products. Salt companies were instructed to add iodine to salt by an act of Congress during World War I. During a large draft call for soldiers needed in the armed services it was discovered that goiter, an enlargement of the thyroid caused by lack of iodine, was rampant among the U.S. population. Since many people didn't live near the ocean, they had no way to obtain iodine. Freshwater lakes or steams don't count; only ocean or seawater has iodine. In those days, salt was considered

Food	*Serving Size*	*Milligrams of Sodium*
Potato chips	1 ounce	170
Baked potato	1 medium	8
2% milk	1 cup	120
American cheese	1 oz	400
Whole-wheat bread	1 slice	150
Biscuit	1 medium	540
Roast pork	3 oz	50
Sliced ham	3 oz	1180
Fresh cucumber	1 large	6
Pickle	1 large	1730

(**Source:** *www.nal.usda.gov/fnic/foodcomp*)

Figure 7–5 Amounts of Sodium Found in Foods

a staple, something that everyone used every day. Since everyone was guaranteed to have some salt every day, it was the logical item to iodize. Salt is iodized to this day. You have to read the label, though, as salt is available both iodized and not iodized. Kosher salt and popcorn salt are usually not iodized. Sea salt does not need to be iodized, since it naturally contains iodine. Some chefs say they can taste the iodine in salt and choose to use non-iodized salt in their dishes.

Sodium is a good-guy, bad-guy kind of mineral. Salt is an essential nutrient and helps maintain fluid balance in the body and is a participant in many reactions, including the beating of the heart. Unfortunately, too much sodium in the body can cause elevated blood pressure (hypertension), can put strain on the kidneys and can even cause an irregular heartbeat. The USDA recommends that Americans eat no more than 2,400 milligrams of sodium per day. This translates into about two teaspoons. Most people would be pretty hard-pressed to limit their sodium intake to this amount. In addition to being a common preservative, salt is a taste that most people enjoy. Chefs rise to the challenge of cutting back the salt with the use of fresh and dried herbs, spices, citrus (your taste buds react the same way to lemon juice as they do to salt), wine and vinegar reductions, and vegetable purees, to name a few techniques. A skillful chef doesn't need salt to make food taste good.

The importance of iron has been known for a long time. Ancient Greek medical writings point out the importance of iron. In medieval France and England, iron, in the form of fine filings dissolved in wine, were given to treat anemia.

Iron is one of the few minerals that is necessary through every stage of life, from infants to senior citizens. Iron is needed to ensure that all the cells of the body are nourished with oxygen. Infants, children, adolescents, pregnant women, athletes, vegetarians, blood donors and senior citizens can all be at risk for iron-deficiency **anemia.** In other words, just about everybody.

Iron deficiency is usually caused in healthy people by poor dietary intake. It can also be caused by excess blood loss and some illnesses. Iron needs can range from 10 to 30 milligrams of iron per day. The typical American diet has only about 6 milligrams of iron for every 1,000 calories eaten. In addition to food, it is thought that using cast-iron cookware may add some iron to the diet.

Of course, nature had to have its joke with humans and iron. Many types of dietary iron are poorly absorbed. Foods containing the highest amount of iron are the least desirable. Organ meats, such as liver and kidneys are high in cholesterol and are despised by a large number of people. Oysters and clams are also good iron sources, but not too likely to be a regular part of most people's diets. Lean beef, pork, veal, and poultry do have some iron. Iron from animal sources is better absorbed than from plant sources.

Which is not to say don't eat your spinach. You'll just need to increase your intake of dark green leafies, such as kale, collards, mustards, and beet greens along with spinach. Dried fruit, dried peas, nuts, enriched breads and cereals, and blackstrap molasses also contain iron.

Iron has some friends and some enemies. Vitamin C helps, high acid in cast iron helps, plant foods and iron complement each other. So, sprinkle some tangerine sections on that spinach salad or prepare a tomato sauce in a cast iron pan. Both techniques will assure you lots of vitamin C and iron.

On the other hand, the following foods prevent the body from absorbing iron: egg yolks, calcium-containing foods, tea and soy. Zinc found in multivitamins and in sore throat lozenges can also inhibit iron absorption. So, have a spinach salad for lunch and wait a couple of hours before having that frozen yogurt or tofu smoothie. Order a glass of wine or some sparkling water instead of iced tea with that spinach salad, as well.

THE COMMON COLD AND NUTRITION

There is no cure. Turn the page. Discussion over. Well, maybe we can talk about it a little bit.

There are more than 250 viruses that can cause the common cold. They find their way into the body by way of airborne droplets spread by sneezing. The droplets can land on a surface, such as a table or an apple. An uninfected person touches the surface, then transports the droplets into the body through the eyes, mouth, or nose. Children can have six to ten colds per year and adults two to four. People suffer from at least one billion colds per year in the United States alone.

Cold weather does not cause colds. Seasonal weather changes in humidity can, however, provide a better breeding ground for viruses. Low humidity, such as that in overheated homes or cars, is a favorite of viruses. So, cold season is not so much caused by the cold temperatures as it is to the lack of moisture in the air. This means you haven't got a good excuse to avoid inventorying the walk-in freezer.

Herb	*Properties*
Black cohosh	may help with PMS or menopause symptoms
Cascara sagrada	laxative
Catnip	promotes sleep, may ease menstrual cramps
Chamomile	may sooth stomach and headache upsets
Chapparal	can cause liver damage
Dong quai	may help with PMS or menopause symptoms
Echinacea	may reduce severity of cold symptoms
Ephedra	can cause heart attacks and seizures
Ginger	relieves nausea, may soothe sore throats
Ginseng	may increase energy
Goldenseal	may help with sore throats, ear aches
Kava kava	herbal "Valium"
Kola nut	contains caffeine
Peppermint	helps digestion, decreases nausea
Senna	laxative
Willow bark	has aspirin-like make-up

Figure 7–6 Quick Rundown of Herbal Remedies

HERBS AND BOTANICALS

Vitamin C, herbal preparations such as echinacea (a purple daisy originally used by Native Americans as a medicinal tea), or massive amounts of orange juice will not prevent colds. Washing your hands will. The more frequently you wash your hands, the more you lower your chances of exposure to cold viruses (*Preventing the Common Cold,* 3). Getting enough rest helps replenish your immune system, as does drinking lots of noncaffeinated, non-alcoholic beverages. Fluids help nurture the cells of the body and also help to flush out foreign invaders. Antibiotics do not work against colds. Colds are caused by viruses and antibiotics only work on bacteria. Antibiotics are prescribed only when a secondary, bacterial infection sets in.

The best "cure" for colds is prevention, as we've outlined above. Take your vitamin C if you like, but wash your hands and get enough sleep before you do.

But what about all these herbal preparations sold to prevent or cure colds and a thousand other ailments? Many people begin to take **echinacea,** an herbal preparation first used by Native Americans and extracted from the purple coneflower, during flu season. Some research has found that echinacea might boost the immune system. Rather than using pharmaceuticals, some people may turn to **St. John's Wort** to help with depression or **kava-kava** to relieve anxiety. Some beverages and meal-replacement bars have ginseng added as an "energy" enhancer. Consumers have accepted herbs, or botanicals, as an alternate method of handling aches, pains and well-being.

Natural Is Not Always Better

It's important to educate yourself about herbs, as some may help, some may hurt, and some may not do anything but waste your money. Remember that just because something is "natural" does not mean that it is better and can do no harm. For example, willow bark extract, which herbalists may recommend for headaches and muscle pain, contains the same chemicals as aspirin. If you are allergic to aspirin, you will have the same allergic reaction to willow bark. Many pharmaceuticals are merely chemical interpretations of substances isolated from nature. Something else to remember about herbs is that they do not act quickly, but have to be taken over a period of time to show an effect. St. John's Wort, which is sometimes used for depression, takes four to six weeks to change how someone feels. The moral to this story is to not self-diagnose. If you don't feel good, discuss your issues with a health-care professional. If you want to use herbs or botanicals as part of your plan, be sure to mention it. Herbs can interact with some medications or may cause unwanted symptoms or side effects. For example, goldenseal, an herb sometimes taken for colds or sore throats, can cause blood thinning. You wouldn't want to take goldenseal right before or after surgery or if you have problems healing. **Ephedra** is an herbal preparation included in many "natural" diet pills. Ephedra can elevate blood pressure, cause irregular heartbeats, and can lead to liver and kidney damage.

Some Good Guys

On the good side, many herbs and botanicals may help, or at least do no harm. Ginger can be eaten raw or brewed in tea to help soothe sore throats or to relieve nausea. Some people who experience mild motion sickness use ginger to prevent it. The natural properties of cranberries may help to prevent kidney and bladder infections with no side effects. Saw palmetto is thought to help assist in preventing prostate cancer. There have been no reports of negative consequences. Soy foods contain plant estrogens that may be a factor in women's health. It has been shown that populations that have diets high in soy have less heart disease and breast cancer.

Making Your Sugar Toasties Better

For over fifty years, the FDA has required fortification of certain food products with essential nutrients in which the American diet is deficient. You're familiar with that. Tomorrow morning, while you're chomping on your favorite sugarcoated frosty flakes, focus on the milk carton. Notice the "fortified with Vitamins A and D" on the label. Likewise for the cold cereal. It's amazing how many vitamins and minerals can be packed into your cereal bowl.

The rise in consumers' interest in health has lead to the voluntarily use of supplements and the preference for **functional foods** over "regular" food and beverage. Botanicals have become more popular as the population becomes more aware of the link between dietary intake and health.

STANDARDIZATION OF HERBS AND BOTANICALS

According to statistics released by the federal government, $12 billion was spent on supplements and functional foods in 1997. Amazingly, there are no uniform tests for standardization for the botanicals used in the creation of these products. What this means is that lots of consumers are purchasing bottled iced tea with ginseng or tea bags enhanced with echinacea or orange juice fortified with calcium rather than un-enhanced products. Walk down the beverage aisle of a supermarket. You can find water fortified with minerals, soda enhanced with herbal preparations, and juices mixed with "healthy" ingredients. None of these "enhancements" are overseen by government agencies. As natural products, rather than chemical products, minerals, vitamins, and herbs (called "botanicals") can be added to products without scientific substantiation.

Herbal or botanical standardization is an issue because, at this time, standard methods for botanical analysis are not in use throughout the industry and are not required by the government. Many useful and effective methods exist and are used in-house by botanical processors but there is no single source for test selection or implementation, such as is used with pharmaceuticals by the United States Pharmacopoeia (USP). Botanicals are natural products. Without standardization there is no way to know if a consumer is getting 30 milligrams of these herb or one ounce of that herb when using a botanical products.

A Rose is Not Always A Rose

Another reason for standardization is, as with most organic material, all botanicals are not equal. Think of botanicals in terms of roses. All roses have wonderful aromas. But the intensity and the make-up of the aroma varies from rose bush to rose bush according to the rose variety, its age, the time of year it is plucked and the way it is stored (in a florist's refrigerator versus a warm room). In the same way, properties of botanicals may vary from plant to plant, influenced by the species of plant selected, the growing area, the time of year harvested, the age of the plant, and the conditions under which the plant is harvested and processed.

For example, explains Brian Toy, a Canadian nutritional scientist specializing in herb research, echinacea has at least three different species. Currently, there is no consensus as to which species is effective for treatment of various physical conditions. Hypericin, the active ingredient in Saint John's wort (although at the time of this writing another ingredient was being identified as being more effective) is more concentrated when harvested from plants which are in flower and are grown in warmer climates. The active ingredient in American ginseng (gingsenosides) is more concentrated in older plants than in younger plants. Without standardization, it is difficult to impossible to guarantee that the promised ingredient is present in the promised concentration.

Since botanicals are natural products, every aspect of handling and testing influences the final outcome. The flow of handling includes growing, harvesting, processing, specification fulfillment for raw and finished materials, and selection of marker substances.

With today's methods, when a manufacturer receives bulk, raw product the hope is that what arrives is what was ordered. Without standardization, there is no way to know if the correct species was shipped, or if accidental mixing of another botanical occurred.

During processing, the raw material is forced through a screen and a metal detector to get rid of bugs, bits of metal and stones, ground between blades and rollers and placed in an extraction tank where solvents, such as ethanol are used to obtain the desired ingredients. After extraction is complete the solvent is distilled off and the resulting material is shipped wet or dry. At this point, unless there are in-house tests, no standardization analyses are performed, making the guarantee of quality, safety, or efficacy of the product difficult. So, you get the picture. As much as many people prefer "natural" ingredients, it is very difficult to ensure how much of the natural ingredient is actually getting into a product.

At this time, lab analysis methods differ from lab to lab and country to country. Analysis for different **marker substances** are done according to customer demands and the availability of reference standards. Vendors can find it difficult to obtain certificates of analysis for the products they purchase or sell.

A word must be mentioned about marker substances and their role in standardization, as there are several schools of thought on them. One school holds the opinion that attempting to isolate particular constituents in a plant brings botanical standardization closer to pharmacological (perceived as very accurate) evaluation. Another school feels that the concentrating of a particular substance displaces other substances that may or may not be important to the action of the botanical.

Marker substances are used for synthetic medicinal compounds (such as aspirin) to measure purity and activity level. It is easy to do this with synthesized materials, as it is known their exact properties, what concentration levels can be expected and how they will react. This is not so easily done with natural products, which have many unknowns.

Put in another way, plants have many ingredients which interact relative to each other; measuring one particular ingredient may not give an accurate read as to the action of the plant or it may—the jury is still out.

In other words, one school of thought holds that isolating natural-occurring chemicals lead to the making of more uniform botanical products. Another school of thought holds that the interaction of all chemicals in a plant are important and that the capturing of one chemical does not capture the action of the botanical. "Which is better—a Vitamin C tablet or a glass of orange juice" might sum up the marker substance debate.

NATIONAL AND INTERNATIONAL MONITORING OF HERBS AND BOTANICALS

Internationally, many countries in Europe and Japan require full certification of botanicals. In Germany, botanicals are registered drugs that come with full documentation (that covers quality, safety and efficacy) from Commission E.

Commission E is Germany's equivalent of an herbal FDA as is the *AVIS AUX FABRICANTSI* in France. To sell botanicals in these countries they must go through a prescribed process that tests and documents their purity, safety and uses. In Japan, functional foods must be approved through the government. "Foods for Specified Health Uses," or FOSHU are tested for purity, safety and specific health claims.

In the United States, several groups are developing industry standards and seeking to have them implemented. Among them are the Council for Responsible Nutrition, the National Nutritional Foods Association and the Institute for Nutraceutical Advancement, the American Botanical Council, the American Herbal Products Association, the Herb Research Foundation and the Association of Official Analytical Chemists. Along with the USP, these organizations are working towards the "gold standard" in botanical analysis.

The USP, which generally covers pharmaceutical issues, is developing selection criteria for the botanicals that account for 90 percent of U.S. retail sales, including ginger, valerian, garlic, Asian ginseng (panax ginseng), gingko, feverfew, St. John's wort, American gingseng, echinacea, chamomile (matricaria flower), saw palmetto, hawthorn, golden seal, milk thistle, cranberry, nettle root, ephedra (ma huang), kava kava, Siberian ginseng (eleutherococcus), licorice, and angelica. In part, these botanicals were selected because they are widely used by the public, and there was a history of use in traditional medicine.

Listen to the Doc

What does all this mean for you? Some of you may already use some herbal preparations as part of your daily routines and some of you may have friends, employees or customers who use them. Now that herbal or botanical preparations have hit the mainstream and seem to be staying there, you need to know how to make decisions about using or not using them.

"Our understanding of the value of herbal medicine in the prevention of disease is just beginning to take off," said Robert M. Zeit, MD, a specialist in preventative medicine practicing at HealthView, Newport Beach, CA, "I expect that the acceptance of the use of herbs for the prevention of disease will escalate geometrically in the next several years."

Dr. Zeit noted that in his twenty-five years of practice he has seen more and more patients turn to herbals for the prevention of disease. For example, Dr. Zeit sees patients who are interested in the prevention of coronary disease, which means controlling cholesterol. He says his patients are interested in cholesterol control with diet and herbs rather than prescription medications. Many have done their own research and have designed their own regimen of herbs, diet, and exercise.

"In Germany, physicians have to have some training in herbal medicine," according to B. Clair Eliason, MD, Medical College of Wisconsin, Milwaukee, "in other developed countries we find a more rational approach to herbals."

Look It Up

The *Physician's Desk Reference* (PDR) is the bible for prescription medicine information. Published every year, the PDR lists extensive information (use, method of action, indications for use, side effects, current studies, etc.) for every prescription and over-the-counter medication available in the United States. When you go to get a prescription filled, you can ask the pharmacist to show you PDR information about your medication. The PDR for Herbal Medicine, edited by Joerg Gruenwald, Thomas Brendler, MA, and Christof Jaenicke, MD, in its third edition, is available for botanicals used in the United States. The herbal PDR contains information on over 600 herbal medicines, including possible side effects and indications for use, thorough references, and Commission E statements on therapeutic considerations, dosage, and side effects.

ENHANCING VITAMIN, MINERAL, AND BOTANICAL RETENTION IN FOOD PURCHASING AND PREPARATION

Chefs have always used herbs to enhance the aroma, appearance, and flavor of menu items. But how many chefs realized that rosemary contains antioxidants, blueberries might assist in preventing some visual problems, or that naturally occurring compounds in red pepper may help reduce pain? When the chef adds fresh ginger to a dish, is it to turn up the heat on the customer's palate or is it to assist in soothing sore throats or motion sickness? Those garlic and onions may add heart to a sauce, and they may also heal the heart by helping to reduce blood pressure. Food ingredients serve many more purposes than appears on the surface. And you thought those tomatoes and olives on your pizza were there for taste? No way! The tomatoes contain a botanical substance called "lycopene," thought to help reduce the incidence of prostate cancer. The olives contain olive oil, and everyone knows that olive oil is a heart-healthy choice.

Keep It in Balance

Asian and Indian chefs have known and cared about the healthy properties of foods for centuries. Dishes were designed with balances of "heat" and " cold" so that the body could get the maximum benefit from all the foods eaten. There are many "herbal" restaurants in different parts of Asia. Herbal medicine is an important part of Asian medicine. An herbalist might give a customer a combination of herbs to brew in a tea or a soup or might give the customer a "prescription," which could be taken to an herbal restaurant. Chefs in these restaurants are expected to be knowledgeable about herbal remedies and are able to prepare food items that taste good and include your "prescription." We're talking really advanced chicken soup!

Western chefs may not stock a pharmacy worth of herbs in their kitchens, but they can maximize the nutrition experience for their customers. It doesn't cost extra money or use extra labor to ensure that that carrot still has some vitamin A left in it or that that fruit salad has some minerals remaining. As has been discussed earlier in the chapter, there are many ways to keep the nutrients in foods. The process is the same for vitamins, minerals, and botanicals.

Whenever it is possible, purchase the fresh ingredients. Not only will fresh ingredients have more nutrients, they'll have more intense flavors. Think a tomato's a tomato? Think again. Locate a farmers' market in your area and purchase some tomatoes. Compare these against store-purchased tomatoes. No comparison. An extra-added dividend of scoping out farmers' markets is finding produce treasures, such as heirloom tomatoes or varieties that are only available locally.

Cook It Right

Not all cooking methods are created equally. You already know that boiling carrots for hours will cook all the beta-carotene (and flavor and color out of them). Opting for steaming or fast grilling would seem a logical choice. They certainly do help to retain nutrients. Unfortunately for food-service professionals, microwaving has been found to retain the most nutrients when cooking vegetables. Even more interestingly, fresh tomatoes or carrots that are microwaved for a very brief time give up more of their nutrients. The vitamins, minerals, and botanicals in slightly cooked tomatoes and carrots were used more efficiently by humans than were raw tomatoes and carrots. Go figure!

Does this mean you should microwave everything? Not by any means. That would be monotonous and wouldn't do very much for the culinary profession. All foods are not tomatoes and carrots and give up their nutrients just fine when eaten uncooked or prepared with various methods. If you eat a varied diet, you are not relying on one food to supply you with all your daily needs. For example, you can get all your vitamin C by drinking a gallon of orange juice every morning. That could get boring, expensive and does not assure you that that OJ has all the vitamin C it promises. You could have left the carton open to air and light, which would destroy some of the vitamin C. If the orange juice is pasteurized, some of the C could have been lost during the heating process. You would be much better off drinking some orange juice in the morning, tossing some fresh grapefruit sections on to your green salad at lunch, piling on the fresh salsa (tomatoes, peppers, and chilies have vitamin C), munching on some mango or kiwi and adding some strawberries to your frozen yogurt. Eating a variety of foods that all have the same nutrient is a better insurance plan than relying on one food source or cooking technique.

We've covered vitamins, minerals and herbs so far. Now's the time to talk about what you wash them down with, that is, water.

WATER AS A NUTRIENT

Water is an essential nutrient. No, you can't obtain energy from it and it does not directly ramp up the immune system or build better bones. You are, however, about 60 to 70 percent water. Your muscle tissue has about 70 percent water and fat tissue has about 20 percent water. If you are well-nourished, you could theoretically go about 6 weeks without eating food. It wouldn't be pretty, but it's possible. On the other hand, you could only go about three days without water. You can store and conserve energy, but you can't store or conserve water.

We usually take water for granted. It's not interesting and doesn't seem to do very much. In reality, water participates in just about every reaction and function in your body and is a large part of each and every cell.

REQUIREMENTS FOR WATER

Water helps regulate body temperature. If you have ever gone swimming in a lake or the ocean, you'll notice that water changes temperature much more slowly than land. The same thing happens in your body. Water holds on to heat and changes temperature very slowly. By holding onto heat, the water in your body helps you stay warm. When you need to cool down, your body releases water, in the form of perspiration. The perspiration comes to the surface of the skin, where it evaporates. Evaporating water requires energy from heat. So, as perspiration evaporates, heat energy is taken from the skin, cooling it. Just to give you a perspective, it takes about 600 calories to evaporate one quart of perspiration. That's why people who have had high fevers lose a couple of pounds over several days. Do not try this at home. Maintaining a fever is no way to lose weight.

Water is a large portion of your blood supply and other body fluids, such as lymph. Water in these systems, as well as in your muscles and internal organs, help to get rid of waste products. Water is used, and waste products are produced as a result of digestion, exercise, breathing, and all those other things bodies do to stay alive. Water helps dilute the waste products so that the kidneys are not damaged and helps to move the waste products out of your system.

Since you lose water every day, and since you are 60 to 70 percent water, it is important to replenish your supply. Remember, you are even losing water when you breathe! The old rule of thumb was that everyone needed eight glasses (or a half-gallon) of water per day. If you want to be more scientific about it, you need about 1 milliliter of water for every calorie you burn. So, if you think you burn about 1,200 calories per day, then you'd need about 1,200 milliliters, 1.2 liters, or about 5 cups of water per day, minimum.

Sources of Water in the Diet

You don't have to get all your daily water from drinking straight H_2O. You can get water from fruits and vegetables (and their juices), foods that are mostly water or ice, such as soups, gelatin, and sorbets or from drinking herbal teas, decaffeinated beverages or sparkling or flavored waters. Of course, water is still the best source of water.

Caffeine and Alcohol

Caffeine and alcohol are the enemies of water. Caffeine-containing items, such as coffee, green and black tea, cola beverages, sodas to which caffeine is added, chocolate and other products that have been "fortified" with caffeine, as well as alcohol-containing products act as diuretics. Diuretics tell the body to get rid of water even though water is needed. So, theoretically, you could drink caffeinated iced tea all day and wind up becoming dehydrated! In addition to having a diuretic effect, caffeine may have a negative effect on the absorption of calcium, resulting in osteoporosis. We have already discussed the role of caffeine in heart disease in Chapter 3.

Dehydration

Dehydration can have mild to severe symptoms, which can range from headaches and thirst to muscle aches, flu-like symptoms, fever, irregular heartbeat, and even mental confusion. Dehydration puts a strain on all your organs and can cause physical and mental damage if it is allowed to be a chronic condition. This is especially important to be aware of if you are working in a hot environment, like a kitchen! Heat makes you lose water at a faster rate and you need to replace everything you lose. Back off the soda, coffee and beer and turn onto sparkling water, fruit juice smoothies and sorbets.

PROBIOTICS

You know that selecting the right food is important for your health. To go a bit beyond that, let's get into a discussion of foods that some people feel can not just help you when you're sick but can help prevent disease.

Probiotics are microorganisms that live in food and have been found to, possibly, convey some health effects (Koop-Hoolihan,1). The cultures or colonies of microorganisms that live in yogurt would be good examples of probiotics. Some yogurts are inoculated with species of lactobacillus (literally, "milk bacteria"), bifidobacterium and streptococcus strains (the good kind, not the kind that causes sore throats). These bacteria occur naturally in the human digestive tract and help to keep the gut healthy and relatively disease-free. Antibiotics can destroy the balance of bacteria in your gut. Probiotics can help to restore the balance. There is very preliminary research being done to see if eating foods with probiotics can help in eliminating the effects of some peptic ulcers, gastritis, colitis and other intestinal diseases. The jury is still out on the far-reaching effects of probiotics. In the short term, unless you have allergies to certain molds, fungi or foods, eating foods with probiotics shouldn't do any harm and may possibly help. Yogurt, dairy-based drinks, and supplements are currently being sold enhanced with probiotics. However, if you're healthy, probiotics won't give you a "super-gut" able to ward off any or all disease. At best, probiotics will help to keep a good balance, making you a bit better at warding off some diseases. And you must be dedicated if you want probiotics to work. Initially, it may take three to four weeks to establish this balance. To maintain it, you must ingest probiotics on a regular basis.

FYI: THAT CONTROVERSIAL LIQUID REFRESHMENT—WATER

Humans and the planet we live on are mostly water. For that reason, water has always played a large role in where we live, what we eat, and how we feel.

Back in the good old days, water was thought to possess almost mystical powers. Water is so essential to life that it took on magical status in many societies. Water was and is an important ingredient in both social and religious rituals. Until approximately fifty years ago, when a sick person did not make a fast recovery, they were packed off to "stay at the seaside" or at least were sent "to take the waters" at a lake or river. Many resorts began as sanitariums for the chronically ill.

In addition to being near the water, people bathed in the water and drank the water, in the hopes of making a full recovery from their ailment. The springs near Perrier, France, provided "healing" waters to many, as did the springs near Palm Springs, California, and Sarasota Springs, New York.

Think we modern, scientific people are beyond all that? Think about H_2O, a water and oxygen bar in Beverly Hills, California. Owned in part by actor Woody Harrelson, customers may sample over 100 different varieties of water from all over the world. Oxygen can be purchased in metered doses and customers can dine on macrobiotic, raw foods cuisine.

Or check out one of the high-tech waters available on the market. Energy Brands company sells a water "supplement," called Glaceau Wellness Water. It is available in four flavors and is enriched with vitamins, minerals and botanical herbs and is flavored with tropical fruit and tea. It would seem we still believe in the "magical" powers of water in the twenty-first century.

So, what if you can't get to France or Beverly Hills; how will you meet your daily water needs? You know the drill. Non-active adults need about two to three liters of water per day. If you are physically active you increase your need for water. If you eat a high-sodium, high-protein, or high-fiber diet, your water needs increase. Likewise for those that hit the coffeepot or the soda machine a lot; caffeine increases your water needs. Quick consumer quiz. Which canned soda contains the highest amount of caffeine? Excluding sodas that advertise additional caffeine, Mountain Dew™ rates the highest on the caffeine scale. Remember that caffeine is an added ingredient. Don't assume that only cola-flavored sodas contain caffeine. Read the label!

In addition to drinking good, ol' H_2O, you know that you can obtain water through your menu choices. Fruit and vegetables (and their juices), sauces made from fruits and vegetables, hot cereals, puddings and gelatins (made with water and milk), milk and products made from milk, fruit ices, and sorbets are all sources of water. The choices are endless.

So, is it necessary to purchase bottled or distilled water? Many brands of bottled water are obtained from municipal water supplies, just like the cool, clear fluid coming out of your home tap. If you don't happen to like the flavor of the local water (which is influenced by the combination of minerals from the water supply) and you won't drink it, then bottled water is an option. Distilled water, processed so that it is free of all bacteria, is an unnecessary precaution for most people (except for the severely ill). Remember that the minerals in hard tap water can have some health benefits!

So what is tap water, anyway? Your town has a municipal water source, which could be a reservoir, a lake, or wells. The water is filtered to remove contaminants, such as disease-causing bacteria, and may be chlorinated to ensure that bacterial counts are never high enough to cause disease. Some towns fluoridate their water, to improve dental health. Fluoridation was a *huge* controversy in the 1950s. Many people did not understand the concept of fluoridation and thought that it was a government plot! It took several years to convince people that fluoride was a safe addition to water and was not a "mind control" drug!

Water will continue to be absolutely essential to life, and the various forms in which it is marketed will probably continue to be controversial. Make your choice to drink it from a glass, a bottle, or a fountain, but be sure and drink lots of it!

For more information on the ways of water, you can visit:

www.perrier.com (for a fast rundown on the amazing array of available bottled water)

www.gatorade.com (for an interesting discussion about Gatorade versus water!)

www.brita.com (for a discussion on home water filtration)

Nutri-Words

Anemia: a condition in which sufficient iron is not present in the red blood cells.

Antioxidants: substances that combine with free radicals and neutralizes them. This reduces the amount of oxidative damage free radicals can do in the body.

Aseptic packaging: a form of packaging, commonly seen in the United States in juice boxes, that reduces nutrient loss during processing.

B_{12}: a B vitamin, also called "cobalamin," plays an important role in assisting folate to function in the body. A deficiency of B_{12} may result in pernicious anemia.

Echinacea: an extract of the purple daisy, used by Native Americans as an antibiotic and an immune system stimulator.

Ephedra: an herbal extract, found in many diet aides; a central nervous system stimulant that can cause irregular heartbeat and cardiac problems.

Fat-soluble vitamins: compounds needed in the diet in small amounts to promote health that are soluble in body fluids, such as vitamins A, D, E, and K.

Fluoride: an essential mineral, known for its role in dental health.

Folic acid-folacin-folate: different forms of the same B vitamin, known for its ability to reduce the incidence of certain birth defects.

Free radicals: a substance produced during normal functioning, such as digestion or muscle use. Free radicals can cause damage to the body's cells. See "antioxidants."

Functional foods: foods that contain health-related properties. For example, tomatoes naturally contain lycopene, a substance thought to help reduce the risk of certain cancers. Some manufacturers add natural substances to products, such as adding calcium to orange juice, to create their own functional foods.

Iron: an essential mineral, known for its role in supporting the red blood cells.
Kava-kava: an herbal extract, known for its calming properties.
Major and trace minerals: organic substances, such as iron, potassium and sulphur, that the body needs to function normally.
Marker substance: a natural substance known to occur in significant amounts in a product. Used to ensure that natural products contain significant amounts of identified substances. For example, echinacea would be a marker substance in extracts of purple daisies.
Megadoses: amounts of vitamins or minerals that far exceed a safe daily intake.
Osteoporosis: "thinning" of the skeleton, secondary to negative calcium balance.
Positive and negative calcium balance: calcium is an essential nutrient in the body. With proper diet, hydration and exercise, the body can maintain an adequate supply of calcium, known as positive calcium balance. If there are not sufficient calcium stores to cover the body's needs, there is negative calcium balance; more calcium is required than is stored in the body.
Recommended Daily Allowance (RDA) versus Reference Daily Intakes (RDI): the RDAs, first established in the late 1960s, are the recommended intakes of nutrients, including vitamins and minerals for healthy people in the United States. The RDIs are based on the highest amount of vitamins and minerals recommended by the RDAs for adults.
Riboflavin: a B vitamin that is more stable than thiamin, utilized most efficiently when obtained from animal products, such as dairy and meat.
Scurvy: a deficiency disease of vitamin C; one of the first documented nutrient-deficiency diseases.
Sodium: an essential mineral, which, if consumed in excessive amounts, may be a causative factor in high blood pressure, fluid retention and kidney problems and cardiac-related issues.
St. John's wort: an herbal extract, known for its antidepressant properties.
Thiamin: a B vitamin that assists the body in obtaining energy from food
Toxicity: a level of intake at which injury occurs.
Vitamin C: also known as ascorbic acid.
Vitamin supplements: vitamins extracted from natural sources or synthesized in the laboratory, reduced to a pill form.
Water-soluble vitamins: compounds needed in the diet in small amounts to promote health that are soluble in body fluids, such as vitamin C and all the B vitamins
Zinc: an essential mineral, important for healthy circulation and eye health.

Whaddaya think?

1. Do you think you, personally, can get all the vitamin and minerals you need from your diet?
2. Why is milk considered a "complete" food?
3. Historically, why do you think people were afraid to eat raw foods?

4. Do you believe the story of how vitamin C was discovered? What's your take on it?
5. What type of food habits could result in vitamin D toxicity?
6. Suggest a one day menu that contains all the necessary B vitamins.
7. Suggest a two-day menu, rich enough in folic acid for a woman planning to start a family
8. What's the deal with vegans and B_{12}?
9. As few as they are, what are the redeeming nutrients found in a cheeseburger and shake meal?
10. How would you store fresh produce to maximize nutrient retention?
11. How would you prepare fresh produce to maximize nutrient retention?
12. How do you stay in positive calcium balance?
13. How would you stay in positive calcium balance without dairy products?
14. Make some suggestions on how to increase iron intake in preschool menus
15. Design a go-for-broke all nutrient dinner, including water- and fat-soluble vitamins, minerals, water, probiotics, and herbs.

Critical Application Exercises

1. Make a list of all the foods you've eaten in the past three days that contain fat- and water-soluble vitamins. How are you doing? Do you need to make any changes?
2. Explain to your employees who are always complaining about being too short of cash how they could save money by eating better and not buying so many vitamin supplements.
3. Design a short training program for your culinary staff. The objective is to enhance the vitamin and mineral content of your menus as much as possible.
4. Do a survey. Find out what types of herbal remedies your buddies believe in to promote health. Record your observations.

References

Koop-Hoolihan, L. (2000). "Prophylactic and Therapeutic Uses of Probiotics: A Review," *Journal of the American Dietetics Association*, February, 101: 2, pp. 229–231.

Neergaard, L., (2001). "New Vitamin Guidelines Confuse," *Los Angeles Times*, January 16, p. C3.

Preventing the Common Cold (1999). National Institute of Allergy and Infectious Disease, pamphlet, Bethedsa, Maryland.

Rubin, Karen (1992). "Everything You Should Know About Minerals," *Food Service Director Magazine*, March 15, 50:3, p. 92.

Rubin, Karen (2000). "Water-Soluble Vitamins: Their Role in Disease Prevention," *Food Service Director Magazine*, February 15, 50: 2, p. 70.

Squires, Sally (2000). "With More and More Supplements, It's Easy to Succumb to 'Vitamania.'" *Washington Post*, December 12, p. B25

Chapter 8

Nutrition and Activity

Chapter Overview

Energy Balance and How to Get There
- *Positive*
- *Negative*

Hunger
Satiety and Appetite
Calorie Needs and Use
- *Athletes*
- *Men and Women*

Ideal Body Weight
- *Calculations*

Body Fat Percentage
- *A BMI is Not a Sports Car*
- *Water Displacement*
- *Bioelectrical Impedance Analysis (BIA) and Air Displacement*

Obesity and Related Conditions
Weight Management
- *Dieting Theories*
- *Surgical Interventions*
- *Culinary Clues*
- *Super-Sizing*
- *Diet Revolutions*
- *High-Protein Diets*
  - *Dr. Atkins and Dr. Sears*
- *High-Carbohydrate Diets*
  - *Dr. Ornish*

Menu Planning for Athletes
- *Take a Pill, Run Faster?*

FYI: The Freshman Five or Fifteen

Chapter Objectives

After reading this chapter, the student should be able to:

1. *Contrast historical and modern theories of energy needs.*
2. *Explain why men and women have different energy needs.*
3. *Calculate an ideal body weight.*
4. *Compare hunger, appetite, and satiety.*
5. *Speculate as to which type of body fat percentage assessment procedure will be effective in different settings.*
6. *Discuss the effect of obesity on health.*
7. *Suggest methods for profitable food services without supersizing.*

8. *From a culinary and nutrition standpoint argue the pros and cons of high protein diets.*
9. *Plan a restaurant level menu using the Ornish plan as a guideline.*
10. *Suggest how to stock the pantry for a restaurant serving an Olympic running team.*

Introduction: Changing Theories on Energy Needs

So, how much do your favorite sports figures earn per year? Are their performances important? Do the food and beverage they choose impact their performance?

Twenty years ago, preparing breakfast for a college football team meant a dozen eggs, a pound of bacon, and one or two steaks for each player, with large pitchers of whole milk on the tables. Today it could mean egg white omelets filled with grilled vegetables, fresh fruit salad garnished with nuts, and whole-wheat muffins. My, how times have changed! We're seeing more and more endurance-sport athletes leaning towards a plant-based diet.

In this chapter we will discuss when and how much energy is needed and how to assess your energy intake. We'll figure out the difference between ***hunger*** *and* ***appetite*** *and how to balance the two. We'll determine various methods used to assess your overall fitness and some of the diet plans that claim they will get you there. We'll also explore ways to get your food service operation in tune with the latest diet plans and how to plan your menus accordingly.*

ENERGY BALANCE AND HOW TO GET THERE

Feeling and staying healthy is based in part on the amount and type of energy you shovel into your body. Sufficient amounts of the right type of energy will allow you to maintain all your systems in a great working manner.

Positive

Energy balance is what you are looking for. Energy intake is the relationship between energy intake (what you eat) and energy output (what you burn up). If energy in equals energy out, then you are in energy balance. This is a great state to be in. It means that you are eating just the right amount and type of food to maintain your weight and to perform all the tasks you want to do, which includes basic body functions, exercise, and day-to-day activities. If you take in more energy than you put out, then you are in **positive energy balance.** This means that your body can open a savings account in your liver and fatty pads (doesn't that sound attractive!) and that you will gain weight.

Positive energy balance is a good place to be if you are growing, as in childhood and adolescence, repairing, as in recovering from a broken leg or the flu, or during pregnancy. The body is able to call on the stored energy supplies as needed. Positive energy balance is not such a good thing if you are fully grown and in good health. Too much stored energy can lead to **obesity** and its related diseases, such as diabetes and heart disease.

Negative

If you take in fewer calories than you need, you'll be in **negative energy balance.** You'll see weight loss but may also feel tired and have depressed immunity, to name a few problems. The moral to the story is that the body likes to be in balance. Think of your body as a car. When all the fluid levels are correct, the oil and gas tank are filled with high-quality products and the belts are all properly tightened, then your engine just purrs along. Your body is the same way. It likes to stay in balance. An energy-balanced body will reward you with great performance. Selecting the correct amount of food, fluid, and exercise is the key.

Every person is in either negative or positive energy balance sometime throughout the day. After a good night's sleep, you are well-rested, but are very low in useable energy. You are in negative energy balance. Another example would be if you woke up too late to grab breakfast. It's now two o'clock in the afternoon and all you've had time for today was coffee. You'll be feeling the effects of negative energy balance, including headache, fatigue, and lack of energy. Just about everybody is in positive energy balance during the holiday season or after a big birthday dinner. Both types of energy imbalances are easily correctable.

If you are constantly in energy imbalance, you will see variations in weight and changes in energy levels you need to assess your intake to avoid these situations. Let's look at what tells you when and how much to eat.

HUNGER

So what makes you hungry or tells you to stop eating? Hunger (feed me) and **satiety** (okay, I'm full) are a real team effort, with different parts of the body reacting in different ways. When you're awake, if the stomach goes without food for three or four hours, it starts to contract, hence, the growling stomach. A part of your brain, the hypothalamus, gives you cues about when to stop and start eating. Being exposed to cold seems to trigger the hypothalamus to send out "eat" messages. This is a good survival instinct. When you eat, your metabolic rate increases, helping you to generate heat and also increase your fat stores that provide insulation. When protein, fat, and carbohydrate levels in the blood get too low, your liver sends messages to your brain to go on a search-and-seek mission.

There is an interesting connection, or non-connection, between tasting, salivating, chewing, swallowing . . . and satiety (a feeling of having eaten enough). Normally, when you eat, food passes through your esophagus into your stomach and small intestines. They become distended and send messages to your brain that say, "Enough already, turn it off!" This makes sense. However, research was done with people who had certain medical conditions that prevented food from entering the stomach, such as having a hole in the esophagus. These people chewed and swallowed food that never reached their stomach. They reported a feeling of fullness and a sense of satiety. Just goes to show you how intricately the different parts of your body are interwoven. It also means don't wolf down your food. If your body doesn't get a chance to register that you've eaten, you'll never feel satiated. This will result in overeating, which will result in excess weight gain and the whole ball of wax that entails.

SATIETY AND APPETITE

Just to add some extra factors when it comes to eating, there is the concept of "appetite." Appetite has very little to do with physiological sensations of hunger. Appetite has to do with the psychology of hunger. To put it another way, hunger is a basic, physical response to the need for fuel. Appetite has to do with nonphysical responses to eating, such as your mood, the time of day and your cultural background. If you eat when you are not physically hungry, then you are responding to your appetite. That extra slice of pizza or that dessert you thought you were too full to eat are examples of appetite. Appetite can be related to cultural background and to social "rules." For example, many people think "cold, sweet cereal" when they head for the breakfast table. If they are met with barbecued ribs, although they are physically hungry, their psychological appetite says "no way."

Appetite can be taught. You've heard of **behavior modification.** Small children are told "finish your broccoli and you can have dessert" or "sit quietly for 15 minutes and I'll give you a cookie." Both examples teach children to respond to appetite, not hunger. Child psychologists and nutritionists will tell you that food is not a good reward. Remember that when you promise yourself a pint of ice cream if you can just finish reading this chapter.

CALORIE NEEDS AND USE

Once you've figured out the right amount of calories to keep you in energy balance, it's always interesting to know how those calories are being used. Since adults can take in anywhere from 1,200 to 2,500 calories per day, it's obvious from looking at energy expenditure tables that most people are not burning the majority of their calories from exercising.

Athletes

Energy needs increase when the outside temperature is extremely hot or cold, when you have a fever, if you drink caffeinated beverages or smoke, if you are pregnant or if you have a very **lean body mass** (like an Olympic runner). Some medications and some medical conditions can also increase energy needs. As you get older, your energy needs decrease; this is just a natural aging process. When you sleep, your energy needs go down.

Men and Women

Mother Nature designed it so that women have less energy needs than men do. This is related in part to the ratio of lean muscle tissue to fatty tissue. Lean muscle uses more energy than fatty tissue. Put another way, women have less muscle than men do. This does not mean that all women are fat, or that women athletes are not muscular. It just means that ratio-wise, women are less able to "bulk" up the muscles. This relates to childbearing and the energy

Table 8–1 Feel the Burn

The table below gives you an idea of approximately how many calories you can burn during various activities

Gym Activities					
	Approximate Calories Burned Per Hour				
Activity	100 lb. Person	125 lb. Person	150 lb. Person	175 lb. Person	200 lb. Person
Aerobics, Step: high impact	480	600	720	840	960
Aerobics, Step: low impact	336	420	504	588	672
Aerobics: high impact	336	420	504	588	672
Aerobics: low impact	264	330	396	462	528
Aerobics: water	192	240	288	336	384
Bicycling: 12–13.9 mph	384	480	576	672	768
Bicycling: 14–15.9 mph	480	600	720	840	960
Bicycling: 16–19 mph	576	720	864	1008	1152
Bicycling: > 20 mph	792	990	1188	1386	1584
Bicycling: BMX/mountain	408	510	612	714	816
Bicycling, Stationery: moderate	336	420	504	588	672
Bicycling, Stationery: vigorous	504	630	756	882	1008
Bowling	144	180	216	252	288
Calisthenics: moderate	216	270	324	378	432
Calisthenics: vigorous	384	480	576	672	768
Circuit Training: general	384	480	576	672	768
Elliptical Trainer: general	432	540	648	756	864
Gardening: general	216	270	324	378	432
Golf: carrying clubs	264	330	396	462	528
Golf: using cart	168	210	252	294	336
Gymnastics: general	192	240	288	336	384
Handball: general	576	720	864	1008	1152
Heavy Cleaning: car, windows	216	270	324	378	432
Hiking: cross-country	288	360	432	504	576
Hockey: field & ice	384	480	576	672	768
Ice Skating: general	336	420	504	588	672
Kayaking	240	300	360	420	480
Moving: carrying boxes	336	420	504	588	672
Mowing Lawn: push, hand	264	330	396	462	528
Mowing Lawn: push, power	216	270	324	378	432
Operate Snow Blower: walking	216	270	324	378	432
Racquetball: casual	336	420	504	588	672
Racquetball: competitive	480	600	720	840	960
Raking Lawn	192	240	288	336	384
Rollerblade Skating	336	420	504	588	672
Rope Jumping	480	600	720	840	960
Rowing, Stationery: moderate	336	420	504	588	672
Rowing, Stationery: vigorous	408	510	612	714	816
Running: 6 min/mile	792	990	1188	1386	1584
Running: 7 min/mile	696	870	1044	1218	1392

Gym Activities

Activity	Approximate Calories Burned Per Hour 100 lb. Person	125 lb. Person	150 lb. Person	175 lb. Person	200 lb. Person
Running: 8 min/mile	600	750	900	1050	1200
Running: 9 min/mile	528	660	792	924	1056
Running: 10 min/mile	480	600	720	840	960
Running: 11.5 min/mile	432	540	648	756	864
Running: 12 min/mile	384	480	576	672	768
Scuba or skin diving	336	420	504	588	672
Shoveling Snow: by hand	288	360	432	504	576
Sitting: reading or watching T.V.	54	68	81	95	108
Skateboarding	240	300	360	420	480
Ski Machine: general	456	570	684	798	912
Skiing: cross-country	384	480	576	672	768
Skiing: downhill	288	360	432	504	576
Sleeping	30	38	45	53	60
Snow Shoeing	384	480	576	672	768
Stair Step Machine: general	288	360	432	504	576
Stretching, Hatha Yoga	192	240	288	336	384
Swimming: backstroke	384	480	576	672	768
Swimming: breaststroke	480	600	720	840	960
Swimming: butterfly	528	660	792	924	1056
Swimming: crawl	528	660	792	924	1056
Swimming: general	288	360	432	504	576
Swimming: laps, vigorous	480	600	720	840	960
Swimming: treading, vigorous	480	600	720	840	960
Tennis: general	336	420	504	588	672
Walk/Jog: jog <10 min.	288	360	432	504	576
Walk: 13 min/mi	240	300	360	420	480
Walk: 15 min/mi	216	270	324	378	432
Walk: 17 min/mi	192	240	288	336	384
Water Polo	480	600	720	840	960
Water Skiing	288	360	432	504	576
Weight Lifting: general	144	180	216	252	288
Weight Lifting: vigorous	288	360	432	504	576

efficiency needed to do it. We may live in the modern world, but our bodies and metabolism are still living in a cave.

This still does not account for all the calories you take in every day. Even the hardest physical labor or the toughest sports don't account for the 2,000 calories of the average adult intake. It may not seem like it, but you've got a pretty high maintenance engine going there. About 60 percent of all the calories you eat go to basic physiological functions, such as breathing, keeping your heart beating and your blood circulating, your eyes blinking, digesting and absorbing food, eliminating waste products, maintaining the correct body temperature and keeping muscles toned (we're not talking biceps here, we're talking muscles in places like the lungs or the small intestine). Another 30 percent is used for physical activity, like walking, chewing, speaking, and oh yes, working and going to the gym. The remaining 10 percent is the amount of heat you burn by processing food. It takes energy to break popcorn down into glucose and sushi into amino acids. If you want to get fancy about it, this is called the "thermic effect of food."

IDEAL BODY WEIGHT

Weight, weight, weight. An **ideal body weight** is the weight at which you feel your best with consideration given for your height, bone structure, and muscle development at age 25. Where your weight is in reference to your ideal weight is often used as a health check, because it can be done quickly and easily and does not require complicated equipment.

Calculations

If you promise not to faint, we'll tell you how to figure out your ideal weight. For women, you get 100 pounds for your first five feet of height. For every additional inch, you get 3 pounds. For men, you get 105 pounds for the first feet of height and then 5 pounds for each additional inch of height. To create a weight range, you add or subtract 10 percent. So, a woman who is 5 feet, 3 inches should weigh somewhere around 115 pounds, with the range for a 5-foot, 3-inch woman between 103 to 126 pound. A 5-foot, 7-inch guy would have an ideal body weight of 140 pounds, with a range of 136 to 144 pounds. After figuring out your ideal weight, how many of you just need to be taller?

A very fast, but not terribly accurate way to figure out approximately how many calories you need per day is to add "zero" to your desired weight. For example, if you wanted to weigh 120 pounds, you would need approximately 1,200 calories per day. This is a very, very rough estimate and does not take into consideration lifestyle, medical condition, etc. It's just a convenient way to "guestimate" about where your calorie intake should be every day.

BODY FAT PERCENTAGE

Why are men and women's weight and calorie needs calculated differently? Because men and women differ in muscle mass and in energy needs. Women tend to be smaller than men and, pound for pound, have less muscle mass. This means that women should be lighter in weight and should require fewer calories. The less muscle you have and, really, the less body you've got, the less energy you should require. Oh, that it were so! Remember the difference between hunger and appetite. Although a woman might "feel" she needs the same portions of food at mealtimes, the reality of the situation is that a 70-inch woman, no matter how lean she is, still requires less energy to run her body than a 70-inch man does. The man has many more square inches of muscle to fuel and probably has a bit less fatty tissue. Mother Nature's cruel joke, but women must deal with it.

Many different techniques measure just what type of shape you are in. Most scientific techniques attempt to ascertain what percentage you are fat. Since excess fat can lead to poor health condition, scientists and health professionals have tried for years to measure a person's body fat. There are lots of different methods, some involving being immersed in a tank of water, others involving electrodes.

A BMI Is Not a Sports Car

The **BMI,** or **body mass index,** only involves a ruler, a scale, and a chart. Remember that simply weighing someone does not really give a good picture of what condition they are in, since the percent of fat to muscle is not known.

The BMI is more useful than a height-for-weight chart. You're familiar with those charts. You look up your height and then see what you're supposed to weigh. That's okay, but does not take into account how much of you is muscle, and, more importantly, how much is fat. What you weigh is not as important as how much of you are fat. Why? Because muscle equals healthy living, and fat equals risk of high blood pressure, diabetes, cancer, circulatory diseases, and other undesirable things. Consider this another way. A person who includes weight-lifting, skiing, and swimming in his or her regular exercise program will probably be mostly lean muscle. And that person will probably show up as **overweight** on a height-for-weight chart, as muscle is denser and weighs more than fat.

The BMI has ranges for height and takes other factors into consideration. Another perk of the BMI is that it can be used for all ages. Other charts, such as insurance tables, are geared specifically to adults or children.

See Table 8–2 for a BMI chart or go to *www.shapeup.org//sua/bmi/chart.htm* for "Shape Up America's" BMI Chart. Shape Up America is a cooperative effort between the federal government, local agencies and national spokespeople to get Americans off their butts and onto the exercise arena. Locate your height and then your weight. Look to the top of the chart for your BMI. A BMI of 25 is usually considered to show a healthy weight, 25 to 30 is considered overweight and over 30 shows obesity. If you're not into charts, Figure 8–2 shows the way to calculate your BMI.

Water Displacement

Okay, so you don't want this wimpy pen and paper measurement stuff. You want to measure fat and other assorted stuff like the science guys do. You're absolutely right. Body composition isn't just about weight. What you're really looking for is the amount of lean body mass (think: muscles, tissues, and organs) versus the amount of body fat. Health is not so much about total weight as it is how much muscle and how little fat you have. You can guestimate that on paper, but you really need to do some physical tests to get an accurate answer.

First you find yourself a *big* container of water. **Water displacement measurement** is a fairly common way to calculate body density. Body density is the body mass divided by the body volume. Fat and lean tissues have different densities. By using one of those magic formulas that scientists have,

Table 8–2 Body Mass Index Table

	Normal							Overweight				Obese					
BMI	*19*	*20*	*21*	*22*	*23*	*24*	*25*	*26*	*27*	*28*	*29*	*30*	*31*	*32*	*33*	*34*	*35*
Height (inches)	Body Weight (pounds)																
58	91	96	100	105	110	115	119	124	129	134	138	143	148	153	158	162	167
59	94	99	104	109	114	119	124	128	133	138	143	148	153	158	163	168	173
60	97	102	107	112	118	123	128	133	138	143	148	153	158	163	168	174	179
61	100	106	111	116	122	127	132	137	143	148	153	158	164	169	174	180	185
62	104	109	115	120	126	131	136	142	147	153	158	164	169	175	180	186	191
63	107	113	118	124	130	135	141	146	152	158	163	169	175	180	186	191	197
64	110	116	122	128	134	140	145	151	157	163	169	174	180	186	192	197	204
65	114	120	126	132	138	144	150	156	162	168	174	180	186	192	198	204	210
66	118	124	130	136	142	148	155	161	167	173	179	186	192	198	204	210	216
67	121	127	134	140	146	153	159	166	172	178	185	191	198	204	211	217	223
68	125	131	138	144	151	158	164	171	177	184	190	197	203	210	216	223	230
69	128	135	142	149	155	162	169	176	182	189	196	203	209	216	223	230	236
70	132	139	146	153	160	167	174	181	188	195	202	209	216	222	229	236	243
71	136	143	150	157	165	172	179	186	193	200	208	215	222	229	236	243	250
72	140	147	154	162	169	177	184	191	199	206	213	221	228	235	242	250	258
73	144	151	159	166	174	182	189	197	204	212	219	227	235	242	250	257	265
74	148	155	163	171	179	186	194	202	210	218	225	233	241	249	256	264	272
75	152	160	168	176	184	192	200	208	216	224	232	240	248	256	264	272	279
76	156	164	172	180	189	197	205	213	221	230	238	246	254	263	271	279	287

Source: Adapted from *Clinical Guidelines on the Identification, Evaluation, and Treatment of Overweight and Obesity in Adults: The Evidence Report. www.nhlbi.nih.gov*

if you know a person's volume and weight, you can calculate the ratio of fat to lean. Once you've done that, you can figure out how healthy a person's body composition is. Women should look for body fat percentages from 20 to 25 and men should look for 12 to 25 percent fat. Anything over 25 percent should set off an alarm that hypertension, diabetes, and heart disease could be waiting in the wings. Water displacement weighing uses the above-water

1. Divide your weight (in pounds) by your height (in inches).
2. Divide your answer from #1 by your height (in inches).
3. Multiply your answer from #2 by 703. This is your BMI. For good health, it should be 25 or under.

For example: if you are 5 feet 3 inches (63 inches) and weigh 110 pounds:

1. $110 \div 63 = 1.746$
2. $1.746 \div 63 = 0.0277$
3. $0.0277 \times 703 = 19.4$ BMI

Figure 8–1 Figuring Your BMI

Table 8–2 Body Mass Index Table

				Extreme Obesity														
36	*37*	*38*	*39*	*40*	*41*	*42*	*43*	*44*	*45*	*46*	*47*	*48*	*49*	*50*	*51*	*52*	*53*	*54*
Height (inches)				Body Weight (pounds)														
172	177	181	186	191	196	201	205	210	215	220	224	229	234	239	244	248	253	258
178	183	188	193	198	203	208	212	217	222	227	232	237	242	247	252	257	262	267
184	189	194	199	204	209	215	220	225	230	235	240	245	250	255	261	266	271	276
190	195	201	206	211	217	222	227	232	238	243	248	254	259	264	269	275	280	285
196	202	207	213	218	224	229	235	240	246	251	256	262	267	273	278	284	289	295
203	208	214	220	225	231	237	242	248	254	259	265	270	278	282	287	293	299	304
209	215	221	227	232	238	244	250	256	262	267	273	279	285	291	296	302	308	314
216	222	228	234	240	246	252	258	264	270	276	282	288	294	300	306	312	318	324
223	229	235	241	247	253	260	266	272	278	284	291	297	303	309	315	322	328	334
230	236	242	249	255	261	268	274	280	287	293	299	306	312	319	325	331	338	344
236	243	249	256	262	269	276	282	289	295	302	308	315	322	328	335	341	348	354
243	250	257	263	270	277	284	291	297	304	311	318	324	331	338	345	351	358	365
250	257	264	271	278	285	292	299	306	313	320	327	334	341	348	355	362	369	376
257	265	272	279	286	293	301	308	315	322	329	338	343	351	358	365	372	379	386
265	272	279	287	294	302	309	316	324	331	338	346	353	361	368	375	383	390	397
272	280	288	295	302	310	318	325	333	340	348	355	363	371	378	386	393	401	408
280	287	295	303	311	319	326	334	342	350	358	365	373	381	389	396	404	412	420
287	295	303	311	319	327	335	343	351	359	367	375	383	391	399	407	415	423	431
295	304	312	320	328	336	344	353	361	369	377	385	394	402	410	418	426	435	443

weight, the submerged weight and the amount of water displaced during submersion. You don your bathing suit and are lowered on a scale that resembles a receiving scale for meat, into a special tank. You have to exhale completely, hold your breath and remain motionless while you are completely submerged. The measurement lasts as long as it takes for the scale to be steady and the water to be still. As you can imagine, this technique is not for everybody.

Bioelectrical Impedance Analysis (BIA) and Air Analysis Displacement

Two dry techniques are also available, although fairly expensive. Bioelectrical impedance analysis (BIA) looks something like an EKG measurement. Electrodes are placed on the ankles and wrists. The way electrical current bounces off various parts of your body shows the technician how much fat and lean tissue you have. Lean tissue conducts electric current very well while fat stops, or impedes, electrical current. Some gyms and health centers offer BIA analysis. We enjoyed watching an air displacement measurement in the **BodPod.** The BodPod is a chamber of a known volume of air. The victim, we mean the person, is sealed in the BodPod for a minute or two and air displacement, rather than water displacement is measured. Both BIA and air displacements are a lot easier to perform and in which to participate.

There's always lots of speculation about the causes of obesity. Some say genetics, others say environment, and others say not enough pushing away from the table. Here are some current thoughts:

1. Soda: A British study concluded that the more soda children drank, the more they increased their chances of becoming obese, regardless of activity level, TV watching, or even initial body weight.
2. Mom: children who's mothers had gestational diabetes (diabetes only during pregnancy) tended to become obese later in life. It's thought that this could be because of high levels of fetal sugar exposure.
3. Genes: Just can't seem to beat 'em. For example, the level of leptin, a hormone that tells you "you're full" could be a genetic thing. If you lack the chromosome that tells you to produce leptin, then you might overeat because of poor signaling.
4. TV: people who watched more than five hours of television per day were more likely to become obese.
5. Hormones: women with syndromes associated with high levels of testosterone are usually obese.

Figure 8–2 Current Theories on the Cause of Increased Obesity

Why all this thought and discussion on weight? Because, unfortunately, the world is getting bigger, and we mean around the waist, not around the ocean. As food technology improves the availability of products, the citizens of industrialized nations go up in belt and dress sizes. Obesity, formally an issue with the over-forty set, has inched its way down to very young children. Being overweight, or more specifically over-fat, brings with it all types of health issues. Diabetes, high blood pressure, heart, kidney and liver disease, and certain types of cancer have been linked to obesity.

OBESITY AND RELATED CONDITIONS

Of course, there's overweight and then there's overweight. Actually, "overweight" is thought to be anyone who has a BMI of 25 to 30 or is 10 to 20 percent over ideal body weight. Someone is considered to be obese if their BMI is over 30 or they are over 20 percent above ideal body weight. Someone is considered to be morbidly obese if they are over 100 percent of their ideal body weight. Morbid obesity is just what it sounds like. A body carrying around so much excess fat to the point where it is life-threatening.

> FOOD FOR THE MIND
>
> Four calories per gram in all carbohydrates
>
> Four calories per gram in all proteins
>
> Nine calories per gram in all fats
>
> Seven calories per gram in all alcohol

On the other side of the scale (pun intended), there are people who are underweight. "Underweight" is thought to be anyone who is 15 to 20 percent below his or her ideal body weight. Although much less common than overweight, underweight carries its own set of problems, such as decreased ability to fight off disease and poor growth (for children). Plain and simple, the body likes to be in balance, not too much and not too little.

Personalize your own trendy diet, by selecting one from each of the categories: (Note: Following this diet may result in heart disease, high blood pressure, diabetes, loss of bladder and bowel control, stroke or liver damage, but, what the heck, you'll look great!)

1. YOU CAN LOSE UP TO:
   10 pounds   20 pounds   30 pounds   most of your body weight
2. IN
   just two days   just five days   the time it takes to read this
3. WITH THE UNBELIEVABLE
   low carb   high carb   low and high carb   no carb   all carb
4. DIET!!!! ALL YOU NEED IS
   lots of money   lots of laxatives   only minutes a day   total ignorance
5. YOUR SPECIAL DIET FORMULA HAS
   an amazing amount of sugar so you'll always feel good   chemicals that have been used by some countries for chemical warfare   a form of rat poison   don't ask
6. DEVELOPED BY
   a group of disgruntled home economists   someone who flunked freshman chemistry—twice   former drug smugglers   several fraternities
7. SO SEND
   lots of U.S. currency   for our amazingly upbeat factless video   your brother-in-law Ralph
8. AND JOIN THE
   thousands   millions   one remaining person without medical damage
9. WHO HAVE BEEN
   hospitalized   damaged beyond repair   fled the country
10. BY THE AMAZING
   pseudo-diet   scam parading as a health plan   snake-oil copy

Figure 8–3 The Super-Fantastic, Lose-All-the-Weight-You-Want-Overnight Trendy Diet

WEIGHT MANAGEMENT

Weight gain or loss can be aggravating or scary, depending on the circumstances. Sudden weight loss can be a symptom of diabetes mellitus and some cancers, but can also mean you are not eating sufficient calories. Sudden weight gain can be an indicator of some types of heart disease or cancers, or it means you've been eating more calories than you can use. You know how you eat and what you need.

Calories in equals calories out. Period. No magic. It takes about **3,500 calories** to lose or gain a pound. That means 3,500 calories per week (7 days × 500 calories per day) must be cut out to lose a pound a week or 3,500 calories added to gain a pound. Makes you wonder about those "miracle" diet plans that promise a twenty-pound weight loss in a weekend. Do the math.

As we've just said, overweight or underweight is not desirable. Your body likes to operate like a well-oiled machine, with perfect calibration. If you are underweight, you may have problems fighting off infections and illnesses. If your body has to use all its energy just to get the basic systems running, it won't have reserves to assist in warding off bacteria and viruses.

Overweight can bring on diabetes, high blood pressure, and heart disease, and puts undue strain on your back, legs, and circulatory system. You wouldn't try to get top performance out of your car by adding sandbags to the trunk! Overweight people are not necessarily well-nourished. They may still suffer from vitamin and mineral deficiencies. Why and how is that possible? Just because you eat a lot of food doesn't mean you eat foods that contain the nutrients you need. Let's face it, very few people gain too much weight overeating fresh fruit salad, baked sweet potatoes, or grilled vegetables. Cookies, beer, hot dogs, and chocolate cake all may taste great, but have very little nutrition.

So how is it that some people can chow down fifteen times a day and some people only have to look at food to gain weight? There are many theories about the cause of obesity. Some theories look at heredity and genes, some look at social influences and others look at anything from evolution to blood type. We don't really know what predisposes some people to obesity. What we do know is that obesity is dangerous.

This brings us to weight management. There are lots and lots of weight loss systems available today. Some are self-help books and products, some are counselor-driven, some are done under medical supervision and some are run like a twelve-step recovery program. There is no one system that works for everyone. Some of these weight management programs are based on good science and firm nutrition theories and some are based on—well, we're not sure what they're based on. Remember that weight loss is a long-term commitment and any successful plan will include behavioral changes, eating pattern and menu selection changes and physical activities.

Weight management is not just for people who are overweight. People who are chronically underweight have to make a conscious effort to maintain weight. Weight gain may be difficult for people with chronic medical conditions. If you don't feel good, you don't feel like eating. Drug therapy may interfere with the ability or the desire to eat or may interfere with the body's ability to absorb nutrients. Psychological or emotional stress may contribute to weight loss or weight gain, depending on the individual.

Dieting Theories

Maintaining a good weight is a lifelong program. The reason fast weight loss programs don't help people to keep weight off for extended periods of time are because they don't teach people anything. You can restrict your calories for several weeks and lose weight. When you return to your "normal" eating pattern, the one that helped you gain the weight in the first place, your body says, "All right! now we're home!" and goes right back to putting extra calories, translated into fat, into all the nooks and crannies in your body.

Some people have a cycle of losing weight, gaining it back, and then losing it again. This is called **"yo-yo" dieting**. After a while, it becomes almost impossible for a yo-yo dieter to lose weight. The body becomes so efficient at saving the calories it's given that you can't restrict calories to a low enough level to lose weight. The body says "I don't know if you're starving me or fattening me up this week, so I'm not taking any chances. I'm saving all the calories I can" (Rosenfeld, 4) (Rubin, 5).

Surgical Interventions

People who are morbidly obese, people who may need to lose one hundred pounds or more, sometimes use a technique commonly called "stomach stapling." You do not need the entire area of your stomach to function normally. In stomach stapling, a portion of the stomach is surgically partitioned, so that food cannot reach it. This effectively reduces the size of the stomach, making you feel fuller faster. People who have had stomach stapling must reduce their intake, as they have a reduced capacity. If they overeat they suffer great discomfort, including severe cramps, vomiting and diarrhea. Nutrition counseling is recommended for people who undergo stomach stapling, as they must learn how to eat to maintain a correct weight.

Maintaining a proper weight has become a national issue. Everyone seems to be discussing it and doing something about it (Squires, 6).

Culinary Clues

If you work or go to school in the culinary field, then tasting is inevitable. For some reason, people tend to taste-test the hollandaise sauce and the paté more than the seasonal fruit salad. For this reason, more and more culinary students and professionals have become interested in fitness.

The Culinary Institute of America (CIA) at Hyde Park (New York) recently built a nine-million-dollar recreation center, ironically just five hundred yards from the pastry kitchens. Students and faculty can attend "butt and gut" workout classes or create their own exercise regimen. Johnson and Wales University (Rhode Island) has also opened a recreation center on its culinary campus. Both schools require students to attend stress management and fitness classes (*Los Angeles Times*, 1).

1. Use low-fat cooking methods (see Chapter 4).
2. Avoid extreme calorie restrictions. Don't skip meals or fast.
3. Eat at least 1,200 calories per day. Balance, with 60 percent CHO.
4. Lose weight slowly, one or two pounds per week, remember, 3,500 calories/pound.
5. Select a diet that fits your lifestyle and food preferences. Plan for special events.
6. Exercise! At least thirty minutes most days.
7. Be realistic. Look at your body type and heredity.
8. Forget the scale; weigh yourself once a week at most.
9. Reward yourself with something other than food!

Figure 8–4 Experts' Suggestions For Permanent Weight Loss

Many universities and community colleges offer culinary arts majors. As part of their general education requirements, all students must take a certain number of physical education classes. Culinary employers are getting into the fitness idea. Many companies are offering culinary staff and employees fitness center memberships as part of their benefits package. Where available, staff and employees are being encouraged to take advantage of on-site exercise facilities.

CIA had always been interested in health, but from nutrition, not an exercise standpoint. The St. Andrew's Café, opened in 1986, is an on-campus restaurant and training classroom offering four course meals that contain 1,200 calories or less. CIA students knew they needed more than healthy cooking and pushed for fitness facilities.

The old philosophy was "never trust a skinny cook." Not so true today. Culinarians are learning that running marathons and making a mousse are not mutually exclusive.

Chefs all over the country are aware of the need to watch the scales. Diane Forley, the chef owner of Verbena, in New York, says she makes a conscious decision to be aware of everything she eats. She realized that most people who work in restaurants don't sit down to proper meals, but "grab and graze." Forley eats a regular breakfast and avoids snacking in the kitchen while she is working. She tries to carbo-load rather than eating a lot of meats. She makes time to exercise three times a week.

Scott Cohen, chef of Las Carnarias restaurant in San Antonio, Texas, lost a good friend several years ago. This got him thinking—and losing weight. Cohen found that he didn't overeat that much on the job. Rather, he found he and his fellow chefs overate more after hours. They ate and drank too much after work in order to relax and unwind. Now he exercises, goes to nutrition counselor, eats less, rather than a complicated diet, focuses on times of day he's eating, and tries not to eat four to six hours before bed. He cites as a reason that he wants to be there to see his kids grow up.

Mark Strausman, Campagna, New York, lost seventy-five pounds by learning when and how to eat. He constructed an eating plan that resembled a diabetic diet, using the Exchange Lists for Meal Planning. He's kept his weight off by biking. His motivation? "I don't want to die" (Parseghian, 3).

On the other hand, it seems as if some portions of the food industry are trying to make weight loss pretty difficult.

Super-Sizing

"Would you like to super-size that?" is a common question at fast-food outlets and convenience store food counters. We live in a wonderful world, where fifty cents can increase your meal from 1,000 to 2,000 calories and beyond.

Super-sizing is an excellent merchandising tool. **A National Restaurant Association (NRA)** survey indicated that customers feel like they're getting "real value" and "more for their money" when they **super-size.** These feelings will bring customers back for more and more and more. The NRA survey also showed that super-sizing accounted for about one-third of sales on certain items, such as French fries, beverages, and sandwiches (Lempert, 2).

The food-service industry knows that customers appreciate and search out bargains and good deals. Look through newspapers and magazines or listen to radio advertisements for the multitude of two-for-one meals or beverages, get a free (fill in the blank) with the purchase of a meal, and "all you can eat" offers.

Although many offers encourage the scarfing of more calories than are needed, super-sizing really helps tilt the scales. We can delude ourselves that customers will choose free soup or baked potato or will select wisely from a buffet. But super-sizing pinpoints the fat, sugar, and empty calorie items. It's the world we live in. After all, how "sexy" does this sound: Super-size your green salad, sir?

See Chapter 4 for a discussion on the link between childhood obesity and the increase of Type 2 diabetes. Too many calories, especially from fat and sugar, help to put on the pounds and keep them there. It takes 500 extra calories a day to gain a pound a week, using the calculation of 3,500 calories contained in one pound. It's been estimated that most Americans are eating at least 200 extra calories a day. That translates into about a weight gain of about fifteen to eighteen pounds per year. And its not just the cosmetics of fat we're concerned about but also the increased risk of heart disease, high blood pressure, stroke, gallbladder disease, and certain cancers.

So, a 16-ounce glass of cola has about 200 calories and about 45 grams of sugar. The 32-ounce super-size version whomps up to 400 calories and about 95 grams of sugar. Do the French fry math. An average order of fast food French fries has about 350 calories and about 16 grams of fat. Supersize that and you can get up to 600 calories and 30 grams of fat. Just as a reference, an average, moderately active adult male should eat about 2,500 calories and 85 grams of fat. An average, moderately active adult female should have about 1,800 calories and 60 grams of fat. Better enjoy that super scoop of fries as they contain one-third to one-half of most people's fat needs for the day.

Fast-food dessert fares no better. No, that baked apple pie does not count as one of your five daily serving of fruit. But it does add to your calories and fat. One of those innocent-looking pies has about 250 calories and 14 grams of fat.

Serving sizes are a tricky business. People's perception of what they eat is usually quite different from what they actually eat. This works with both more and less. Anorexic patients tend to overestimate what they ate, listing a half sandwich as a "feast." Healthy or overweight people tend to underestimate their intake. Estimates of portion sizes tend to be a combination of social background, degree of hunger, time of day eating, food packaging suggestions, and restaurant-size servings.

Those spoilsports known as nutritionists and dietitians suggest guidelines that most people tend to disregard (or disdain). A serving of meat should be no bigger than a deck of cards. Entrée plates should be equally divided into thirds, with one third for vegetables, one-third for carbohydrates, and one third for the entrée. You get the idea. For more details, you can check *www.eatright.org* (the American Dietetic Association's site) or *www.aicr.org* (the American Institute for Cancer Research's site). Both sites go into detail about portion sizes.

Until customers start to accept an extra glass of juice or a bunch of grapes as a super-size option, you face a conundrum. If you offer healthy serving sizes, customers don't feel they're getting value for their money. If you super-size portions, then you're contributing to the "larding" of America.

This puts the culinarian in an awkward position. Value marketing, such as super sizing, seems to be what the customer wants. But the customer also seems to want healthy meals as well.

Diet Revolutions

While this book was being written, one out of five Americans was overweight. The diet industry is a billion-dollar industry at this point, one of the largest sectors in the food industry. At least 50 percent of women and 25 percent of men are trying to lose weight at any one time, but only 10 percent keep it off for over a year. Why the weight regain?

We've mentioned the "yo-yo" effect of dieting. Your body is efficient and learns to extract every calorie it can from the food you give it. If you go on starvation cycles, the body craves high fat to replace lost body fat.

What's worse is that the body redeposits fat in the abdominal area (stomach) when it can. Fat above the waist is easier to lose than fat below the waist. This is simple physics. Your heart has to pump blood to all areas of the body. Gravity helps the heart with the distribution of fluid. Anything above the heart is more work, as it makes the heart work against gravity. Anything below the heart requires less work. You've probably known someone who is dieting. The first noticeable place they lose weight is usually in their face. The body works from the top down, getting rid of the weight in areas that require more work to maintain. So, if there is extra fat, the body is going to deposit it below the waist, where it doesn't require so much work. You thought you had a choice where you lost your weight? Think again. There is no such thing as "spot" reducing.

So is all hope lost? Should we just give up? Don't be ridiculous! Remember the basic tenet of weight—calories in equals calories out. You have to come up with a plan that you can follow, with allowable exceptions, for the rest of your life that allows for the right amount of calories for you. Look at how and what you like to eat and work with that to devise a comfortable eating plan.

Behavior changes with regular exercise and a healthy lower-fat diet are what have been found to work over the long haul. You'll be watching for fat, not calories. Low-fat diets are more effective than low-calorie diets. Foods with less fat have fewer calories! Counting calories and depriving yourself are not as effective as eating more of lower-fat foods. In other words, have the pizza. Rather than saying you're only "allowed" one-half slice of a sausage and pepperoni pizza, how about "allowing yourself" three slices of a vegetarian pizza, heaped with three kinds of peppers, four kinds of mushrooms and some olives. Remember the whole satiety and hunger thing. If you feel full, you'll feel satisfied and more likely to continue on the plan. Anyway, let's get real: Who's going to eat a half slice of pizza?

High-Protein Diets

Cheeseburgers, hold the bun? Steak and potatoes hold the potatoes? BLTs, hold the L, T, and the toast? Is this any way to diet? The biggest diet books of the last decade preach the gospel of bacon, hold the pasta. Dr. Robert Atkins created a "diet revolution" and *Sugar Busters,* and *Protein Power* all preached the power of high-protein, high-fat, low-carbohydrate, low-sugar diets. With an **Atkins-style diet,** you eliminate almost all fruit, vegetables, grains, breads, pastas, cereal, and starches, and you eat mostly meat, fish, poultry, eggs, and dairy products. Review protein digestion and the concept of "ketoacidosis" to understand the high-protein concept (Turner, 7).

Yes, eating out is much more fun when you're on a high-protein diet. Steak houses and hotels are offering "Atkins" menus to attract more clientele. It's much easier for the food-service staff to serve a bacon-wrapped steak, hold the potato, than it is to create an interesting seasonal vegetable grill with quinoa pilaf served on a tomato and pepper reduction.

In the short-term, there is weight loss on a high-protein diet. There is also ketoacidosis, as your unleaded body attempts to burn leaded fuel. Depending on genetics and lifestyle, in the long-term there could be **arteriosclerosis,** high blood pressure, diabetes, and heart disease. The weight loss is mostly artificial. Carbohydrates hold onto water. If you don't have any carbohydrates, you hold onto less water. Eating fat makes you less hungry and eventually you may reduce the amount of food you are eating every day. In the end, the pounds come back, as no one can maintain this eating style over the long run.

Some people attempt to lose weight by eating only once a day. People who eat only once a day have a very low resting metabolism. This means they need fewer calories. Their body has adapted to the idea that it won't be getting very much, so it reduces its needs. Their metabolism rises after each meal to burn calories. Unfortunately, they probably also find themselves with very little energy, as their blood sugar levels are so low for most of the day. It would be almost impossible to get all the nutrients needed at one meal a day. If people following this eating pattern ever decided to eat several times a day, they'd see a weight gain, as their bodies would store all the extra, unneeded energy.

The moral to the diet story is that different people will need different weight-loss diets and pattern. Remember that weight loss is lifetime gig. There are no "quick fix" diets that continue to work over time. Dietary regimes need to be continued over a lifetime.

So, why do these "miracle" diets work at all? Although they get at it in different ways, all these diets require that certain foods be eliminated or reduced, which means that, by hook or by crook, calorie intakes are reduced. But once calories or the eliminated foods are returned to the daily intake, the pounds also return.

High-protein, high-fat, and low-carbohydrate diets, such as Dr. Atkins's diet or the Zone diet have gotten very popular. As we've said previously, the theory behind a high-protein, low-carbohydrate diet is that eating carbohydrates triggers the body to release insulin to help in using up the carbohydrates. If too many carbohydrates are eaten, then the body will overproduce insulin and insulin tells the body to store extra energy as fat. Dr. Atkins take on this is to have people eliminate carbohydrates from the diet, forcing the body to look to protein and fat for energy. Your body is not designed to do this very efficiently, so it has to work harder (translation: burn more calories).

Dr. Atkins and Dr. Sears

Lots of people lose weight on the Atkins or Zone diet. Fats tend to "stay with you," that is, they tend to keep you feeling full for long periods of time. Perhaps small amounts of fat help some people to eat less, since they feel satisfied.

This sounds like a dream come true. Eat all the protein and fat you want and lose weight. Think about an eating pattern as a marriage you plan on keeping for life. Are you prepared to go through life eating bacon, burgers, and beef, hold the bread, potatoes, and tomatoes? If you said an emphatic "yes!" consider the consequences. Depending on your genetics, you may be losing weight but eating yourself into early coronary artery disease, hypertension, diabetes, or arthritis. The excessive amounts of cholesterol and saturated fats in the Atkins and Zone diets can lead to clogged arteries that can in turn lead to heart attacks or strokes. High-fat diets can be constipating; isn't that something you want to look forward to for the rest of your life? And because of the limited amounts of carbohydrates, there are very few nutrients and little fiber in these diets.

Dr. Barry Sears's Zone diet is a little less extreme, allowing 40 percent of calories to come from carbohydrates in the form of fruits and vegetables, but limited amounts of grains and cereal products. The 30 percent protein component is supposed to come from lower fat fish, chicken, and yogurt or cottage cheese. This is a more reasonable approach than Dr. Atkins, but it is still limited in calcium and fiber and has more protein than is recommended by the USDA and the American Dietetic Association. Eating elevated amounts of protein for extended periods has been linked to kidney and liver disease and may cause certain vitamin deficiencies. As culinarians, you should be familiar with this diet. At its peak, there were "Zone" restaurants in most major cities. Dr. Sears has expanded his Zone philosophy to include soy. One of his current books is "The Soy Zone." This addition to the Zone repertoire allows vegetarians or people who don't want to eat animal products to follow a high-protein, plant-based diet.

High-Carbohydrate Diets

People who design diets like to experiment with many types of nutrient combining. We spoke earlier in the chapter about high-protein, low-carbohydrate diets. We'll now examine some high-carbohydrate, moderate-protein diets.

It's very interesting that both high-protein and high-carbohydrate diets promise the same end result—weight loss.

Dr. Ornish

At the other end of the spectrum is the **Ornish diet.** Proposed by Dr. Dean Ornish, a cardiologist, the Ornish diet is extremely limited in fat; actually it is practically fat-free. Dr. Ornish's diet plan is almost vegan, with fruit, vegetables, grains, and beans and legumes as the main ingredients for daily use. There are limited amounts of nonfat cottage cheese and yogurt, but no meat, poultry, or seafood. The diet is very "bulky" so people feel full after a meal. Dr. Ornish also recommends a regular routine of weight-bearing and stress-reducing exercise. The Ornish diet does work, and it has helped people with risk factors for heart disease to lower some of their risk. However, the Ornish diet takes a lot of commitment, as all foods have to be prepared from scratch and there needs to be time every day for exercise and stress reduction.

How about something in the middle? The **Mediterranean diet** (see Chapter 1) is an eating pattern that has worked for centuries for many people. The Mediterranean pyramid includes lots of enjoyable foods that are familiar and easy to prepare. Combine this with the Asian pyramid and you've got a real plan! The point is to construct a moderate eating plan, one that you can follow and enjoy and one that allows for gradual weight loss.

When it comes to losing weight and keeping it off, there's no easy, painless solution. Any diet pattern that contains 1,400 to 1,500 calories or less per day will produce short-term weight loss in most adults. You can live on 1,500

A NUTRI-BAR

The Nine Commandments of Healthy Eating (as proposed by the USDA)

1. Aim for a healthy weight: a reasonable guideline is a waist measurement of less than forty inches for men and thirty-five inches or less for women.
2. Exercise every day: children should be physically active for at least sixty minutes every day, adults thirty minutes.
3. Use the Food Guide Pyramid as your diet plan.
4. Include lots of fiber every day, including whole grains, fruits, and vegetables.
5. Be a safety guy (or gal): Be sure foods are stored and prepared in a safe and sanitary way.
6. Keep the calories from saturated fat and cholesterol as far down as possible.
7. Back off from foods that are high in sugar.
8. Resist the urge to shake: the salt, that is. Experiment with lemon, herbs, and seasonings instead of salt.
9. Avoid excessive salt. Twenty-four hundred milligrams of sodium a day is considered to be the outer limit of daily salt intake. That's about a teaspoon.

calories of chocolate and bacon and lose weight (please do not try this at home!). However, you'll probably wreck your health; you'll be real skinny for a couple of months and look just great sitting in the cardiologist's office. Most diets, no matter how weird, produce some weight loss for a short amount of time. After that, weight comes back with a vengeance, as your body attempts to stabilize its metabolism.

When all is said and done, eat your vegetables, have a piece of fruit, try for a balanced diet and exercise. You'll get healthy, look and feel good, and save a lot of money on all those diet products and books you don't need.

MENU PLANNING FOR ATHLETES

If you are in the hospitality field, then you are bound to have patrons or guests who will be attempting to vacation or travel on business while counting calories, considering that there were over sixty-million Americans who attempted to diet last year. You and your staff will have to have a team plan as to how to please the steak-and-potatoes people along with the salad-and-fresh-fruit people. More on that in Chapter 11. Start thinking about it now.

On a happier note, you may be asked to be the food-service professional in charge of a nationally acclaimed basketball team. In Southern California, some of the amateur bicycle clubs have become so organized that they hire chefs to cater meals at the end of their rides. The same goes for a lot of sports across the country.

When selecting foods that are going to be used to power amateur and professional athletes, let the Food Guide Pyramid lead you. Carbohydrates are your friend, with 60 percent of calories from them. Fats, at 30 percent play a supportive role, and proteins, at 10 percent play the distant stranger. Energy is the most important part of a hard-training athlete's diet. The major source of energy should come from carbohydrates with fat being a secondary source.

Just a note about fat intake among athletes. Although fats should not play a major role in a healthy diet, they should not be excluded or reduced to almost nothing. Several studies have shown that athletes who ate diets that were less than 15 percent fat (about half of the recommended amount) had more incidences of inflammatory disease, like arthritis, and had depressed immune responses (Squires, 5). Translated into English, this means that vigorously training athletes (college runners and swimmers were the main people studied) increased their possibility of sore and inflamed muscles and joints and left themselves open to colds, flu, and other contagious diseases. When the athletes increased their fat intake to 30 percent of daily calories (the current recommended amount), their problems disappeared. The moral to the story? Balance, don't restrict, nutrients (Venkatraman, 8).

You've all probably heard about **carbo-loading,** and you may be asked to design menus that accomplish this, so let's discuss it. To fully understand the body mechanics of carbo-loading, return to Chapters 3 and 4 and review carbohydrate digestion and absorption.

Glycogen, an end product of the body's processing of glucose, helps muscles work harder and longer during exercise. That's because glycogen is the storage form of carbohydrates in the body. That said, consider that getting more glycogen to muscles only seems to help in activities that require aerobic exercise for ninety minutes or more. Athletes who engage in aerobic activities that are less than ninety minutes in duration do not seem to get any benefit in carbo-loading. So, forget the spaghetti dinner on bowling night; it won't improve your score. But do think about carbo-loading when going for that fifty-mile bike ride or that five-mile swim.

If you are planning menus for marathon runners, cross-country skiers, competitive swimmers, triathlon participants, or time-trial cyclists or rowers, then carbo-loading is in order. Carbo-loading is achieved by increasing carbohydrate calories to 60–70 per cent of daily calories while slightly decreasing workout duration and intensity several days prior to competition. This regimen increases the store of glycogen in the muscles and liver, offering extra energy on race day.

Carbo-loading is generally considered to be safe, although individual medical status should always be considered. The downside to carbo-loading is a temporary weight gain. Every gram of stored glycogen grabs about three grams of water. The resultant weight gain is usually lost during competition, but some athletes say that even a slight weight gain throws off their timing.

Aerobic exercise helps your body to metabolize fat. When an athlete trains, there is more oxygen pumped to all the muscles, which, in turn, can burn more fat as fuel. Fat is used as the main source of fuel in low and moderate intensity workouts. However, the more in shape an athlete is, the body favors fat less and carbohydrates more as energy. Thirty percent should be the top number for athletes' diets. High-fat meals are usually lower in carbohydrates than an athlete needs and this limits the amount of glycogen that can be stored for competition energy. High-fat meals may contribute excess calories and saturated fats while giving little in the way of energy needs.

Protein should not be used as a source of appreciable energy for anyone, athletes included. Protein does help in the maintenance and repair of muscles, but it does not "build up" muscles. Rippling biceps are a result of a balanced diet, adequate hydration (translation: drink that water!), and lots of exercise. Although some sports do require slightly higher levels of protein, we're only talking about three or four more ounces a day. For the metric among you, endurance athletes and serious strength-training athletes require about 1.2 to 1.4 grams of protein for every kilogram of body weight. Athletes in extreme training may require up to 2 grams of protein per kilogram for short periods of time. We mere mortals require only about 1 gram of protein per kilogram. Good sources of protein for an athlete's menu include low-fat items, such as egg-white omelets, lean poultry, beef, pork and veal, poached, steamed, grilled or broiled (just not fried) seafood, nuts, soy products like tofu, soy cheeses, tempeh, and all kinds of beans and legumes.

High-protein diets can be dangerous, as we discussed in Chapter 6. Once again, increased protein intake will not add to muscle bulk or improve muscle tone. Eating too much protein encourages the body to get rid of water

Breakfast
8 ounces cranberry orange juice
2 cups cold cereal (like Shredded Wheat, Rice Krispies or Cherrios) or oatmeal with raisins, chopped dried apricots and fresh chopped apples
8 ounces nonfat milk or nonfat fortified soy or rice milk
2 slices banana bread with fruit preserves

Snack
Toasted bagel with skim milk mozzarella and tomato sauce and tomato slices
8 ounces orange juice
8 ounces sparkling water

Mid-day Meal
Veggie and lean meat (3 ounces sliced turkey, chicken or beef) submarine sandwich heaped with shredded lettuce, sliced bell peppers, shredded carrots, sliced radishes and onions; 1 ounce mayo-type salad dressing
Fruit basket (two pieces fresh fruit, like peaches, tangerines, apples, etc.)
12-ounce fruit juice smoothie (made with fresh fruit juice, banana and ice)

Snack
4 peanut butter or oatmeal raisin cookies
4 ounces frozen yogurt or ice milk topped with fresh or frozen berries

Evening Meal
1 cup of Caesar salad with 1-ounce salad dressing
4 ounces herbed grilled chicken or turkey breast
1 cup rice pilaf or 1 large baked sweet potato with 1 ounce of butter or sour cream
1 dinner roll
1 cup grilled vegetable brochettes (mushrooms, cherry tomatoes, bell pepper, sweet onions, summer squash, fresh fennel)
Angel food cake topped with sorbet and fresh fruit
8 ounces milk "shake" (nonfat milk or soy milk blended with frozen strawberries and ice)

Snack
2 cups popcorn (flavored with chili or herb blend)
8 ounces sparkling water

Figure 8–5 A Sample for a Carbo-Loading Menu Designed for Athletes with Extended Training Programs

or may be high in fat, since many protein sources come wrapped in animal fat. Too much protein makes the kidneys work harder and, if done over extended periods of time, can lead to mineral loss in bones, osteoporosis, heart disease, and even certain types of cancers.

Vitamins and minerals are needed in normal amounts for the athlete. Athletes have to be sure they are planning their meals so that they are getting adequate amounts of vitamins and minerals. Female athletes can be at a higher risk for iron deficiency, as can endurance or marathon runners. The type of impact done in running can cause increased red blood cell breakdown and signals the kidneys to excrete these broken blood cells. This can result in sports or runner anemia. This is not a true anemia and can be solved with a few days rest with adequate diet and hydration.

Fluids are very, very important for athletes. Exercise requires energy and energy burning means fluids are being used up. A hard-training athlete can lose up to 6 to 10 cups per hour.

You sweat to keep your body cool. Sweating rates vary, depending on the type of clothing you're wearing, how hot and humid or cold the weather is and how fit you are. Your blood also helps to cool the body. When you start heating up, blood flows to the surface of the skin to get "cooled off." This can interfere with muscle efficiency, as the heart has to divide its power between pumping blood to muscles or pumping blood to the skin surface. It also requires more fluid.

It's easy for an athlete to become dehydrated. As we said in Chapter 7, signs of dehydration are headache, feeling of inappropriate tiredness, decreased energy or performance, inappropriate elevated heart rate, and infrequent urination. When possible, athletes should drink fluids during exercise and should certainly take lots of drink before and after exercise.

Hey, how about some alligator sweat to quench your thirst after a workout? One of the first and still very popular **sports beverages** was developed by a leading university in Florida. The formula is based on the components of human perspiration. Hmmm.

Are special sports beverages necessary? Actually, water and a banana or an orange will do the same job as most sports drinks. What you're looking for before, during and after exercise is a source of water, carbohydrates, and a small amount of potassium, sodium, chloride, and phosphorus (the minerals lost in sweat). For most weekend warriors, water and fruit is adequate.

When you are speaking about exercising more than four hours at a time, then you may need a balanced sports drink that contains all of the water and nutrients listed above in a rapidly available form. Fructose, which is the sugar found in most fruit and fruit juice, can cause cramping when taken in large enough amounts to rehydrate someone who is completing an Iron Man triathlon. Mineral needs may be higher than can be met with straight fruit or fruit juice when exercise lasts more than four hours.

Take a Pill, Run Faster?

What about all those neat-o herbal and "natural" supplements available to enhance athletic performance? You've heard that ginseng will help reduce fatigue, chromium will increase your fat-burning ability, and sodium bicarbonate (baking soda or Alka Seltzer) will reduce muscle cramps. Maybe, no, and absolutely not! See the discussion on herbal preparations in Chapter 7. If you want to improve your performance, eat right, hydrate well, get enough rest, and concentrate on your workout. That'll do it, won't cost you extra money and may keep your heart, kidneys, and liver from working overtime.

There are some very serious side effects when athletes use odd supplements or engage in extreme or very fast weight loss or fast muscle building. We've discussed the supplements. We're sure you have read about or heard stories about athletes who have developed serious physical impairments from using unsavory supplements.

Some athletes may be in sports that require specific weight categories. Some athletes feel that weight loss is necessary for better performance. Extreme or unrealistic weight loss combined with hard training can result in premature osteoporosis and eating disorders, such as anorexia nervosa. Female athletes who decide to do extreme dieting and weight loss can develop amenorrhea, or loss of menstruation. This probably occurs because of the combination of low body weight, increased physical activity, inadequate energy intake, and low body-fat levels.

But you're not going to let that happen to you or any of the athletes you know.

You're the culinary nutrition person, and you're going to fix them right up with the fluids, carbs, protein, fats, minerals, and vitamins they need! In Chapter 11, we'll discuss even more how to plan menus that appeal to athletes while helping their performance.

FYI: THE FRESHMAN FIVE OR FIFTEEN

Going to school, full- or part-time, can wreak havoc with your schedule. We're speaking about your dining and exercise schedule, that is.

We're sure that prior to entering college you exercised at least three or four times a week and were a member of the "five a day" club. That is, you planned your meals, snacks, and grazing so that you had at least five servings of fruits and vegetables a day.

Unfortunately, as you start your college schedule, you may become a member of another "five" club. It is estimated that most college freshmen gain at least five pounds their first semester of school with many gaining as much as fifteen pounds.

The first week of school was probably a very hectic time, adding classes, finding the library, purchasing books. What could skipping a few days of exercise hurt? And meals? Ha! Pizza counts as a vegetable, right?

Things will quiet down the second week and then you'll get back to a healthy routine.

Week two dawns with the realization that you have twelve papers due, daily quizzes, and it takes at least an hour to find a parking space. Well. Running to feed the meter a couple of times a days counts as exercise, doesn't it? Do you find you know the menu selections in the on-campus vending machines too well?

So, you're three weeks into the semester. Carrying those books and a heavy knapsack does not constitute weight-bearing exercise. You can chart your daily intake from the fast-food wrappers on the floor of the car. Well, at least you're drinking water!

Does this sound vaguely familiar? Along with many other college traditions, the "Freshman Five" continues, a long-standing and unfortunate historical fact. This can be attributed to an increased workload, trying to balance employment and studying and irregular hours.

Here's an astounding statistic: according to the Pizza and Pasta Institute (there's a research council for everything) in the year 2000, high school and college students in the United States and Canada ate over sixty-million slices of pizza. Fast food and pizza are a mainstay of college food. It's quick, it's easy, it can be relatively inexpensive, and it's available almost around the clock. It will take some planning to find foods that are so easy and accessible. Let's face it, if it's fried or greasy, it's probably higher in fat than most people need.

Try to go grocery shopping once a week and stock up on "fast" foods that you enjoy and can make in a minute. This can include fresh fruit and nuts, cold cereal (go for the grains, leave the sugar behind), low-fat granola, sparkling and still water, herbal and decaffeinated tea, fruit and vegetable juices, flavored and plain yogurt, cottage cheese with fruit, lean sliced meats, such as turkey and ham, pretzels and crackers, to name a few. If you have a microwave, then go for the low-fat/low-sodium popcorn, individual rice bowls, lower-fat/lower-salt soups, veggie burgers, and rice mixes.

Stress can affect the way you eat. Some people will eat everything in sight when they feel stressed and some completely lose their appetite. Neither scenario is desirable.

Organization and exercise can help reduce stress. All-night study sessions are a stressful tradition that you can live without. In addition to losing a good night's sleep, you'll feel tired and jittery on test day from all the caffeine you consumed. Wave your magic wand and try to squeeze in study time when you can.

Keep a Palm Pilot or a good old-fashioned day planner notebook up to date. Knowing where you're supposed to be and when you're supposed to be there will help make things less hectic.

While you're scoping out the campus, try to find a quiet place where you can escape for at least a couple of minutes a day. If this isn't possible, keep a pair of headphones or earplugs to occasionally tune out and chill out.

Exercise is a fantastic stress-reliever. Not only does it tell your body to release lots of feel-good chemicals, it gets your mind off your problems. Feeling a little tense? Take a fast walk around campus. Feeling really tense? Take a kick-boxing class. Feeling stressed and hectic? Check out a yoga class. Want more info? Surf *www.teachhealth.com*.

Here are some Web sites that will give you more info:

www.dietsite.com/nutritionfacts/index.htm A site that lists food label information for over two thousand food items.

www.fastfood.com A site that lists the calories, fat, and other cheery news about popular fast foods.

www.cyberdiet.com This site was developed by registered dietitians, is easy to navigate, has assessment information, resources, and support groups. Diet information is based on the Food Guide Pyramids.

www.dietsite.com This site was developed by registered dietitians, follows the Food Guide Pyramids and has sports nutrition info, nutritional info for people with medical conditions, and "has been created to enhance the efficiency and effectiveness of nutrition and diet."

www.collagevideo.com This site offers a free "Guide to Exercise Videos."

www.acefitness.org The American Council on Exercise site has ideas for all levels of exercisers. You can ask online exercise questions of certified exercise professionals.

Nutri-Words

3,500 calories: the number of calories that have to be eaten to gain a pound of weight or restricted to loss a pound of weight.

Appetite: both a physical and psychological trigger for eating. Appetite can be learned and modified with behavioral techniques.

Arteriosclerosis: the build-up of fatty deposits, called plaque, on the interior of veins and arteries, which can lead to severe blockage of blood flow.

Atkins diet: a diet made popular by Dr. Atkins, requiring dieters to derive the majority of their daily calories from protein. The Atkins diet severely restricts carbohydrate calories.

Behavior modification: a form of training that can be used to change eating patterns.

Body Mass Index (BMI): a ratio comparing height, weight, and other factors to derive a healthy weight gain.

Carbo-loading: an eating style used by athletes to store energy for competitive events. It entails increasing the daily percentage derived from carbohydrates above 60 percent.

Hunger: a physical response to low energy stores.

Ideal body weight: calculations used by health care professionals to ascertain if a person is within what is considered to be healthy weight norms.

Lean body mass: the weight of the body that includes muscle, tissue, and bone, and excludes fat and fluid.

Mediterranean diet: a diet that follows the typical eating patterns of Mediterranean countries, such as Spain, Italy, Turkey, and Greece, with an emphasis on whole grains, fresh fruits, and vegetables, fat from olive oil and seafood.

National Restaurant Association (NRA): The NRA is a professional organization whose membership consists of food service and culinary professionals and educators.

Negative energy balance: every body requires a certain amount of energy to perform all necessary tasks. If you consume less energy than your body requires, than you are in negative energy balance, and may begin to be unable to perform necessary tasks.

Obesity: defined by health-care professionals as being 20 percent or more over ideal body weight.

Ornish diet: a diet made popular by Dr. Dean Ornish. Originally designed for patients with severe heart disease, the Ornish diet combines a very low fat, mostly vegetarian diet with regular exercise and stress reduction.

Overweight: defined by health-care professionals as being 10 to 20 percent above ideal body weight.

Positive energy balance: every body requires a certain amount of energy to perform all necessary tasks. If you consume more energy (in calories) than your body needs to perform these tasks, you have excess energy in reserve. This is called "positive energy balance."

Satiety: a physical response to having consumed sufficient calories, especially triggered by consuming fat-containing foods.

Sports beverages: commercially marketed beverages that are supposed to replenish fluids and electrolytes (minerals) lost during strenuous exercise.

Super-size portions: restaurant portions that exceed standard portion sizes.

Water displacement measurement: a technique to measure the percentage of fat and lean body mass, requiring total body immersion.

Yo-yo dieting: a cycle of weight loss and weight gain. Thought to be an unhealthy practice that makes weight maintenance difficult.

Whaddaya think?

1. How's your energy balance?
2. Can you explain the physical mechanisms for hunger?
3. What do you pay attention to: hunger, appetite or satiety?
4. What's your BMI? How do you rate?
5. Why are there different energy needs for men and women?
6. If one of your food-preparation staff wanted to lose thirty pounds, what type of information would you supply?
7. What's your solution to super-sizing?
8. Work both ends of the spectrum: Design both an Atkins and an Ornish three-day menu for your hotel.
9. Suggest a breakfast buffet for the football team at a local college.
10. Now, make it adhere to the Mediterranean diet!

Critical Thinking

1. Calculate your ideal body weight:
   a. Now calculate the approximate amount of daily calories you need.
   b. Design a one-day menu that meets these calorie needs (use the Exchange Lists for Meal Planning).
2. If a healthy active friend asked for some information about losing a couple of pounds, what types of diet and exercise would you suggest?
3. Your hotel is adding a spa section:
   a. Design a three-day Dr. Atkins–style menu for those clients following a low-carbohydrate, high-protein diet.
   b. Design a three day Dr. Ornish–style menu for those clients following a vegan, low-fat diet.

References

"At Chef School, Good Work Goes to Waist," (2000). *Los Angeles Times,* December 1, p. A49.

Lempert, Bill (2000). "Dining Well in a Jumbo-Portion World," *Los Angeles Times,* December 18, p. S2.

Parseghian, Pamela (2001). "Keeping Fit and Healthy is Weighty Task for Chefs," *Nations Restaurant News,* January 1, p. 52.

Rosenfeld, Isadore (2001). "Which Diet is Right for You?" *Parade Magazine,* March 18, pp. 4–5.

Rubin, Karen (1993). "Avoid the Yo-Yo Syndrome," *Food Service Director Magazine,* February 15, p. 74.

Squires, Sally (2001). "When It Comes to Long-Term Weight Loss, There's No Magic Bullet," *Los Angeles Times,* January 15, p. A24.

Turner, Richard (1999). "The Trendy Diet That Sizzles" *Time Magazine,* September 6, p. 60

Venkatraman, J. T. and Leddy, J. (2000). "Dietary Fats and Immune Status in Athletes: Clinical Implications," *Medicine and Science in Sports and Exercise,* 32: July, 389–392.

Chapter 9

Food Safety

Chapter Overview

Chapter Objectives

As a result of reading this chapter, the student should be able to:

1. *Decide between the health benefits and health hazards of food additives.*
2. *Trace the history of food technology.*
3. *Explain the process of canning.*
4. *Explain the process of irradiation, including consumer concerns about irradiation's safety.*
5. *Describe the uses of food additives.*
6. *Identify the difference between "clean," organic, and natural foods.*
7. *Relate the reasons for the development of biotechnology and bioengineered foods.*

8. *Define "GMO" and explain how these products are developed.*
9. *Describe how food safety is achieved on an industry level.*
10. *Describe how food safety is achieved on a facility level.*
11. *Explain how to implement HAACP procedures in a food service operation.*
12. *Prepare a food service operation for a health inspection.*
13. *Relate current legislation to consumer concerns about food safety and health.*
14. *Develop a personal philosophy about food safety and its relation to health and nutrition.*

Introduction

How do nutrition, culinary arts, and ***food safety*** *interact? Lots of ways. If you are planning to go into the food-service industry and feed the public, remember that the public reads and listens to media reports. You'll need to be ready with a* ***clean*** *and* ***sanitary*** *property and lots of answers to consumer questions.*

Almost all food products originate from natural products. Even that over-processed cream-filled dessert cake was once wheat, growing in a field. Our food supply is both nutritious and safe. You need to know how it gets that way.

Food safety on a restaurant level has to do with the day-to-day cleaning operations and the ordering and receiving of safe food from reputable sources. How is that food kept safe? Through ***HACCP*** *(****Hazard Analysis Critical Control Points****—discussed later in the chapter) procedures in the processing plant and in your kitchen. Some foods have chemicals added to them to further ensure safety. What do you know about these chemicals and how will you answer customer questions about them?*

Agency	*Responsibility*
APHIS	Oversees control of disease in animals used for food Animal and Plant Health Inspection Service
CDC	Investigates and monitors all reported causes and Centers for Disease Control incidences of food borne illness
EPA	Establishes water quality, regulates use of pesticides, Environmental Protection Agency and pesticide levels
FDA	Safety of all foods sold across state lines (except Food and Drug Administration meat, poultry and eggs), oversees animal feed, including added drugs and hormones, oversees all processed foods, including food plants and imported foods, oversees and enforces use of food additives, such as color and preservatives
FSIS	Oversees standards for wholesomeness and quality of Food Safety Inspection Service red meat, poultry and eggs; part of the USDA
National Marine Fishery Service	Has a voluntary inspection and grading system for fish products; part of the Department of Commerce

Figure 9–1 Food Safety Agencies

A NUTRI-BAR

Resources for Food Safety

Need some support materials for your food safety sessions? The following agencies offer a wide variety:

American Red Cross (offers food safety courses, have posters and printed material)

Local Health Departments (offer printed material, safety signs; many will have sanitarians available to give short presentations)

National Restaurant Association (*www.edfound.org* or 800-765-2122 for the national offices or use your state chapters—materials range from college-level texts to training videos (in English and Spanish) to food safety bingo games to illustrated posters)

NSF (National Safety Foundation) International (*www.nsf.org*—offers posters, printed material, safety check lists, information on food thermometers)

The Food Marketing Institute (*www.fmi.org*—offers consumer and industry safety materials)

Daydots International (800-321-3687—offers colored dot systems for food labeling and rotation, color-coded cutting boards, food storage bags, food safety demo kits)

USDA (*fsis.outreach@usda.gov* or fax to 202-720-9063—newsletters and education kits on food safety)

FOOD SAFETY AND CHEMICALS

For example, many foods contain added preservatives and have had them added for hundreds of years. The fine art of **charcuterie,** making sausages, has used preservatives to prevent the growth of foodborne illnesses for centuries. A real bad guy, ***Clostridium botulinum,*** has a particular affinity for sausage, including some of America's favorite sports and junk food, like hot dogs, hot links, and sausage and pepper sandwiches. In fact, *Cl. botulinum* takes its name from the Latin word for sausage, *botulus.* The practice of adding preservatives, in the form of **nitrites,** to sausages has virtually eradicated causes of botulism food poisoning in these products.

DO ALL FOOD ADDITIVES CAUSE CANCER?

But there's a catch. About twenty-five years ago, some researchers thought they had found a link between consuming nitrites and the risk of certain cancers in adults. To understand this claim, we have to give you a little human science about how the body handles nitrates and nitrites.

Nitrates are found naturally in vegetables and water. They can also be synthesized and added to foods as a preservative. About 95 percent of the nitrites you consume are from "natural sources," such as broccoli or drinking water and about 5 percent come from chemical nitrites added as preservatives.

When nitrates hit your saliva, some of them are broken down by bacteria in the saliva to form nitrites. It is thought that about 20 percent of all nitrates get converted into nitrites. Up until a couple of years ago, it was thought that nitrites traveled to the stomach and reacted with some proteins to become cancer-causing substances called **nitrosamines.** Preserved meat was pointed to as the villain and pressure was put on the meat industry to reduce the amount of nitrates added to food.

But think about this. Most nitrates come from vegetables and water, and we can be pretty sure that neither one of those items cause cancer. In fact, they are thought to help keep you healthy. Humans had been consuming vegetables and water, with high nitrate contents for years without large incidences of cancer. Only a small percentage of nitrites were coming from preservatives.

Reducing nitrites in preserved food also presented a dilemma. We know that *Cl. botulinum* is a very harmful bacteria, capable of causing death. That will get you for sure. Nitrites were thought to *possibly* cause cancer, used over a long period of time. So which will it be? Certain death from botulism right now or the possibility of death from cancer caused by nitrites many years from now?

Some recent studies have shed some interesting light on this issue. One group of thought was that it was not the nitrites' fault, but the fault of the bacteria in the mouth causing cancer-producing substances. In studies where certain oral bacteria were reduced, the amount of carcinogenic nitrite substances were also reduced (Young, 8).

Some even more interesting research found that not only did dietary nitrites not cause cancer, but actually had a protective effect against several food-borne bacteria that tended to establish itself in the stomach, including **salmonella,** shigella, ***E. coli*** and yersinia (Young, 8). It was noted that when people took antibiotics they tended to get more infections of the mouth and gut. The antibiotics reduced the amount of salivary bacteria that turned nitrates into nitrites, reducing nitrites protective effect against bad bacteria. Nitrites have also been shown to kill off *H. pylori,* a stomach bacteria linked to both stomach ulcers and stomach cancer.

WHEN DOES FOOD SAFETY OUTWEIGH POSSIBLE HEALTH RISKS

In 2000, a national review board announced that there had been little evidence to support that nitrites caused cancer. However, interpreting the research in a different way, a small group of scientists still believed that nitrites could cause cancer. So where does this leave the culinarian? You'll have to make that decision for yourself and your customers. The important thing is to have an understanding about these issues, so that when a customer accuses you of serving unsafe food, you can enter into an informative discussion, based on fact and science.

You'll find that lots of people are concerned about cancer. Cancer is frightening. Many of your customers will be preparing foods at home that they believe will help reduce the risk of cancer. They'll appreciate ordering the same categories of food when they dine out. We asked several health-care professionals what they would recommend in terms of eating healthy to reduce cancer risk. Here is their consensus answer:

1. Have a plant-based diet with lots of fresh fruits and veggies, beans and legumes and whole grains.
2. Exercise for an hour every day (this includes running around at work) and keep your weight where it should be.
3. Really attempt to have five servings of fruits and vegetables every day.
4. Limit alcohol—two drinks per day for men and one for women.
5. When you have a choice, fish, poultry, and game (venison, duck, etc.) is better than red meat.
6. Watch the fat and keep it below 30 percent of daily intake.
7. Watch the salt and keep it below two teaspoons per day (that's a hard one!)
8. Eat safe foods that are handled properly—and stay away from puffer fish (a popular sushi fish, that, if not prepared correctly, can be lethal).
9. Think about the water you're drinking—is it from a safe source?

(Reference: *http:/www.cdc.gov/foodsafety*)

1. Campylobacter bacteria is beginning to develop some antibiotic-resistant strains. Resistant strains have been isolated in developing countries and from undercooked poultry.
2. According to the Foodborne Disease Surveillance Report 1993 to 1997, 68 percent of all foodborne illness outbreaks are caused by "unknown." Many times breakdowns in the diagnostic chain (lab techniques, collecting samples, late reporting, etc.) prevent outbreaks from being pinpointed.
3. Gotta protect people from themselves. In a recent survey, both young and old people with compromised immune systems continued to eat risky foods, especially undercooked, or runny, eggs. In the survey, this at-risk population reported eating more potentially disease-causing foods then their healthy counterparts.
4. Don't try this at home: An FDA survey done in September 2000 of 900 commercial and noncommercial food establishments found the following to be the most often occurring food service food safety mistakes:
   a. Incorrect temperatures and time for holding food.
   b. Cross-contamination of equipment.
   c. Poor personal hygiene.

On the bright side, cooking temperatures were generally found to be adequate, and food was obtained from safe sources

Figure 9–2 Micro-Trivia

1. As soon as you've gathered all the who, what, why, where, and how, report the incident to the appropriate agency. Time is important to prevent more incidences, so report right away.
2. The FDA handles problems relating to adverse reactions to food (except for meat and poultry) and foodborne illness. The nonemergency number is 800-332-4010. For matters requiring immediate attention, call 301-443-1240.
3. Meat and poultry problems are reported to the USDA. The USDA hotline number is 800-535-4555.
4. The Adverse Reaction Monitoring System, a division of the FDA handles incidences related to food additives. They can be reached by mail at: ARMS HFS-636 FDA 200 C Street, NW, Washington, D.C. 20204
5. The Consumer Product Safety Commission handles hazardous household products, including cleaning materials on a federal level. Report incidences to the state department of consumer protection as well.
6. False or deceptive advertising should be reported to the state's department of consumer protection. On a federal level, report to the Federal Trade Commission.
7. Air and water pollution, as well as improper pesticide use should be reported to the state's environmental protection department. On the federal level, it's the EPA.
8. Unsafe or unhealthy restaurant practices should be reported to local health departments.
9. Grocery stores are responsible for selling safe food. Return unsafe food to the store and they will track down the problem, reporting it to the proper agency.

Source: *www.fda.gov/opacom/backgrounders/problem.html*

Figure 9–3 Reporting Unsafe, Unsanitary, Mislabeled, or Deceptive Food Products

FOOD TECHNOLOGY

Many of the foods we eat are not eaten in their natural state. Baked potatoes are nice, but you like a potato chip now and again. A bowl of oatmeal is great in the morning, but an oatmeal cookie really does it in the afternoon. Food safety entails **food processing** as well as safe food handling.

Brief History

We can thank Napoleon for kick-starting the whole food technology field. Napoleon came to power by having a large army. As we all know, armies travel on their stomachs. During Napoleon's time, there were very few methods of **food preservation.** No **canning,** no freeze-drying, no frozen food, no MREs (meals-ready-to-eat, the modern version of the military C rations). The only way the army ate was to conquer a village and to take all the village's food.

This didn't work very well when you're talking about Europe in the winter. Most villages subsisted on a small amount of grain, some root vegetables, and fresh eggs and milk (if the animals produced in cold weather). Not the type of diet on which to conquer the world. Soldiers would get tired of being hungry and cold and take off for more hospitable climes. No soldiers, no army, no taking over new countries.

Canning: A Royal Proclamation

Napoleon declared a reward and all kinds of official prizes for anyone who could invent a means by which to feed the army. In 1810, Nicholas Appert invented a process that he very modestly named "appertization," known today as canning. He placed potted (boiled) beef in an airtight bottle and heated it. The meat's shelf life was extended, the army was fed and Appert won 12,000 francs.

Appert's attempt at using tins instead of glass was not such an immediate success. He cooked some meat with wine and sealed it in a tin can. To seal the can Appert used the solder material of the day, which was lead. Tin and lead are fairly soft metals and reacted with the acid from the wine. In addition to giving the meat a "tinny" flavor, the acid-lead reaction gave a lot of soldiers lead poisoning. The troops were well-fed, but tended to drop dead after a steady diet of tinned foods. Back to the drawing board. This event may have caused the birth of quality control in the food industry.

Today, canning is considered to be the "grandaddy" of all food processing, with greatly perfected techniques. Canning is usually done in glass, plastic or aluminum with sufficient heating to destroy food-borne illness microorganisms. Cans are sealed with inert materials, materials that will not react with canning materials or food ingredients.

Irradiation or X-Ray Zombies from Mars

Irradiated food has been around for at least forty years, but consumers are just beginning to hear about it. Irradiated food is not an "x-ray zombies from Mars" invention. Most people don't want to hear "food" and "radiation" in the same sentence. "Radiation" is nuclear reactors. "**Irradiation**" is the preservation of foods. Different method, different rays, different outcomes.

Many insects, parasites, and foodborne bacteria, such as *E. coli*, salmonella, staphyloccus, and listeria, resist traditional food preservation techniques, like drying or refrigeration. Irradiation, which involves bombarding foods with high-powered x-rays or electron beams, is able to destroy many more disease-causing pathogens. Because it does the same job as traditional (hot) pasteurization without using heat, irradiation is also called **cold pasteurization.**

Eating irradiated food does not cause cancer or genetic damage and does not make food radioactive. There is just enough energy used to disrupt the protein in parasites and bacteria but not to make anything radioactive. Irradiation causes the same change in food as cooking does. In other words, cooking causes chemical changes in food and so does irradiation. Because there is no heat, there are fewer changes made to food. That means that irradiated foods can taste and look fresher than traditionally preserved foods. Developing countries have been using irradiation for years to ensure an adequate supply of food for their citizens. You have eaten irradiated food if you have used certain brands of flour, spices and poultry (Leibman, 4).

FOOD FOR THE MIND

Food for (Irradiated) Thought: The CDC (Centers for Disease Control) says that treating meat and poultry with gamma rays or nonradioactive electron beams has the possibility to help prevent close to a million cases of foodborne illness and their related hospitalizations, or possible deaths, every year.

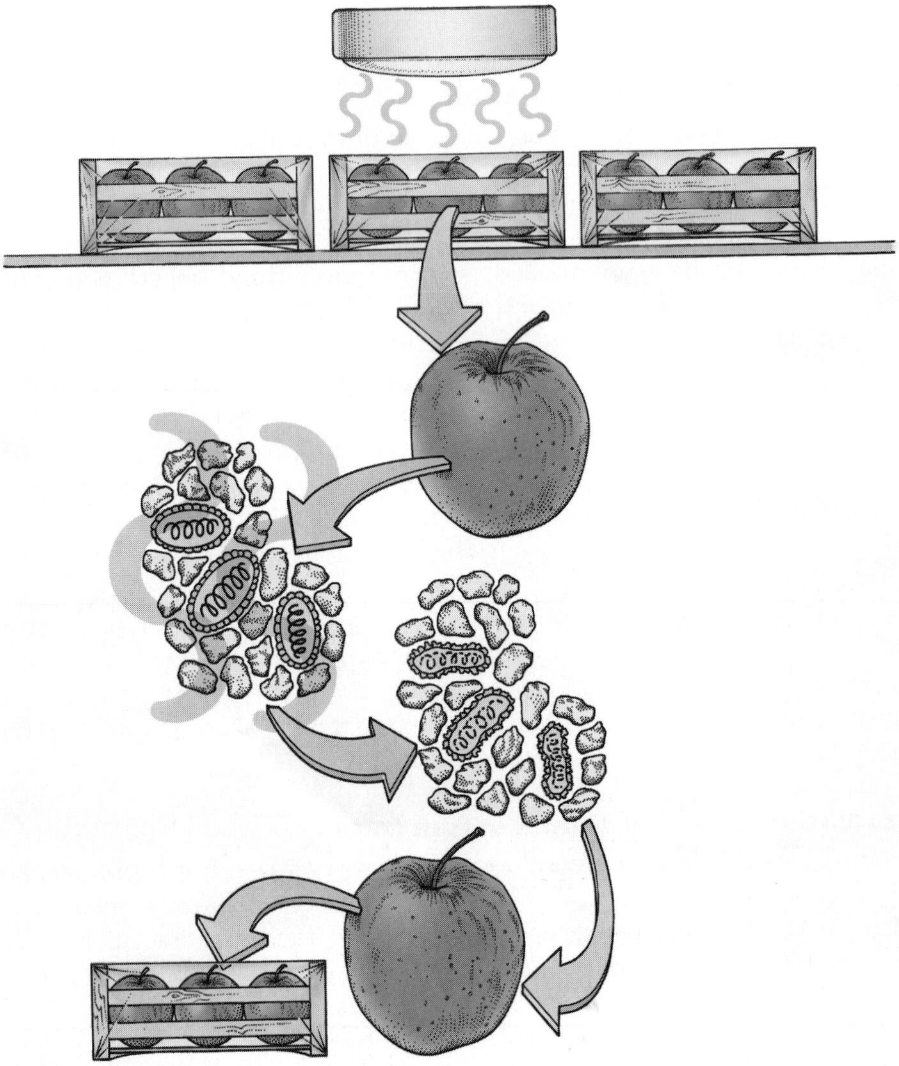

This diagram outlines apples being irradiated to prevent spoilage. The crated apples are sent through a processing tunnel where they are bombarded with gamma rays.

The USDA conducted a survey of over 20,000 consumers in 2000. Half the people surveyed indicated they were willing to purchase irradiated meat, but only 23 percent said they'd only be willing to pay more. If you'd like to read some or all of the survey, go to *http://www.cdc.gov/foodnet* and click on "publications and presentations."

Irradiation got a leg up several years ago when there was an outbreak of hoof-and-mouth disease in Europe, developing simultaneously in the United Kingdom, France, and Germany. General food hysteria ensued, and it became a world issue. Canada refused shipments of beef from Argentina because Argentina had obtained some beef breeding stock from Europe. Imports and exports of meat and products produced from animals, like cheese and gelatin were halted and economies were affected.

The moral to the story: The world has gotten so small it's hard to isolate food borne disease. Whether we like it or not, we may have to learn to like some modern technology.

Additives

Another method of preservation is the use of **food additives.** Loosely defined, a food additive is any item that intentionally or unintentionally becomes part of a food product. There are over 4,000 substances used today as intentional food additives and at least 10,000 more substances that find their way into food (Lehman, 3).

Intentional additives need to fit into one or more of the following categories:

1. Assist in processing or preparation. These substances may help to give body or texture, control acid content, prevent lumping, help products to flow or change the freezing point. For example, monoglycerides are emulsifiers that can help to make margarine smooth and to keep peanut butter from separating. Calcium silicate and silicon dioxide help to keep salt and powdered sugar flowing and prevent clumping.
2. Maintain or improve nutritional value. Many foods have vitamins and minerals added as either a replacement for nutrients lost during processing or to enhance the quality of the food. Nutritional fortification of food began in 1924, with **iodine** added to salt to prevent goiter. Since then, milk, flour, juices, and many other products have been enriched or fortified to improve the quality of the American diet.
3. Maintain freshness. Bacteria and mold can cause food to spoil and exposure to air can cause foods to discolor. Additives are necessary to extend shelf-life and to prevent organisms that can cause illness from growing on food. Not all preservatives are chemicals. Vitamins C and E are natural antioxidants that will prevent foods from turning brown. Salt pre-

Year Approved	*Food*	*Reason*
1963	Wheat flour	prevent mold
1964	White potatoes	inhibit sprouting
1986	Fresh pork	prevent Trichinosis parasite
1986	Selected produce	increase shelf life
1986	Dried herbs & spices	prevent contamination
1990	Poultry	reduce bacterial pathogens
1997 & 2000	Meat	reduce bacterial pathogens
2000	Shell eggs	reduce salmonella
2000	Selected shellfish	reduce contamination

Source: *www.cdc.gov/ncidod/dbmd/diseaseinfo/foodirradiation.htm#whatis*

Figure 9–4 Foods Approved by the USDA for Irradiation

vents bacterial growth. Some chemical preservatives that you will see on food labels can include potassium sorbate, BHA and BHT.

4. Make food more appealing. Everything looks better with a cherry on top. Some foods lack appealing colors, and some foods have bland flavors. Sugar, salt, corn syrup and food color are the additives most used today. There are thirty-five approved colors allowed to be used in foods today; over half of them are synthetic. Herbs and spices would be considered food additives, as would soy sauce. **Flavor enhancers,** such as MSG (monosodium glutamate), are still very popular, despite their high salt content. Flavor enhancers help the taste buds to "perk up" and taste more effectively. If a food is flavored with a very subtle substance, such as natural vanilla or fresh raspberry extract, flavor enhancers add an exclamation point effect, underlining the natural, but weak, flavors (Durant, 2).

NATURAL FOODS

Some people want **natural foods,** and want to stay away from additives altogether. You can't really give a hard-and-fast definition of "natural," as the government does not regulate it at this time. Most people would assume that natural foods have none of the types of additives we have listed above. However, if you want to stretch it, potato chips could be considered a natural food, since they are made with "natural" potatoes, "natural" vegetable oil, and "natural" salt.

Organic Foods

Speaking of additives, let's talk about **organic food,** which is newly regulated by the government. A scientist will look you in the eye and tell you that all food is organic because the scientific definition of an "organic substance" is any substance that contains carbon. Everything that is alive or was once alive contains carbon. You wouldn't want an inorganic food, as you would be talking about chewing on things like a hunk of iron or a piece of meteorite. In this sense, even coal or petroleum are organic, as they are created from the fossils of animals and plants that lived many eons ago. All plants and animals contain carbon, which makes them scientifically "organic." Ever wondered how scientists figured out how old a dinosaur or an old plant fossil is? You may have heard about carbon-14 testing. Through a series of chemical and biological tests, scientists can figure out how many years ago the carbon in a sample was formed, which allows them to put a year of origin on the sample.

Food people tend to go beyond the carbon issue when discussing organic. In a general sense, "organic" has come to mean plants and animals that are grown without the use of chemicals or foods that have been processed from organic crops without the use of chemicals, such as synthetic preservatives, artificial flavor or artificial color. In other words, a loaf of bread that is labeled "organic" should tell the customer that the wheat was grown without the use of pesticides or chemical fertilizers and was processed without using stabilizers, artificial caramel color or synthetic butter flavor.

Techniques

Some naturally occurring products can be used as preservatives, colors or flavors in organic products. Vitamin C and vitamin E, which can be made from organic sources, such as citrus fruit or nuts, are naturally occurring antioxidants. Both Vitamins C and E can be added to beverages, dessert mixes, or baked goods to keep them from turning brown. Both sugar and salt are "natural" products and can help in the preservation of canned and refrigerated foods. Many herbs and spices, such as rosemary, garlic and cinnamon may have an antibacterial effect on food. Natural colors and flavors can be gotten from fruit and vegetable extracts as well as spice extracts, such as turmeric, saffron and parsley. Organic processors will make use of these products rather than using synthetic ingredients (Chapman, 1).

Current Legislation

Organic farms and food processors were self-regulated until several years ago. There were many private consortiums that would inspect farms or processing plants to ascertain if organic standards were being met. The Organic Trade Association was a national organization formed to promote the cause of organic agriculture and food processing. Although there were many people passionate about ensuring the purity of organic foods, there were no consistent standards. The federal government got into the organic act by passing the "National Organic Standards" in December 2000. These standards sought to cover every step of the food process, from seed selection through farming to harvesting, processing, and packaging.

The federal organic standards do not allow growers or food processors to use genetic engineering for plants or animals, irradiation as a method of preservation or sewage sludge (pasteurized and treated by-products of sewage processing with the nutrients left in and the illness-causing bacteria taken out). Processed foods, like canned goods or bakery mixes, may be labeled "organic" if they contain at least 95 percent organic products. The remaining 5 percent must also be organic products, if such products exist. For example, if you want to add 2 percent mango nectar to your organic Tropical Salad Marinade and there is no organic mango nectar anywhere around, federal standards allow you to go ahead with the traditionally grown mangos. If your Tropical Salad Marinade is not made exclusively with organic ingredients, you may label it "made with organic ingredients" if it has at least 70 percent of its ingredients from organic sources. If you decide to offer an organic chicken burger at your restaurant, your chickens must have been fed 100 percent organic chicken feed and processed without preservatives.

Pesticide residues were a hard item to tackle. The private organic commissions had regulations that were a lot tougher than the government's. In fact, many organic producers continue to adhere to the stricter private regulations, considering the federal regulations as too lightweight. In general, private organic commissions have a zero-tolerance policy of pesticides. If your products test positive for even a trace of pesticide, you can't obtain organic certification. This is handled by allowing producers to label their products

transitional, meaning that you are on your way to organic and have stopped using chemicals and pesticides. Traces of chemicals can linger in soil, groundwater, or even trees for many years. If a producer has a farm or ranch in between two traditional growers, the wind can carry chemicals to his crops. The federal guidelines are a bit more lenient. If a producer can prove that only organic techniques were used and pesticide residues on products do not exceed 5 percent of the **EPA (Environmental Protection Agency)** limits, then organic certification is possible.

By the time you read this chapter, the organic standards and regulations will have been modified several times. This is a very hot topic and will be open for political discussion for years to come. Food is always political, and the tussle over organic is not different.

Many traditional growers fear that consumers would perceive organic foods as higher in quality or more nutritious and fought the federal government's bestowing of organic labeling. They felt as if the government would appear to be endorsing organic foods over traditionally grown foods.

As a food person, you will have to decide whether or not to purchase organic foods for your business. In and of themselves, organic foods cannot guarantee more nutrition, higher quality, or fresher products. Organic designation only guarantees that the lowest possible amount of chemicals is available in a particular product.

Somewhere between organic and traditional growing techniques is **sustainable agriculture.** Many chefs back this form of agriculture and try to purchase as much as possible from sustainable farms. Starting about thirty years ago, sustainable agriculture was a response to the problems seen with the overuse of land and the improper use of chemicals. Sustainable agriculture attempts to promote environmental health, economic profit, and even socioeconomic improvement. An example of socioeconomic improvement can be seen in developing countries where a vast amount of crops are raised and harvested by women. Sustainable agriculture techniques allow them to raise crops that will succeed, need fewer chemicals and give greater yields (Omaye, 5).

How is sustainable agriculture done? If you grow a crop one season that depletes the soil of nitrogen, then rotating the crop next season replaces the depleted nitrogen. If you grow crops that are appropriate for your area, you don't use all the water and other natural resources; the same idea applies to raising animals. Trainers would visit developing countries and instruct female farmers in these techniques. Sustainable agriculture was a great success. People were able to feed their families without exhausting the land and water.

We will give you more details on **biotechnology** in a moment. Biotechnology is thought to help sustainable agriculture (science meets nature). Biotechnology helps to develop drought-resistant crops or plants capable of breaking down pesticides, so the soil is cleansed and there's no pesticide residue. Crops have been developed that have increased yield but require little tillage, so less machinery or man or animal power are needed. With increased yields, less land is needed, so there's less deforestation. These are some of the reasons why some people are not making too big an uproar about biotechnology.

1. 100 Percent Organic: these foods contain only organically grown and processed ingredients. Irradiation or other excluded methods cannot be used.
2. Organic: these foods must contain 95 percent organically grown and processed ingredients. Five percent consist of nonagricultural substances (such as synthetic vitamin C) approved by the government or nonorganically grown products not commercially available as organic products.
3. Made with Organic Ingredients: Can contain 70 percent organic ingredients, with the remaining 30 percent nonorganic products. Cannot have used irradiation or other excluded processing methods.

Figure 9–5 Organic Labeling Requirements (*Reference:* USDA Web site, March 2001)

Some organic producers are very much into offering the best possible, freshest, most nutrition-retaining foods without polluting the planet. So are some traditional producers. Remember that label claims are just that . . . claims. You will have to sample, taste, cook with, and get to know the producers of the food you purchase to make an informed decision (Sloan, 6).

A NUTRI-BAR

Frankenfood or Just Fine Fruit

Heirloom produce, such as apples, pears, melons, tomatoes, beans, and nuts grown from traditional seed, are gaining in popularity. Ever notice that there are only one or two types of tomatoes in the produce section? Once upon a time, there were many, many regional varieties of all fruits and vegetables. Chefs and consumers are showing increased interest in restoring heirloom produce to its former popularity.

Responding to the chefs' push, animal producers are feeding their livestock grass and grain, not hormone-laced feed, supplying clean water and allowing them to roam free rather than penning them "Healthier and happier" seems to be on the agenda for crops, livestock, and consumers.

Interestingly enough, biotechnology has eased its way into the clean movement. Consumers responded in the affirmative for biotechnology to be used for lowering fat in foods, foods that prevent disease, foods that taste better, stay fresher longer, and decrease price. Some egg producers are creating eggs that are lower in cholesterol and higher in vitamin E and omega-3 fatty acids (thought to be good for heart health). They're doing this by altering the poultry feed. Broccolini is a hybrid of Chinese cabbage and flowering broccoli, resembling deep green asparagus with tiny broccoli florets; chefs and consumers love it. This is biotechnology that chefs and consumers seem to accept.

BIOTECHNOLOGY

Beyond organic, many culinary and non-culinary people are concerned about the various methods being used to "improve" the food supply. We're talking about biotechnology and **genetically modified organisms (GMO).**

GMOs

Talk about politics! Several European and Asian countries decided they didn't like the idea of GMOs in American food products and refused to allow shipment of certain food products that contained GMOs, such as fruit, vegetables, soy products, and rice into their countries.

So what is this Star Trek–sounding technique we're speaking about? Biotechnology is the area of science devoted to modifying food crops to use less water, be more pest-resistant, require less nutrients from the soil, etc. In some ways, bees and butterflies practice biotechnology by cross-pollinating the different crops on which they land. The earliest farmers saved the seeds from the best producing plants, crossing them with other hardy plants to produce what they hoped would be huge crops undaunted by pests. Food technologists and lots of scientists have embraced biotechnology as a way to keep ahead of the world's population growth and increasing urbanization.

Biotechnology has given the world drought-resistant grain and "golden" rice, a variety of rice with a large supply of beta-carotene (a forerunner of vitamin A that is crucial for eyesight). The grain helps feed starving populations in sub-Saharan developing countries, and the rice helps to diminish the number of undernourished children in the world who suffer from vision problems or nutrition-related blindness. Not too many people have a problem with that.

FOOD FOR THE MIND

Both Sides of the Story

Want to be convinced that biotechnology is a good thing? Go to *www.whybiotech.com*, the website for the Council for Biotechology Information. Want to be convinced that biotechnology is not so hot? Go to *www.greenpeace.usa.org* for the Greenpeace side of the story. In addition to their biotech philosophy, this site lists food products that contain biotech ingredients.

Current Uses for GMOs

What raises eyebrows (and sometimes fists) is the GMO products that seem frivolous or are really fooling around with Mother Nature. For example, by taking a gene from one animal or plant and putting that gene in another plant or animal, we can get fresh tomatoes with a three-week shelf life, oats that require less water to grow, strawberries that are juicier, vegetables that are resistant to insect attacks, or molds and soy beans that yield more oil. Some people say "hooray," and point to increased profits for growers and producers with fewer demands on land and water. Others point to the "Frankenfood," created by tinkering with genetic material. They argue that damage to future

A NUTRI-BAR

AMA says "Biotech Okay" (Sort of)

The American Medical Association's Scientific Affairs Council's report on biotechnology stated that "the potential benefits offered by genetically modified crops and foods are many." The Council suggested that government regulation of GMOs should focus on environmental effects and the intended uses of plants. If you need a little light reading, you can view the whole report at *www.ama-assn.org/ama/pub/article/2036-3604.html*

A NUTRI-BAR

The Center For Science in the Public Interest Says, "Embrace Biotech"

The Center For Science in the Public Interest (CSPI), the same organization that warned you about the evils of saturated fats in movie popcorn and Italian food and who would like to see soda and candy banished from store shelves has put its seal of approval on biotechnology. CSPI's executive director, Dr. Michael Jacobson, suggested that biotechnology is a good tool to increase food production, help to protect the environment and to improve the health content of foods. Dr. Jacobson suggested that food-service people should stop being such namby-pambies about GMOs and start to like them and use them. Want to read all about it? Check out the January 25, 2001 issue of the *Wall Street Journal.*

generations cannot be predicted. The arguments may be moot, as most of the corn crops in the United States are either grown from GMO seed or have been cross-bred with GMO seed via wind, water, and insects.

Clean Foods

With all this discussion of organic, GMOs, and biotechnology, many people are pushing for what have been called **"clean" foods.** Consumers and culinarians are looking for fresh ingredients and processed foods that are GMO-free, have no preservatives or additives or are truly organic. We're talking back to nature or down on the farm. According to many industry experts, clean foods will be a strong market for many years to come. When you consider that the natural food sales for the year 2000 were $28 billion and that organic food sales are increasing at a rate of 24 percent per year, the experts may be right.

You may want to consider clean foods for your menu or even start your own Internet company. Of those $28 billion dollars in natural food sales, over $5 billion were sold over the Internet.

People have different reasons for purchasing or using "clean" food. Promoting health seems to be the biggest reason, either to get healthy or to stay healthy. Clean foods may also be perceived as being fresher, having a higher nutritional value or helping the environment. A poll done by *Prevention* magazine showed that Generation-Xers and Baby Boomers were very interested in eating clean foods and African-Americans and Hispanics were more interested in clean foods than whites. The most popular clean food was produce, followed by cold cereal (quinoa flakes, anyone?), breads, pasta, organic poultry, eggs, canned soups, and milk. Culinarians and chefs have become very involved in the clean foods movement.

Many high-profile chefs have gone to the media to explain their reasons for cooking with organic produce and meat. Chefs are demanding an increase in the variety and quality of organic products. Because chefs have popularized it, growers are responding with both new and heirloom varieties of organic fruits and vegetables.

FOOD SAFETY

Industry Level

The most carefully grown ingredients can prove unsafe if not processed, transported and shipped properly. Here are some of the techniques the food industry is doing to ensure a safe food supply:

Purchasing food ingredients has become a global enterprise. Fresh raspberries may have been grown in California's Central Valley or may have made the long trip from Chile. Canned or dried mushrooms may have been harvested in Washington State or packed and shipped from Malaysia. The variety and availability of products is a boon for the food-service industry.

As the complexity of the food system grows, new safety challenges arise. Along with the variety of food products may come a variety of biological, chemical and physical hazards. Because of this, food production, distribution, and preparation have come under intense scrutiny from government agencies, from consumers and from the industry itself.

Food producers, on the front line of food safety, have formed alliances with educational and research institutions to protect the food supply from start to finish. Producers of beef, pork, poultry, dairy, eggs, and produce are aware that the food-service professional and the consumer must trust the food supply.

The United States has made great strides in agriculture in the past decade. In answer to customer demands, the food service industry continues to use a large amount of produce for healthy, innovative menus. **Fresh-cut**

A NUTRI-BAR

Fat Tom

Here's an easy way to remember what bacteria needs to grow (and how to eliminate bacteria from the food you eat):

F = food: no food, no growth, so keep it clean!

A = acid or pH: bacteria which cause food-borne illness grow in a neutral environment, such as is found in protein foods, cooked grains, and rice and dairy products. Pay extra attention to their handling.

T = time: 4 hours is the maximum time for perishable foods to be in the temperature danger zone (40°F to 140°F). Perishable foods are high-protein foods or foods that have meat, cheese, dairy, eggs, or soy as an ingredient.

T = temperature: bacteria grow best between the temperatures of 41 to 140°F, so, keep hot foods hot (above 140) and cold foods cold (below 41).

O = oxygen: know which bacteria need air (such as *E. coli*, listeria and salmonella) and which live without air (such as botulism) and handle foods accordingly.

M = moisture: uncooked rice does not support bacterial growth, but add water, and watch out; bacillus cereus, here we come!

produce, produce that has been cut, peeled or trimmed and packaged, allows food-service operators to offer fresh produce that is labor-efficient and convenient. Last year fresh-cut produce sales were 10 percent of total fresh produce sales in the United States, topping $8 to 10 billion; packaged salads alone sold $1.2 billion.

The International Fresh-cut Produce Association (IFPA) is a consortium of growers, processors, and distributors of fresh-cut produce. You're familiar with fresh-cut produce as bagged carrot sticks or bagged salad kits. Knowing that the availability of produce throughout the year depends upon safe national and international programs, the IFPA is aggressive in its educational programs. For example, the IFPA's training materials suggest that all cut produce be vigorously washed as many as three times with refrigerated, sanitized water and put into special packaging to preserve freshness and be refrigerated between 33 to 41°F. The IFPA has published HACCP plans for cut produce, guides to chlorination of produce washwater and shipping point and market inspection guidelines. Growers and processors can access IFPA safety information on the Web *(www.fresh-cuts.org)*, attend regional seminars, or obtain safety update periodicals.

According to Carma Rogers, pork information specialist with the National Pork Producers Council *(www.nppc.org)*, based in Clive, Iowa, trichinosis is virtually nonexistent in American commercially grown pork. "This is due to controlled production conditions," said Rogers, "trichinosis has not been a threat to the consumer from commercially grown pork for several decades."

Production methods to control foodborne pathogens in pork can include periodic health checks of the animals, maintaining clean living environments, and ensuring that feed and water are sanitized. A three-state pilot herd certification program is currently in place, a coordinated effort of the National Pork Producers Council and several USDA agencies, including the Food Safety and Extension Service and the Cooperative States Research, Education and Extension Service. Even though trichinae infection from pork is practically nonexistent, the pork industry felt that this type of program would reassure consumers and assist with the development of the pork export market. The pilot included on-farm testing of pigs and sampling of pork from selected slaughterhouses. The Pork Council is happy to report that of 221,000 carcasses sampled no **trichinella**-positive meat was found.

Once beef and pork animals have been sold, slaughtering, processing, and transporting are the areas that may be a weak link in the chain of food safety. Both the beef and pork councils work with their members to form alliances with transportation companies and meat processors to ensure the safe shipping and handling of the finished product. Although the federal and state government provide inspection of transporting vehicles and of processing plants, many companies handling pork and beef have in-house inspections. Very often, the in-house inspections have more rigorous guidelines than the government regulations. For example, where a government inspection might allow a meat product to "pass inspection" with a numerical grade of 85 or higher, many in-house inspections require grades of 92 or higher.

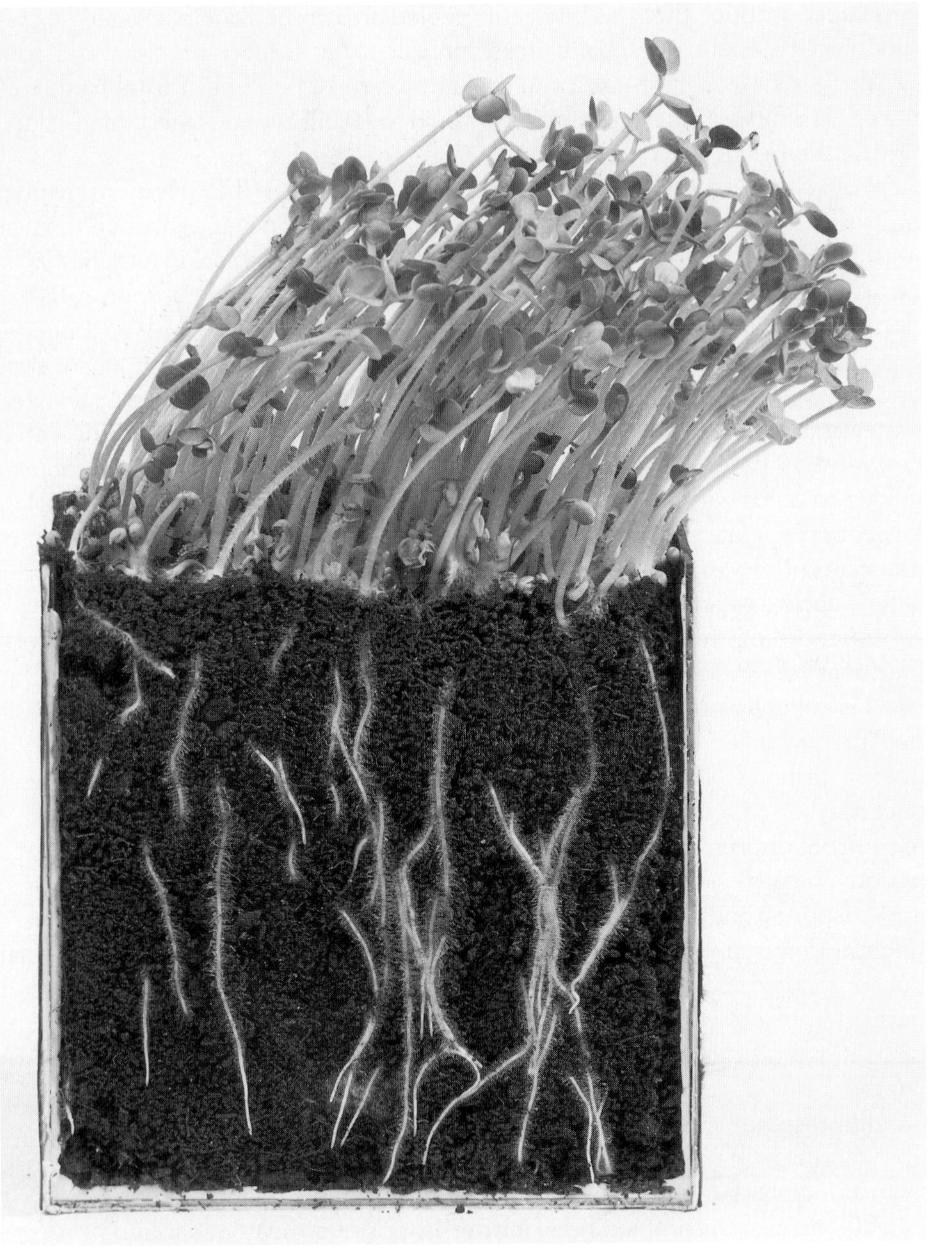

What are your suggestions for preparing these watercress sprouts in a sanitary way?

Both the Beef and Pork Councils note that food irradiation has been approved by the FDA for meat and poultry. Most meat producers have not added irradiation to their procedures, staying more with conventional safety methods. At this point, the Councils are providing consumers information about irradiation, for future reference.

"Poultry producers have a lot of control over the end product," says Bill Renigk of the National Chicken Council, based in Washington, D.C., "the producer starts at the beginning with a live bird and sees it all the way through to end processing."

Renigk explained, "The poultry industry is vertically integrated, that is, one organization is breeding, feeding, overseeing and processing the product. This leaves minimal opportunity for mistakes. It leaves less room mistakes and makes it easier to reach the ultimate goals of reduced numbers of foodborne pathogens."

Stephen Pretarik, Director of Science and Technology for the Chicken Council added, "We are very excited about the Council's Food Safety Initiative. Our members have dedicated themselves to researching and implementing new interventions focused on reducing the number of food illness pathogens."

Interventions, such as cleaning and disinfecting above and beyond current standards or adding organic acids to the poultrys' drinking water, are tested by Council members. Successful interventions are researched and polished. The Council then works with the FDA to obtain approval for the new techniques.

Before the chicken came the egg (we think). And the egg industry is doing its bit to ensure that eggs are a safe food ingredient. Several egg producers have developed safety checks and processes that are being adopted by the industry. In-shell pasteurization of eggs, is being done on a limited basis by several egg producers. Dr. Rakesh Singh, Purdue University, explained that the process is a combination of heating with hot water and microwaves.

"The bacteria within the shell is cooked, but not the yolk or the white," explained Singh, "there is no coagulation or loss of function, just loss of bacteria." Singh hopes to see this process used widely by many producers, as it will help to eliminate any health threats posed by eating undercooked eggs.

The Pennsylvania Agricultural Council developed the Pennsylvania Egg Quality Assurance Program (PEQAP) in 1994 to ensure the safety of eggs produced in the state. Producers enrolled in the program monitor and test eggs at five points and maintain the eggs at 45°F from production to sales. PEQAP participants purchase only salmonella-negative chicks, use an intense rodent monitoring system and clean and disinfect between flocks. Any eggs that test salmonella positive are diverted to a pasteurizing facility.

For humans, being under pressure is a bad thing. For oysters, it could be one of the very best things that has ever happened. Pressure inactivation of food-borne pathogens is a non-thermal (no heat required) procedure that can be used in high moisture food products.

Oysters can sometimes contain *vibrio* bacteria that cause foodborne illness in humans. *Vibrio* is usually destroyed with heat, but many consumers like to eat their oysters raw. Hydrostatic pressure treatment can solve this issue. Fresh oysters in the shell are subjected to high levels of pressure for prescribed amounts of time. Look for UHP procedures to be applied to more seafood products in the future.

The pressure not only kills off microorganisms but also cuts down on labor and enhances the appearance of the raw oyster. Oysters that have been treated with UHP (ultrahigh pressure) open more easily, making oyster shucking easier and safer. The enclosed oysters slide out of the shell easily and are intact without any attachments. The pressure does not change the flavor, taste, or color of the oyster.

Milk is one of the most rigorously tested food products and was one of the first foods that used technology to reduce the numbers of food borne pathogens. The same components that make milk good nourishment for humans are also an excellent component for bacterial growth. The minute it leaves the cow, milk can become a playground for bacteria. For this reason, rigid procedures exist for every step of milk production.

The Pasteurized Milk Ordinance (PMO) is a set of requirements for product safety, milk hauling, sanitation, equipment and labeling specified by the US Public Health Service, a division of the FDA. The PMO covers milk from production at the farm to shipment from the processor.

Milk is sampled, according to PMO guidelines, on a state-by-state basis. Samples are tested for pesticides, antibiotics, and pathogens. The EPA and other federal agencies may also get involved in the testing.

Pasteurization has been an established process for over one hundred years and is required for all interstate-shipped milk. The most common pasteurization technique is to heat milk for 30 minutes to 145 degrees or for 15 seconds at 161 degrees. Two newer forms of pasteurization are **UHT** and ultrapasteurization. UHT (ultra-high temperature) products are heated to 300 degrees for 4 to 15 seconds and packaged in aseptic boxes (popularly used as juice boxes). The UHT process and special packaging allows the milk to be safely stored at room temperature, with no loss of flavor or nutrient value. Ultrapasteurization heats milk to 280 degrees for 2 seconds. Although they have to be refrigerated, ultrapasteurized products have an extended shelf life of 14 to 28 days.

Nowadays, every aspect of the food industry is concerned about food ingredient safety. Jami Yanoski, of the National Honey Board *(www.honey.com)* notes that the Board has developed informational brochures on honey safety. Because of its physical makeup, honey does not support the growth of "headline" bacteria, such as salmonella, *E. coli,* listeria, or campylobacter. It can contain some botulism spores, but this is the exception, not the rule.

"The Center for Disease Control states that the safety of honey for older children and adults remains unquestioned," says Yanoski, "but children under one year of age may not be able to process it."

As a natural product, honey has always contained bacterial spores and yeasts, as do other natural products such as bleu cheese or fruit juice. Honey can cause a rare, but serious disease called infant botulism. Food service providers serving children under the age of one should keep that in mind.

"Honey does not contain many of the food-borne pathogens that are a concern for other foods," explained Marcia Cardetti, Director of Scientific Affairs for the National Honey Board, "it is heat treated to delay the growth of natural yeasts. This extends the shelf life and delays crystallization."

The foundation of food safety continues to be HACCP, education, and vigilance. Food safety is a chain with many links. The people in the production, processing, and distribution "links" are constantly developing new

Want to get up close and personal with the microbe world? Here are some Web sites: *www.extension.iastate.edu/foodsafety/Lesson/L1/L1p8.html*: this site covers all the big, nasty guys, including clostridium botulinum, clostridium perfringens, camplybactor, *E. coli*, listeria, Norwalk virus, staph, and salmonella. Included for each organism is a picture and a family background, such as symptoms, prevention, and incubation time. *http://microbeworld.org* The American Society for Microbiology has a "stalking the mysterious microbe" and lots of information on the miniature beasts. *http://www.nbif.org/outbreak* This site from the National Biotechnology Information Facility, New Mexico State University, may go a little over the top. Their game (they call it an "interactive teaching tool"), entitled "Outbreak!" guides you through identifying causes of foodborne illness outbreaks. Lots of gory bacterial pictures. *http://falcon.cc.ukans.edu/~jbrown/bugs.html* Sponsored by Professor Jack Brown at the University of Kansas, this site has a "What the Heck is" section that has consumer information on *E. coli*, viruses, and GMO (genetically modified organisms), to name a few.

Figure 9–6 Bugs, Ughh!

technologies and interventions to assure the continued safety of the food supply.

Involvement of Professional Organizations

Professional organizations are involved with the production of safe food products as well. The American Dietetic Association (*www.eatright.org*) has published a position paper on safety in the food industry. The paper outlines the ADA's stance on food handling procedures, food processing techniques, such as irradiation and cold pasteurization, and the impact that a safe food supply will have on a healthy America.

The Institute of Food Technologists (*www.ift.org*) recently hosted an international conference to address food safety and quality. Food processors, quality assurance personnel, food exporters and importers and growers attended the three day conference and exhibit to address such topics as the safety of fruits and vegetables and fish and shellfish in the United States and Latin America, implementation of cooperative HACCP programs in the United States and Latin America and rapid testing methods for chemicals, pesticides, and allergens.

The American Culinary Federation (*www.acfchefs.net*) requires that all certified chefs successfully complete an initial thirty-hour course in food safety and sanitation, with an eight-hour refresher course update every five years. Many professional food organizations require that their members maintain local and federal sanitation credentials.

With all the media attention and newly-passed legislation about food safety, you know that you'll have to do your part to maintain a super-duper, bells-and-whistles clean food service operation.

Food-Service Facility Level

Cleaning, and its cousin sanitizing, are the least sexy operations in the kitchen. About the only time we've seen anyone willingly volunteer to do something like scrub pots is when the executive chef has had it "up to here,"

1. Make careful purchasing selections. Don't buy canned or packaged foods from the "fire sale" rack. Do be sure that cans are not dented, leaking, bulging or missing labels. Check expiration dates on refrigerated and frozen foods and on nonperishable foods that have them. Select refrigerated and frozen foods from the back of the case to ensure proper refrigeration. Make the market your last stop before you return home.
2. Store foods properly. Keep cold foods cold. Perishable foods need to go into the freezer or refrigerator immediately. Rotate foods so the first in is the last out. Put a thermometer in your freezer and refrigerator and check at least weekly. Don't jam foods into the refrigerator or freezer. No air circulation means no chilling. Store nonperishable foods, like rice, pasta, crackers, and spices in airtight containers. Keep them off the floor and away from heat.
3. Wash and sanitize everything! Keep a dilute solution of chlorinated bleach and water in a spray bottle to wipe down knives, cutting boards, tables and other food equipment. Wash your hands frequently. Throw the sponge into the dishwasher to get rid of at least some of the bacteria growing in it. If you use cloth kitchen towels, don't cross-contaminate with them; wash them frequently.
4. Cook properly. Cooking foods thoroughly gets ride of most parasites, viruses and foodborne illness bacteria, such as *E.coli* and salmonella. Medium rare might taste good, but it could get you very sick.
5. Chill it! Leftovers should not be allowed to sit out in the kitchen. Refrigerate them as quickly as possible so that uninvited guests can't start growing on them.
6. 165 is the number. All leftovers should be reheated to 165°F before serving.

And just in case. . . .

The golden rule of food safety: when in doubt, throw it out!

Figure 9–7 HACCP for the Household

and humanely decides to perform physical violence on some sauté pans instead of the sauté cooks. This is not, however, a reliable way to get cleaning tasks accomplished on a regular basis.

Correct kitchen cleaning is a mandatory and essential fact of life. It makes no difference how great your cuisine is if your plates are dusty and your pots encrusted (not a pretty picture). It also seems to be a fact of life that everyone on a kitchen staff has to clean, and everyone attempts to avoid it like the plague (which could result if everyone gets away with not cleaning!).

HOW TO'S OF FOOD SAFETY IN FACILITIES

Cleaning entails the basic why, where, who, what, and when of any good mystery. Everyone needs to understand what he or she is to clean, when they are to clean it, with what tools and chemicals they are to accomplish the cleaning and how the cleaning should be done. Even before that, everyone must be playing by the same cleaning rules, so chemicals are used properly and equipment is cleaned carefully. We've listed our tried-and-true rules:

1. Store chemicals in their original containers—this is not just our rule, it is a law in most states. Chemicals can only be transferred to new containers if the new containers are being used in the application of the chemical. For example, small amounts of glass cleaner that comes in a ten-gallon container can be transferred to spray bottles, specifically designated and labeled for that use. Remind employees that chemicals are never to be returned to a container once they have been taken out.
2. Never mix chemicals. As a manager, attempt to purchase chemicals that do not need mixing before use. You don't want the mop sink to become someone's junior chemistry set. Water is the only acceptable substance to mix with chemicals, if appropriate, remembering to add chemicals to water, not the other way around (this keeps down the chance of chemical splashing or flaring).
3. Keep the cleaning equipment clean. Who thinks to scrub out the pot sink, delime the dish machine and sanitize the mop buckets? Your staff, we hope, with quiet prompting from you. You can't get something clean if you're using dirty equipment to clean it.
4. Air-dry everything. Dishtowels are those precious embroidered confections from home-ec class. Your kitchen is the big time and there's no place for ribbons and lace. Pots, pans, glassware, etc. need a sanitized area where they can dry, inverted, in peace. Drying even with single-use towels could mean cross-contamination. This goes for rubbing the spots off eating utensils and glassware—throw out the towels and check the rinse cycle on your dish machine.
5. Unplug it. Be sure to unplug electrical equipment before beginning to clean it.
6. The right tool for the right job. Be sure you have stocked your kitchen (and dining room) with all the right tools in the right number for the cleaning you want done (see side bar). There's nothing more frustrating than having to spend ten minutes hunting for the right brush to scrub out the floor sinks.
7. Your mother doesn't work here, so clean up after yourself. Even with properties that have a full stewarding retinue a kitchen has too many spills and drips to "let someone else get it." "Clean as you go" has got to be your slogan for both sanitation and physical safety.
8. If all else fails, follow the schedule. A well-written cleaning schedule lets everyone know the who, what and when and eliminates the "I thought the night cook did that" syndrome. Be sure to post a clearly written, easy-to-follow schedule that delineates everyone's cleaning responsibilities.
9. Clean and sanitize. We tend to abbreviate "clean and sanitize" to just "clean." Remember that all food surfaces, be they cutting boards, dining-room tables, salt-shakers, or utensil holders have to be both cleaned and sanitized.
10. Safety first. Know how to use cleaning chemicals and equipment, post instructions and manuals, provide safety equipment and enforce safety-in-cleaning rules.

HACCP

With HACCP in full swing, remember that it is a food operator's responsibility to keep Material Safety Data Sheet (MSDS) files up-to-date and accessible in a food-service operation. MSDS information must include the chemical name of all products used in the kitchen, the physical hazards of the chemicals, health hazards, and how to protect against them (such as the use of gloves and goggles for a chemical that can be a skin irritant) and emergency procedures.

MSDS information is made available through the manufacturer and is a valuable training tool (See Rules 2 and 10 above). The MSDS is another way to reinforce the concept of safety in cleaning as well as to have the right chemical used for the right purpose. Take some time to go through the MSDS file. Understanding why particular precautions need to be taken with particular chemicals can prevent your employees from hurting themselves and harming the equipment. Did we tell you the one about the enthusiastic but ill-informed employee who "polished" our brand-new reach-in with degreaser and a wire brush??? Not only did we wind up with a permanently scarred walk-in but also with a wheezy employee (fortunately, the harm done to the employee was temporary).

Cleaning and Sanitizing

We speak a lot about cleaning the kitchen, with the assumption that sanitizing goes hand in hand with cleaning. Remember, clean is the absence of visible dirt and sanitized is the absence of harmful bacteria. Anything that touches food or food utensils must be both clean and sanitized.

Heat was the original way to sanitize and is used in high temperature dishwashers. Rinse water is heated to 180°F, usually by a booster heater. If you have the capability, manual high-heat sanitizing is also possible. Equipment or ware is immersed in water that is 170°F to 195°F for 30 seconds. Large pieces of equipment, too large to immerse, can be exposed to live steam, which is at least 200°F.

A NUTRI-BAR

Stock It and They Will Clean

Be sure you have at least one from each of the following categories represented in your "cleaning closet":

- Handwashing soap (antibacterial is a plus)
- All-purpose detergent (for floor washing and general cleaning)
- Degreaser (for ovens, floors and heavily used equipment)
- Automatic dish- and warewashing soap (and appropriate rinse aids)
- Manual dish- and warewashing soap
- Glass cleaner
- Abrasive cleaner
- Sanitizer (be sure to have a test kit to check levels)
- Polish (steel, wood, and others, as appropriate to your property)

Issues with heat sanitizing are the cost of equipment and utilities (putting a booster on the dishwasher, increased gas or electric bills, etc.), maintaining the heat to provide effective sanitizing and employee safety. Heat sanitizing in an automatic dishwasher is easy to do, as the heat is contained in the machine with minimal human contact. Manual heat sanitizing exposes employees to constant high heat and requires many precautions.

Many facilities may choose to use heat sanitizing with machines and chemical sanitizing when manual washing is done. Remember that sanitizers are chemicals and you must have an MSDS for all of them.

No matter which chemical sanitizer you choose, you will have to test the levels frequently; if there is not enough concentration of sanitizer then the job isn't being done. Test kits can be obtained from your chemical supplier; testing is usually as simple as running a test strip of paper through your rinse water for several seconds. All sanitizers work well in *warm* water, not hot water. In fact, very hot water will inactivate sanitizers; optimum temperatures for sanitizers are 75°F to 120°F. Train yourself to avoid the "double or nothing" sanitizer syndrome, that is, don't fill the rinse sink with steaming hot water and then add sanitizer. Chances are the hot water will be just hot enough to inactivate the sanitizer but not hot enough to heat sanitize, so you've paid for two sanitizing techniques and gotten none. You lose on the money front and your customers lose on the exposure-to-foodborne-illness front.

The most common sanitizing chemicals used in food service are **chlorine,** iodine and **quaternary ammonia** (not the same stuff as the window-cleaning ammonia). Use the following information to decide which is best for your property:

1. Chlorine: easily identifiable, inexpensive; 50 to 100 ppm (parts per million) required for immersion for one minute for effective sanitizing. Can be corrosive to some material, tarnishes silver, is quickly inactivated in overly dirty water, functions okay in hard water.
2. Iodine: 13 to 25 ppm required for one minute. Is not corrosive, doesn't do well in dirty water, not affected by hard water, needs a low pH (5.5)—translation: keep your rinse water clean.
3. Quaternary ammonia: 200 ppm for one minute. Noncorrosive doesn't work well with hard water; okay with some dirty rinse water. Caution: Chlorine and ammonia interact. If you choose quaternary ammonia as your kitchen sanitizer, be sure to read labels for other cleaning products that may contain chlorine. Instruct employees in the appropriate use of these products.

Sanitizers work well with minimum effort as long as you follow the rules: keep rinse water clean, keep rinse water warm (not hot), expose dishes, pots, etc. for at least one minute to the sanitizer and keep sanitizer levels adequate. And no, sanitizer does not have to be rinsed off.

After you've decided what needs to be cleaned and who's doing it, walk through your kitchen and compile a list of needs for cleaning supplies. Here's a head start:

A NUTRI-BAR

Sanitation Checklist

The following checklist is the *minimum* of what the food-service manager should be looking at every day.

WORK AREA	Yes	No	Comments
1. Does fast look give indication of frequent cleaning of equipment and facilities?			
2. Are floors well-repaired?			
3. Are floor drains clean and fast-draining?			
4. Are walls and ceilings in good repair and clean?			
5. Do doors and windows have screens?			
6. Is there adequate lighting in prep and storage areas?			
7. Are handwashing facilities well-located and stocked?			
8. Is the pest-control program effective?			

PERISHABLE AND NONPERISHABLE FOODS	Yes	No	Comments
1. Are all foods ordered from reputable purveyors?			
2. Are all containers stored off the floor?			
3. Are all perishable foods stored below 41°F?			
4. Are all frozen foods stored below 10°F?			
5. Are all foods thawed in the refrigerator?			
6. Are all containers labeled?			
7. Are all foods labeled and dated and tightly covered?			
8. Are cleaning supplies isolated from food supplies?			
9. Are personal items stored out of the kitchen?			

MANUAL AND MACHINE WASHING	Yes	No	Comments
1. Are all dishes and silverware scraped and presoaked?			
2. Are correct detergents, rinse, and sanitizers used in the proper amount?			
3. Are temperatures taken and logs kept for dishwashers?			
4. Is water in pot sinks and machines changed at regular intervals?			
5. Are dishes, silverware, and pots allowed to air dry?			

TRASH DISPOSAL	Yes	No	Comments
1. Are garbage receptacles covered tightly?			
2. Are garbage receptacles and liners nonabsorbent?			
3. Are garbage receptacles washed regularly?			
4. Are garbage areas kept clean?			

PERSONNEL	Yes	No	Comments
1. Are employees made aware of cleanliness and health requirements?			
2. Are employees wearing clean uniforms, aprons and head coverings?			
3. Is appropriate footwear worn?			
4. Is frequent, proper handwashing stressed?			
5. Are locker areas adequate for personal hygiene needs?			
6. Are employees made aware of HACCP procedures?			

EQUIPMENT AND WORK TABLES	Yes	No	Comments
1. Are all equipment and food-handling surfaces made of correct material?			
2. Are all utensils and equipment in good repair?			
3. Is all equipment clean to the touch?			
4. Are cleaning procedures and schedules posted?			
5. Are thermometers available and are employees trained in their use?			
6. Are equipment and utensils stored in clean areas, off the floor, protected from contamination?			
7. Are there adequate facilities for keeping hot food hot and cold food cold?			
8. Are cleaning materials available?			

Grill Area: grill bricks, scrapers, abrasive cleaner, degreaser, wire brushes, grill pads

Oven Area: degreaser, cleaning cloths, safety goggles, heavy-duty gloves, all-purpose detergent, scrapers, brushes

Prep Area: mop, wringer and bucket, all-purpose detergent, sanitizer, scrubbing pads

Dining Room: all-purpose detergent, cleaning cloths, sanitizer, glass cleaner, stainless steel polish, polishing cloths

Dish Room: automatic detergent and rinse sanitizer, manual detergent and rinse sanitizer, presoak chemicals, abrasive cleaner, scrapers, scrubbing pads, degreaser, delimer.

Health Inspection

Now that you understand how to select safe food ingredients and how to keep the kitchen safe, you're ready for what all food service operators live for: the annual health inspection. Yes, we know this is a nutrition text and you're wondering why so much time is being spent on safety and sanitation. Well, if your kitchen's not clean, you won't be providing any food, nutritious or otherwise. Remember all food facilities, from hot dog carts to cruise ships may be inspected by a multitude of agencies, including local, state, county and federal agencies, including the Joint Commission, the Veterans' Administration, Medicare, federal and state OSHA, private insurers who place patients at health-care facilities and health inspectors from local, state, and county offices.

Never fear. You'll run a tight ship with HACCP procedures posted and understood by your staff. There will be calibrated thermometers everywhere and up-to-date temperature logs kept. Your kitchen supervisors will have completed the necessary sanitation courses and their certificates will be posted or filed. Nonfood items will be separated from food items and cross-contamination isn't even a possibility, right?

Just to review, here are some inspection etiquette dos and don'ts:

Yups:

1. Do walk around with the inspector, noting what he or she notes.
2. Do share files, invoices, and records pertinent to the inspection.
3. Do be sure to have all the appropriate posters and certificates posted where they can be easily accessed. Examples would be Heimlich maneuver posters, business licenses, sanitation certificates, etc.
4. Do provide the inspector with an area in which to work (preparing notes, writing reports).
5. Do have appropriate personnel attend the exit interview.

Nopes:

1. Don't argue or debate with the inspector.
2. Don't give files or records to the inspector and expect him or her to go through them to find the appropriate items.
3. Don't try to cover up or explain away obvious code violations.
4. Don't treat the inspector like an adversary.
5. Don't offer the inspector a meal or any special accommodations.

Inspections are inevitable, so we might as all well learn to benefit from them. Use inspections as a free second opinion (we know, we know, that's our taxpayer's dollars at work) for improvement projects or maintenance you might have planned. An impartial set of eyes is always helpful. Inspections can also be used to prove your point, as it were, with employees and administration. Employees may hear a very good sanitation message from supervisors without fully comprehending the importance of them. An outside voice can be very helpful for reinforcement. A word from an inspector may be the nudge that administration needs to approve repairs or the purchasing of new equipment or supplies.

HACCP (Hazard Analysis Critical Control Points) is an important part of health inspectors' training nowadays. Expect HACCP-style inspections in which you need to prove outcomes for safety and sanitation. HACCP is a federal mandate, so you or your manager will be expected to be conversant with the food aspects of HACCP and be able to explain how to implement HACCP in the kitchen. For example, in the good ol' days, an inspector might have gone into your walk-in refrigerator with a thermometer to see if it was working correctly. Nowadays, the inspector will want to see temperature logs, to ensure that the walk-in is working correctly every day. An inspector might also ask a kitchen supervisor how to calibrate a thermometer and how to properly take the temperature of foods and heating and cooling equipment. Just to refresh your memory, here are the seven steps of HACCP:

1. *Identify the hazard.* A good example would be ground beef, which is a potentially hazardous food.
2. *Identify the critical control points.* Critical control points are the areas that you can control in order to keep food safe. Good examples of critical control points would be receiving temperatures of meat, proper cold storage of meat, avoidance of cross contamination while preparing meat and correct hot holding of prepared meat items for service.
3. *Establish how critical control points will be accomplished.* For example, "calibrated thermometers will be available for receiving personnel; all refrigerated meat will be received at 41 degrees or lower," or "the temperature of foods held on the steam table will be checked every hour."
4. *Establish how critical control points will be monitored.* In other words, how will you prove that critical control point procedures are actually being done. Good methods are temperature logs, food waste logs and manager's logs (which note how each shift went).
5. *Establish how corrective actions will be accomplished.* If you find that critical control point procedures are not being performed correctly, how are you going to correct this situation. Examples could be employee-training sessions, educational posters, viewing of training videotapes, etc.
6. *Establish procedures that will show that the HACCP system is working.* This can also be shown with logs, as in Step 4.
7. *Establish systems of documentation that show the HACCP system is in place and is working.*

Employees don't need to be able to recite HACCP procedures. They just have to know how to do them. A HACCP recipe is a good way to reinforce HACCP techniques. Simply add a column to your recipes that include safety and sanitation information. For example, in a recipe for tuna salad, where you have instructions to "fine dice the celery and onions," your HACCP column would read "wash hands and sanitize work area and equipment prior to beginning. Wash onions and celery and do not cross contaminate with other raw foods. Cover, label and date chopped vegetables and place in refrigerator or on ice until ready to use."

There are many agencies that can provide safety and sanitation information for you to share with your employees; well-trained employees in a well-managed kitchen will pass inspection every time. The USDA publishes a newsletter, *The Food Safety Educator,* which is free to the industry (see side bar for information). Information is given on food safety teaching techniques, updates from the Centers for Disease Control, and even marketing tips for encouraging food safety. "Fight Bac!" is a current USDA teaching instrument (get more info at *www.fightbac.org*) and "Thermy—it's safe to bite when the temperature is right!" is being launched as we speak; visit Thermy the thermometer at *www.fsis.usda.gov/thermy* or 800-535-4555. The material is bright and interesting and will provide good training for your employees (and maybe impress the inspector) (Young, 7).

The purpose of a health inspection is to ensure that you and your employees are running a safe and sanitary operation. That means dotting the "i" and crossing the "T"s. Is all your equipment either National Sanitation Foundation (NSF) or **Underwriters Laboratory (UL)** certified? Can you prove it—are there labels on the equipment or information in the equipment manual? Are all employees properly attired—closed shoes, clean aprons, head covered, no nail polish, etc.? Are all foods ordered from reputable purveyors (and can you prove it with at least 6 months of invoices)? Do you have adequate numbers of cutting boards and knives, and is there enough space to thaw foods in the refrigerator so that cross-contamination is avoided? If required by your state or local law, is everyone in the kitchen current with tuberculosis tests and safety certifications? These are just some of the questions you should be asking in preparation for an inspection. Of course, you don't maintain your kitchen just so you can pass inspection, you do it so that you are producing a safe product.

Health inspectors are important in protecting public health. You know the serious consequences of foodborne illness, to the patient, the employee and the facility. With consistent, constant training and reminders, your employees will understand how to keep the kitchen, the food and themselves safe (and make the inspector's job very, thankfully, boring).

FYI: MOTHER NATURE'S HAND IN FOOD ADDITIVES

Many people say that they would prefer the ingredients included in the food they eat to be chemical-free. We have to assume that they are speaking of synthetic or man-made chemicals.

We assume this because nature is full of "natural" chemicals. As a matter of fact, information from the American Cancer Society suggests that we ingest 10,000 times more natural chemicals, by weight, than synthetic chemicals. It all depends if you want to think of a glass of orange juice as a brilliantly colored, nutritious glass of sunshine or as a combination of mono-, di- and polysaccharides, fructose, ascorbic acid with traces of phosphorus, zinc, and selenium. Semantics are very important when you want to discuss nutrition.

For example, antioxidants, such as ascorbic acid and tocopherol are used in products such as cookie mixes and canned potatoes. They ensure that the product won't discolor or develop off flavors. You know them by their more popular names, vitamin C and vitamin E. So if you add ascorbic acid to a product, are you adding a chemical or a "natural product?"

You know that you put sucrose in your caffeine-containing beverage and sprinkle sodium chloride on your fries, right? So are you loading up on chemicals or just doing what comes naturally? It's your decision.

Oxalic acid, in small amounts, binds calcium. In larger amounts, it can tan your hide. Very small amounts of oxalic acid are found in leafy green vegetables, like spinach and kale. Larger amounts are found in rhubarb leaves. Rhubarb leaves are considered to be poisonous to humans. Just to give you the idea of the intensity of natural oxalic acid, consider that, in days gone by, trappers would use crushed rhubarb leaves to tan animal hides. Oh, but don't worry. Rhubarb stalks, the red part of the rhubarb, are safe to eat. For those of you who have tried it, you know that rhubarb is extremely acidic and is usually served in sweetened dishes, such as pies and preserves.

Mother Nature is just not an entity on whom you should turn your back. Many natural products contain toxins that will do more than curl your hair if taken in large quantities. It is postulated that some plant toxins developed as a protective device; if the plant tastes bitter then predators will stay away. Think if it's natural it's okay? Think again:

Solanine: those green spots and "eyes" on your potatoes are more than extra work for the cook. They contain solanine, which inhibits central nervous system function.

Mushroom: some varieties are poisonous. Eaten in even minuscule amounts, they can cause enough damage to require a liver transplant. Some can cause almost immediate death.

Coumarin: a natural substance found in certain kinds of beans, woodruff, and other herbs. Coumarin is a natural blood thinner that is used to prevent blood clotting in people who have suffered strokes. It is also used in rat poison to cause internal hemorrhaging. It is a very potent and dangerous substance.

Goitrogens: found in raw veggies, such as turnips, cruciferous veggies (cabbage, brussel sprouts, broccoli, etc.) and soy, they can inhibit the proper functioning of the thyroid gland. Fortunately, Mother Nature gives us an out. They disappear when cooked.

Laxatives: senna, cascara, and castor oil all contain plant-based laxatives. Taken in "dieters' tea" or other herbal preparation, these natural laxatives can cause cramps, vomiting, diarrhea, seizures, and death.

Food	*Reason*
Tomatoes	longer shelf-life, improved taste and color, thicker skin, increased fiber (pectin) content
Corn	resistance to herbicides and insects
Squash	resistance to viruses
Papaya	resistance to viruses
Potatoes	resistance to insects
Rice	beta-carotene added as a means to prevent childhood blindess and other diseases linked to Vitamin A deficiencies
Soybeans	resistance to herbicides, increase in fatty acid content (so less hydrogenation is needed during processing leading to a healthier product)
Sunflowers	higher fatty-acid content to reduce hydrogenation

Figure 9–8 Bioengineered Crops

FOOD FOR THE MIND

Feeling (Naturally) Lucky? How about a little paralysis for dinner? Nothing could be more natural than a nice fresh piece of fish, right? Right! Natural and potentially the ultimate (as in last) dining experience. The puffer fish is a delicacy in Japanese cuisine. A nasty little guy, the puffer fish contains a chemical which can block nerve transmission and can result in death. But don't worry! Specially trained chefs, certified in handling puffer fish, know which parts to leave and which to take out. If you're lucky, you'll only feel a little tingle. Some people have mentioned a slight numbness which lasts for 10 to 15 minutes after eating puffer fish. A little tetrodotoxin with your meal?

Tannins: found in coffee and tea (yes, in decaf, too), tannins can bind calcium and iron, so save your coffee for a meal that doesn't have a lot of dairy or green veggies.

Aflatoxin: aflatoxins are molds that especially like to grow on the inside of peanut shells. In large amounts, they can cause cancer. All peanut crops are inspected, as is peanut butter, to ensure that the aflatoxin content is under control.

Safrole: sassafras tea used to be a popular folk cure and is still found in some Creole seasonings, such as file (pronounced "fee-lay") powder. Sassafras used to be added to root beer as a flavoring. In large amounts, the safrole in sassafras can cause cancer.

Glycyrrhizic Acid: found in real licorice (the black stuff, not those red things), this naturally occurring acid can cause elevated blood pressure and irregular heart beat. Natural licorice extract is sometimes found in herbal preparations and special teas, such as dieters' teas.

Saponins: found in sprouts, especially alfalfa, saponins can destroy red blood cells.

Nitrates: man did not think of nitrates, Mother Nature invented them first. Found in dark green leafy veggies, lettuces and some root veggies, such as beets and parsnips, natural-occurring nitrates can be converted, by heat, into nitrosamines. Nitrosamines are carcinogenic.

Does this mean you have permission to scrap fruit, vegetable and whole-grain menu items and live a life of French fries and fried pies? Hardly. It means that a good diet is a diet of variety and moderation. Just as it isn't considered to be good nutrition to exist on chocolate bars and atomic sugar flakes, it's not a great idea to live on just apples and peanut butter. Read labels, include unprocessed foods (fresh fruit and vegetables and juices, whole grain cereals and breads, etc.) and go easy on the packaged stuff. Balance is the key to good nutrition, blending the good with the not so good.

Nutri-Words

Biotechnology: a branch of food technology that seeks to enhance food crops on the genetic level.

Canning: preserving food in airless containers after a period of heating.

Charcuterie: the art of sausage-making

Chlorine: a component of some bleaches; a sanitizing agent considered to be safe to use in food service.

Cl. botulism: an anaerobic bacteria found in underprocessed, low-acid foods.

Clean/sanitary: clean is considered to be only the absence of dirt while **sanitary** is considered to be the absence of dirt and the absence of disease-causing bacteria, viruses and parasites.

"Clean" foods: foods that are not bioengineered or chemically enhanced.

Cold pasteurization: another term used for commercial irradiation of food.

E. coli: A disease-causing aerobic bacteria, found largely in meats and produce and in cross-contaminated food products.

Environmental Protection Agency (EPA): the federal agency responsible for overseeing the use of chemicals and preservation techniques in the national food supply.

FATTOM: The acronym used to remind people of the conditions that disease-causing bacteria need to grow: **F**ood, **A**cid, **T**ime, **T**emperature, **O**xygen, and **M**oisture.

Flavor enhancers: natural or synthetic substances added to food to increase flavor perception. Salt and lemon juice are examples of flavor enhancers.

Food additives: natural or synthetic substances added to foods to increase shelf life, decrease disease-causing bacteria or enhance color, flavor, or texture.

Food preservation: extending ingredient shelf-life through physical, chemical or thermal techniques.

Food processing: taking ingredients from their natural state to increase shelf-life or palatability.

Food safety: processes and procedures used to ensure the absence of microbial, chemical or physical hazards from food.

Fresh-cut produce: fresh produce that has been cut for easier consumer and industry use. such as carrot sticks or packaged salads.

Genetically Modified Organism (GMO): an ingredient or crop that has been genetically altered to improve yield or acceptability, resistance to disease, or to increase nutritional properties.

Hazard Analysis Critical Care Points/Material Safety Data Sheets (HACCP/MSDS): Federal legislation overseeing the safety of many industries, including the food service industry. Food-service professionals are expected to understand how to conduct business following HACCP guidelines.

Heirloom produce: produce grown from formerly popular seed stocks not currently in wide circulation.

Iodine: a sanitizing agent considered to be safe to use in food service; functions best in soft water.

Irradiation: exposing food to gamma rays to increase shelf-life and decrease bacterial counts.

Listeria: a disease-causing aerobic bacteria, found largely in underprocessed or unpasteurized dairy products.

Natural foods: foods served close to their natural state, with minimum processing.
Nitrites: food additives that can stop the growth of botulism.
Nitrosamines: chemicals produced when nitrite-containing foods are exposed to heat.
Organic foods: foods grown and processed without chemicals.
Pesticide residues: remnants of chemicals that have been applied to food crops.
Quaternary ammonia: a sanitizing agent considered to be safe to use in food service; can function well in hard or soft water.
Salmonella: a disease-causing aerobic bacteria, found largely in poultry and egg products and in cross-contaminated food products.
Sustainable agriculture: a system of crop selection and growing techniques designed to obtain good crop yields while replenishing the growing area.
"Transitional" foods: crops grown in fields that have used traditional growing methods and are on their way to becoming organic.
Trichinella: a disease-causing parasite, found in contaminated waters and in wild game.
Ultra-High Temperature Pasteurization (UHT): heat pasteurization done under pressure to reduce the time food products are exposed to heat. UHT minimizes nutrient loss and cooking changes.
Underwriters Laboratory (UL): an independent laboratory used by the federal government to determine the safety of nonfood food service products, such as equipment.

Whaddaya Think?

1. What would be your decision about adding nitrites to your homemade sausage?
2. Can you think of some examples of HACCP techniques you use in your own kitchen.
3. Do you have any concerns about cancer? Do you do anything special about cancer prevention in your diet?
4. Would you purchase an irradiated food product? Why or why not?
5. What's your favorite food additive? Why? What are the safety concerns?
6. Why can vitamins C and E be used as a preservative in organic foods?
7. What's your opinion of processed organic foods? Do you think they're worth the extra cost?
8. Can you think of a sustainable agriculture project for your company or your class?
9. Do you eat any foods that contain GMOs?
10. What do you see as biological, physical or chemical hazards in your kitchen at home?
11. Are you convinced that the U.S. food supply is safe?
12. Give some details about the "hazards" of some of Mother Nature's foods.
13. List all the HACCP issues you can think of for a restaurant serving sushi.

Critical Application Exercises

1. Design a HACCP recipe for a menu item containing meat or fish and eggs:
   a. Find an appropriate recipe and highlight all the "hazards."
   b. Add a column to the recipe entitled "HACCP." This column will include all the information necessary to produce food in a safe manner. For example, " sanitize cutting board, knife and hands after deboning fish."
2. Visit a grocery store and a natural food store. Find food labels that denote "organic," " no GMO," " natural," etc.:
   a. Was there a large variety of these types of products?
   b. Would these products enhance a restaurant's menu?
   c. Do these products seem to be popular?

   If you have time and access, interview a chef who uses organic products.
3. Design a small training program for front of the house staff to ensure that they are maintaining their areas in a safe manner.
4. Obtain dried peaches, canned peaches and frozen peaches:
   a. Compare taste, texture, appearance and nutritional value (from the label).
   b. Does the type of preservation method affect the final product? Comment on these after sampling the peaches.

References

Chapman, Nancy, (2000). "The Long-Awaited Organic Rule," *Prepared Foods Magazine,* February p. 20.

Durant, Dianne, (2000). "FoodNet Follow Up," *Food Safety Educator,* United States Department of Agriculture Food Safety and Inspection Service, Washington, DC, Volume 5, No. 4 3/2000 (also available at *www.fsis.usda..gov/OA/educator/educator.htm*).

Lehman, Phyllis, (1992). *More Than You Ever Thought You Would Want to Know About Food Additives,* FDA CONSUMER, Department of Health and Human Services, Food and Drug Administration, Rockville, MD.

Leibman, Bonnie, (1995). *Carcinogens in Chickens,* NUTRITON IN ACTION, Center for Science in the Public Interest, 22:9 (November).

Omaye, Stanley, (2001). "Biotechnology and Sustainable Agriculture," *Food Technology Magazine,* 55:2, 23–35, February.

Sloan, Elizabeth, (2001). "Clean Foods," *Food Technology Magazine,* 55:2, 18, February.

Young, F. E., (1989). *Weighing food safety risks,* FDA CONSUMER, September, p. 8.

Chapter 10

Ethnic Cuisine

Chapter Overview

Chapter Objectives

After reading this chapter, the student should be able to:

1. *Explain the evolution of healthy ethnic cuisines*
2. *Describe the selection of ethnic food ingredients, herbs and spices*
3. *Suggest healthy ethnic alternatives for traditional menu items*
4. *List and describe ingredients and cooking techniques used in Asian and Indian cuisine*
5. *Develop French menu selections that are low in fat*
6. *Suggest how to use salsas as low fat alternatives for sauces and gravies*
7. *Determine how ethnic cuisines can be used in a healthy menu marketing plan*

Introduction

When consumers think of healthy cuisine, they often think of foods that are either lower in fat, lower in salt, higher in fruits and vegetables, lower in meat or all of the above. Unfortunately, consumers may also equate healthy food with unappetizing food. Just because they are thinking of less butter or less meat does not mean they will accept naked chicken and parched salad.

So, the menu designer may ask, what am I supposed to do? Without adding gravy to the roast or frying the chicken, how can I make a flavorful menu? The answer is simple: think ethnic.

READ YOUR HISTORY

Historically, many ethnic cuisines are inherently healthy. Not because people "back then" were virtuous or particularly health conscious, but because many items were too expensive, too valuable, or just not available. In years past, many West African countries were known for their cattle-raising expertise. Although the herds were plentiful, the majority of the population was vegetarian. Why? Because the number of cattle one owned established where one fit in the social order. Also, products obtained from the animal, such as milk or wool, made the animal more valuable alive. In the same way, many Eastern European and Southeast Asian countries raised fair amounts of cattle, sheep

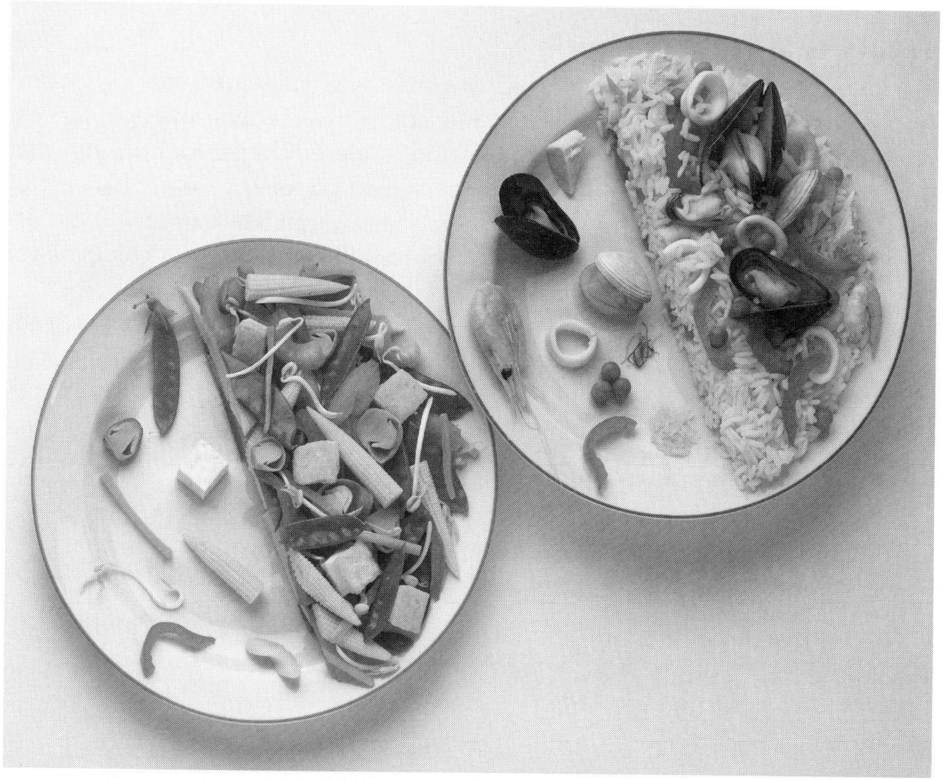

Ethnic foods make an elegant plate presentation.

and water buffalo, but the diet was generally very low in meat products. Animals were needed for their working ability and for the products they yielded. As a result, diets were generally low in saturated fats and high in fiber, something we strive for today (Barer-Stein, 1).

Use What You've Got

Cooking techniques and ingredients were simple because equipment was rudimentary, and fuel was scarce, expensive or both. Ingredients that could not be grown or gathered were used sparingly, as they were expensive or in short supply. If you had to spend several months' income to purchase enough salt for the year, you'd use it sparingly! Ethnic dishes were flavorful, spicy, and interesting, using seasonal ingredients locally grown. Many times they were not high in fat, as meat, dairy or oil were too expensive to use or not readily available. Seems like the perfect combination for today's menu, that is, healthy and cheap.

Not that ethnic cuisines were all wonders of nutritional science. The amount of meat, saturated fat (translation = cholesterol), and salt in your diet depended on where you lived. If you lived near an ocean or a sea, then you got lots of lean protein from fish and seafood, but also got a lot of salt, since it was easily harvested from the saltwater. If you lived in an olive-growing region, then your chief dietary fat was unsaturated, from olive oil. On the other hand, if you lived where the coconuts grew, then your main fat was highly saturated, from coconut, palm and other tropical oils.

Thrifty Is as Thrifty Does

Whatever kind of fat and meat was available was still eaten sparingly compared to today's usage. Both plants and animals were available for harvest seasonally. If you slaughtered an animal and rendered the fat for cooking, that fat had to last several months. The same would go for the yearly harvest of oil-producing plants. Try using cooking techniques that use fat in the most efficient way and you'll get the idea. Respect for all ingredients is a guideline for both ethnic and healthy cuisine.

We are not suggesting that ethnic cuisine will eliminate all the fat, salt, cholesterol, and other so-called villains of the food world. Your goal is not to provide an extremely low-calorie, no-fat, no-salt menu. Ethnic cuisine can offer lower-salt, lower-fat menus that have less meat and dairy and more fruit, vegetables, grains, and starches than traditional American or classical Continental cuisine.

Eat the Pasta, Pass the Burger

Traditional Italian cuisine is a perfect example. As we noted in Chapter 1, the **Mediterranean** Pyramid is a paragon of good health, with its accent on vegetables and grains and its small amounts of dairy and meat. Traditional Italian cuisine was flavorful but sparse because much of the Italian population lived with little material wealth. Vegetables and grains were easier and cheaper to grow than animals and the cuisine developed around that. In Italy, many generations lived on pasta, polenta, whole-grain breads, cooked or marinated greens and vegetables, olive oil, and fresh and dried fruit. The first Italian generation living in the United States had to substitute butter for olive oil, canned vegetables for fresh, and white bread for whole wheat, as that was what was available at the time. You can imagine the weight gain and the ensuing heart disease, high blood pressure and diabetes that resulted as a consequence of the diet change (Kittler, 4).

Conversely, the American diet (as in cheeseburgers and fried chicken) is negatively influencing the health of other countries. Children in Italy, Japan, and Southeast Asia are eating more meat and dairy in the form of fast-food menus. They are also heavier and have higher body-fat percentages than previous generations. Nutrition educators in those countries are attempting to bring back the popularity of traditional foods. Compare the traditional Japanese school lunch which usually includes less than an ounce of animal protein, with lots of cooked and raw vegetables and rice or wheat or rice noodles with the chili dogs and French fries of the American child's lunch.

TAKE A CULINARY TOUR

This chapter was written as a guide, an "ethnic cuisine 101," as it were. Think of this chapter's information as an extended magazine article in a culinary journal. Or think of it as a tantalizing introduction to several world cuisines. As we rhapsodize about spices and exotic produce, you should be thinking about how you will incorporate new flavors and extracts where the butter and the sausage used to be.

Asian Cuisine

Chinese, Taiwanese, Burmese, Tibetan, Vietnamese, Cambodian, and Japanese cuisines are just some of the Asian cuisines that rely heavily on vegetables to flavor and fill up appetizers, soups and entrees. Vegetables are generally low in sodium and fat and high in fiber, minerals and vitamins. But beyond the health aspect, Asian vegetables are an exotic, flavorful addition to traditional or fusion cuisine.

Want Some Gai with Your Fun?

Greens are an important ingredient in **Asian cuisine.** Asian greens are easy to prepare and are attractive on the plate. For customers, Asian greens are exotic enough to be interesting but familiar enough not to be scary. Greens can be spicy, mild, biting or sweet. They add substance to a dish without adding fat or salt. Here's your Asian green vocabulary list:

Bok choy: probably the most familiar of all Asian greens, mild-flavored bok choy is available in large and baby-sizes. The dark green leaves can be used for braising (think chicken stock and garlic) and for garnishing soups (think broth with sliced green onions, minced ginger and shredded bok choy leaves). Use the white stalks for stir-frying and as an ingredient in soups and curries.

FOOD FOR THE MIND

Fusion cuisine is a blending of several traditional cuisines to create new dishes. For example, portabello stuffed won ton with ponzu sauce fuses Italian, Chinese and Japanese cuisine.

FOOD FOR THE MIND

To get a look at some of the exotic produce mentioned in this chapter, surf the Web. Two good sites are *www.freidas.com* and *www.melissas.com,* two specialty produce purveyors. You can also find recipes for specialty produce in the *Purple Kiwi Cookbook* (Kaplan, 3) and *Ethnic Cuisines* (Rozin, 6).

Napa (or Chinese) cabbage: delicately pleated, napa cabbage can be thinly sliced and hurriedly steamed. Once cooked, it can be used as a bed for foods instead of pasta. Add napa to soups, vegetable mixes, and hot salads.

Gai choy (or mustard cabbage): each leafy head grows to only about 10 inches, resembling a miniature bok choy. It can be steamed or stirfried whole and served as an accompaniment dish. Gai choy is a member of the mustard green family and has a tangy flavor.

Ong choy (water spinach): has long, dark-green leaves and hollow stems. It can be used wherever traditional spinach is used.

Gai lan *(Chinese broccoli):* as with bok choy, probably very familiar to American diners. The solid stems, dark leaves and white flowers can be braised in oyster or black bean sauce (in Asian-speak, black beans are black soybeans) as an entrée or braised and used as a side dish (Kaplan, 3).

Asian Basil (also called Thai basil): looks a bit like the usual basil, but has a licorice-like note that gives a Thai, Indonesian, or Vietnamese flair to sautéed or braised vegetables. Think about sautéing spinach with garlic and a little Asian basil.

Asian mint (also called shiso or green perilla): is a cross between basil and mint with a long leaf. In Vietnamese and Cambodian cuisine, Asian mint is used in place of rice paper wrappers for spring rolls. In Japanese cuisine, shiso is breaded and lightly wok—fried just like tempura. Finely chop shiso and add to salads and to stir-fries.

Cilantro: a very international green, cilantro is also known as "Chinese" or "Spanish parsley." Related to parsley and carrots, with seeds that go by the name of coriander, cilantro has a distinctive flavor that may take some getting used to. It can stand up to strong flavors, such as lemon grass, ginger and garlic, and is a perfect garnish or ingredient for dishes seasoned with chili. Cilantro can have a cooling effect on dishes with a bit too much fire.

Eggplant, or aubergine, did not originate in a field of parmigiana, but rather in the woks of Asia. Asian eggplant come in a purple rainbow that begins with palest white and ends in deepest royal purple, with pale greens and lavenders in-between. Asian eggplant shapes start at tiny pea and oval egg, go through to tennis ball, and end at the usual oblong. Pea eggplants are chubby green balls that grow in clusters and add a welcome bitterness to curries and salads.

Thai eggplant can be white and green or all white and all green and resemble veggie golf balls. They are crunchy and tart and appeal to American palates.

Slender eggplants, also called baby or Japanese eggplants are slightly spicy and are usually white-fleshed with purple skin (that is edible). They can be used in soups, stirs, cassoulets, or as a side dish on there own. Japanese eggplant can be tempura-ed to add to the usual carrots, potatoes, squash, green beans and bell peppers.

Asian veggies require little assembly—just a little fast heat, a dash of sauce, and a little liquid. You already have the stock, the ginger, the garlic and the onions and probably the soy sauce. You may want to try some of the following for fast and easy Asian gourmet tastes; not low salt but definitely lower fat than traditional gravies and sauces.

Garam Masala: is a mixture of ground spices, usually containing cinnamon, black pepper, cumin, clovers, cardamom, and nutmeg and carries the flavors of India, Indonesia, and Malaysia

Hoisin Sauce: a thick, red sauce made from soybeans, garlic, sugar, and spices, this adds a tang and sweetness to sautéed greens

Miso: a Japanese staple, made from fermented soybeans and wheat, rice, or barley, miso has a wine-like taste and can be used in sauces and soups. Miso comes in a variety of colors and flavors.

Curry Paste: spice combos are ground and mixed with oil to form fiery flavors. Every country and region has its own curry mixture. Indonesian sambal paste has red chilies, Ceylon curry has fennel, fenugreek, and cumin. Purchase a basic chili paste and add your own signature fire.

Soy Sauce: there are many varieties of soy sauce. Chinese is generally stronger; Japanese soy sauce is more delicate. There are many lower-sodium versions. Have a tasting and match your menu items with your soy sauce.

Don't Forget the Fruit

Mangos and papayas are fruit that can masquerade as vegetables or add a sweet note to savory dishes. Although grown in many tropical countries, mangos and papayas are thought to have originated in Asian countries and have certainly been incorporated into Asian cuisine.

Mangos are available fresh, frozen, in concentrate, and as a frozen or canned juice. Ripe, fresh mangos are wonderful sliced and served as a refreshing dessert or as part of a seasonal fruit salad, or chicken or seafood salad. Ripe mangos can be sliced and served on top of sorbet (or made into sorbet) and incorporated into baked fruit tarts, muffins, and scones. If you find yourself with overripe or frozen mangoes, use them in smoothies and in bar beverages or in savory sauces for grilled seitan or tempeh. Underripe or green mangos can be shredded and used in pasta or green salads or used as a "vegetable" in curries and stirfries.

Papaya is also available fresh and frozen. You are probably accustomed to the pear-shaped, yellow-orange papaya with a million seeds and the peachy-strawberry flavor. Ripe papaya is an excellent dessert, simply halved and filled with a scoop of sorbet or fresh berries. Use papaya cut into pasta or rice salad and even into mixed green salads. Papaya is a colorful way to top sorbet sundaes or to use as an ingredient in soy or rice milk custards. Overripe or frozen papaya can be used in sauces and in fruit shakes.

We tend to forget that pineapple is a tropical fruit, used in Asian cuisine for sweet and sour tastes, as a condiment, and as a dessert. Ripe, fresh

Spice blends, such as this chat masala, can replace the salt in some recipes.

pineapple has a delicate flavor and can be a perfect counterpoint to spicy dishes. Think about a skewer of pineapple with fresh mint served with a fiery Indonesian vegetable curry, barbecued Korean tofu or with garlicky stirfries. Develop pineapple's sugar content by grilling or sautéing it with a touch of rum and serve hot on top of sorbet. Pineapple can be used in both sweet and

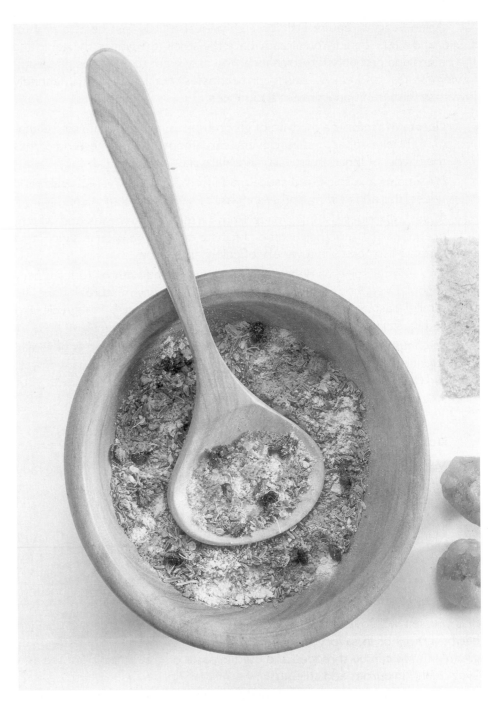

savory sauces, in bar beverages and in bakery items (think pineapple scones or a pineapple pie).

Starfruit, also called carambola, available fresh and dried, looks like a bright-yellow, three-dimensional, five-pointed star. Its tangy sweet flavor, firm flesh, and engaging shape makes it perfect to garnish . . . everything!

Kumquats are available fresh and canned (usually in heavy syrup). Fresh kumquats are an inside-out fruit. Resembling miniature, oval oranges, the kumquat skin is sweet and the pulp is tart. Kumquats can be used whole for garnishes in salads and on desserts or sliced and used in sauces.

Lychees are available fresh, canned and frozen, but the canned are more practical for food service applications. Fresh lychees are very seasonal and have skins that resemble red porcupines and seeds that take up about 50 percent of the fruit. The payoff is that fresh lychees are the roses of the fruit world, highly aromatic with a luscious flavor. However, if you want your staff to continue to speak to you, purchase canned lychees (they're already peeled and seeded) for your property and leave the fresh ones for home. Canned lychees retain a great deal of their flavor and are juicy and smooth. Mix them with tart fruit, such as grapefruit sections, serve with frozen desserts or use in sauces for cooked vegetables.

There are many Asian fruit that are available to the food-service operator, such as the blood orange (a crimson-pulped orange traditionally used for sauces and bar beverages) and the **pummelo,** which resembles a grapefruit on steroids and tastes like a very sweet grapefruit. These are still very seasonal and costs may vary, so include cautiously in your menu.

We feel it is our responsibility to warn you against jackfruit, however. Jackfruit is very popular throughout Asia, although its aroma is so strong that some hotels do not allow guests to bring fresh jackfruit into their facility. Jackfruit usually weigh about ten to fourteen pounds each, are covered with a knobby brown skin (think fruit-flavored armadillo), have a multitude of black seeds and has a flavor that could be compared, when downwind, to overripe meat. If you are still really curious about jackfruit, you can find jackfruit juice (canned) and frozen cubed jackfruit in Asian markets.

A Many-Layered Palette

Asian cuisines rely on the skill of the chef. What it does not rely on are large portions of meat. Traditional Asian cuisine does not use as much oil or deep fat frying as some American interpretations. Dairy is almost nonexistent. The Asian chef selects from a multitude of spices to heighten the interest of menu items. Some seasonings hit the taste buds immediately, some release their flavors gradually and some don't become evident until several minutes later.

The **Chinese five-spice** mixture is a perfect example. Containing dried star anise, black pepper, fennel, cloves, and cinnamon, this mixture is a balance of heat, smoothness, aromatics, and spice. Mix your own or purchase commercial mixtures. To add a Chinese accent to soups, sparingly add five-spice to mushroom broth, along with minced ginger and minced fresh garlic, chopped green onions and snow peas; with the addition of steamed tofu pieces and white rice or rice vermicelli you will have created a delicate yet flavorful appetizer (Rozin, 6).

Indian, Moslem, and Chinese influences can be seen in the cuisines of Singapore and Malaysia. Create a curried mix vegetable dish by steaming summer squash, green beans, green cabbage, and onions, and serving with a sauce made with sautéed onions, tomato and garlic with fresh chili, lemon zest, coconut milk, and vegetable stock. Build this side dish into an entrée by adding rice noodles and pieces of fried seitan or tofu.

Many of the ingredients in American kitchen, such as mushrooms, cabbage, onions, tomatoes, carrots, chopped peanuts, fresh ginger and garlic, and fresh and dried chilies are prime ingredients in Asian cuisine. To capture authentic flavors, you may want to investigate stocking some of the following herbs, spices and condiments:

Chinese Five Spice: a powdered blend of star anise, fennel, black pepper, cloves, and cinnamon. Used to flavor sauces, fake meat dishes, and noodle dishes.

Lemon Grass: is a long-stemmed herb that has a citrus flavor. Fresh lemon grass has the most flavor, and is used in Thai, Vietnamese, and Chinese dishes, such as Thai coconut soup. If fresh lemon grass is not available, use lemon zest instead.

Rice Vermicelli: these dried, thin, glass-like noodles can be soaked and used in stir-fries or soups or can be quickly deep fried for a crunchy garnish or to form an edible basket.

Rice Vinegar: is a clear, mild, and sweet-tasting vinegar, suited to Japanese and Singapore cuisine. If not available, diluted white wine vinegar can be used.

Seitan: called the "wheat" of the meat, seitan has a chewy texture akin to steak. Seitan can be marinated and prepared just like beef or the dark meat of poultry.

Sesame Oil: is a dark brown oil with a nutty, rich flavor. Do not refrigerate, as it will cloud. Use it for Chinese, Korean, and Japanese dishes.

Soy Sauce: there are many varieties of soy sauce; do a tasting and decide which type suits your menu.

Tamarind: sold as a paste, tamarind can be used as a "sour" wherever lemon might be used.

Tempeh: is a soy product one step beyond tofu. Tofu is allowed to ferment to create a chewy, nutty-flavored product that can be used in place of meat.

Wasabi: also called Japanese horseradish, although wasabi is not related to horseradish, wasabi is a river vegetable with a root resembling dark green ginger. Sold as a paste, wasabi is very hot and can be used in soups and as a condiment.

Wrappers: finger food and dumplings are popular in Asian cuisines. Won ton wrappers are small squares of wheat flour and egg dough, so they are not vegan. Spring roll wrappers are a larger version of won ton, or can be made from rice flour. Rice paper wrappers are very thin, made from rice flour and water (and are vegan) and must be brushed with water before using so they become flexible.

Ginger: has got to be the one particular flavor that everyone associates with Asian cuisine. This homely root is probably the key ingredient for boosting the popularity of Asian cuisine in the United States. Ginger's aromatic and "heat" qualities add flavor and intrigue to entrees, sauces, accompaniment dishes and desserts.

No one is really certain where ginger originated or even how old it is because it has never been found growing wild. The earliest ginger cultivators were in India and China; ginger comes from the Indian Sanskrit word for "antlers" (you can see the resemblance) (Batra, 2). During the Middle Ages, ginger was traded as actively as salt and pepper, introduced to Western culture in gingerbread and cookies. Ground ginger was used as a condiment to enhance the flavor of beer in medieval England; this ginger beer was the forerunner of ginger ale.

Fresh ginger has a clean, palate-cleansing property. Used in fish dishes (think: soy-seared sole with fresh ginger and sesame seeds), ginger adds a refreshing, delicate flavor. Fresh ginger, also called green ginger, is essential in Asian and Indian cuisine. It can give a subtle heat to sorbets and dessert sauces (think: ginger-mango sauce for a lemon sorbet) and piquancy and warmth to braised vegetables (think: bok choy braised in mushroom broth with ginger and garlic) and stir frys. To get the most from fresh ginger, peel it and mince, thinly slice or grate it. Large pieces of ginger do not release much flavor and can be too intense if bitten into. Fresh ginger (unpeeled) will last up to one month in the refrigerator.

Dried ginger, usually ground into a powder, is usually a combination of several types of ginger, giving a different flavor and heat to recipes. Ground ginger shows the best in baked goods. Add an Asian flair to your breakfast menu with tangerine-ginger muffins or ginger-kumquat crepes.

Crystallized ginger is a dried, sweetened form of ginger and can be eaten as candy or used in cooking; it may or may not be vegan, depending on the sweetener used. Green ginger is allowed to soak in sugar syrup and is then dried and coated with sugar, creating a sweet-but-hot candy. Crystallized ginger can be chopped into baked goods, used in sauces to provide a counterpoint for fiery entrees (think: three-chili beef stirfry with ginger-pineapple sauce) or can be served with ice cream or sorbets.

Lovers of sushi will recognize preserved ginger. Pretty in pink, preserved ginger is green ginger that has been thinly sliced and stored in light syrup. This salmon-colored ginger has a sharp, concentrated flavor and is traditionally served as a condiment for sushi, but has lots of applications for vegetables and cooked grains, such as rice and couscous (I know, couscous isn't a grain, but a pasta). Serve it on the side instead of a sauce or toss it in at the end of cooking to give a clean Asian flavor.

The Asian Kitchen

When you think Asian, do you think the stirfries, dumplings, and Peking Duck of China, the hot and sour soup and the fire and ice salads of Thailand, the whisper-light tempura and the fresh sushi of Japan, or the noodle soups (phos) and the spring rolls of Vietnam? Or do you lean towards the skewered beef and the marinated fish of Laos, the spicy satays of Indonesia, the empanadas and chorizo of the Philippines or the Indian-influenced curries of Singapore? While you're thinking, don't forget the potato pancakes and hotpots of Korea, the mild curries and fish soup of Burma, and the roasted spices and vegetable fritters of Sri Lanka.

Eat with Your Hands

Asian cuisine has a range of finger foods, served with fragrant teas and cool beers. So, in addition to the dim sum ("little bits") be sure to offer a menu of teas and beers to complement the multiple flavors.

Spring rolls are large won ton, filled with an assortment of chopped and wok-fried or steamed vegetables, meat or fish. For a Thai flavor, add fresh ginger, garlic, cilantro, fresh chili and brown sugar. For a Vietnamese taste, use Asian basil, lemon grass and fish sauce. For Chinese, use bean sprouts, soy sauce, garlic and black pepper. Spring rolls can be fried or steamed and should be accompanied with dipping sauces.

Won tons have traditional names, such as chicken money bags and son-in-law pouch. Fill with the same ingredients as spring rolls and steam or fry, offering several different types on one plate. Small tomatoes or peppers can be stuffed with chopped pork or shrimp, garlic, onions, mushrooms, and egg and quickly fried or steamed.

Dipping All the Way

A small bowl of dipping sauce can heighten the enjoyment of Asian finger foods and of fresh vegetables without adding a lot of extra calories. Ranging from a small dish of soy sauce to complex sauces, dipping sauces can be served with won ton, spring rolls, noodles, tempura, and satays (skewered, thin sliced chicken, beef, pork, or fish). Dipping sauces are lower in saturated fats then traditional gravies or sauces and are generally used in smaller amounts than their Continental cousins.

Have a tasting of commercial dipping sauces and serve as is or add your own signature ingredients. To whip up some fast sauces, try the following:

Sesame Seed Sauce: toast sesame seeds in a dry pan until seeds are golden brown. Grind the seeds in a food processor and add oil until a paste is formed. Flavor with soy sauce, sugar, miso and white pepper.

Soy and Ginger Sauce: Combine minced fresh ginger, soy sauce and sugar. Mix well and serve immediately (this does not hold up well when stored).

Lemon and Garlic Sauce: Combine fresh lemon juice, fish sauce, chopped red chilies, chopped fresh garlic and a small amount of sugar. Serve immediately.

Cilantro and Chili Sauce: Combine fish sauce, chopped fresh cilantro, chopped red chilies and a small amount of brown sugar. Serve immediately.

Thai Peanut Sauce: Sauté chopped onions until soft and slowly stir in peanut butter, chopped garlic, minced fresh ginger, chili powder and coconut milk. Stir until thickened, add ground cumin, lemon juice, garnish with chopped peanuts and serve hot.

A Spicy Bowl

Yum is a flavor unique to Thailand, combining sour, salty, spicy, and aromatic all in one bowl. This taste bud heaven is made with fish sauce, lime or tamarind, fresh chili, lemon grass and fresh ginger. Cooked into a chicken stock with a little coconut milk and some shredded cabbage, *Tom Yum* is the Thai answer to that comforting bowl of chicken soup. Not only will it comfort, but it will also surprise, delight and cheer with very little fat.

Chinese chicken and sweet corn soup is almost an entrée in a bowl. A creamy appearance is made with creamed corn and corn flour, with no dairy present. Chicken pieces are chopped and folded into whipped egg whites. This is added to boiling chicken stock, stirred, and thickened with creamed corn and corn flour. Flavor comes from soy sauce and fresh green onions.

Japanese Udon noodle soup can be made from prepared miso broth to which is added soy sauce, minced green onions or leeks, paper-thin cut chicken or pork and udon noodles (thick, wheat noodles). This soup can be garnished with scrambled eggs and fresh peas.

From Burma we get Twelve Varieties Soup. Chicken broth is loaded up with chicken pieces, mushrooms, garlic, onions, ginger, green beans, cauliflower, cabbage, spinach, bean sprouts, and green onions, and flavored with fish sauce, cilantro, soy sauce, and lime!

Korean dumpling soup uses rice paper wrappers to enrobe minced chicken, garlic, cabbage, bean sprouts, mushrooms and onions that are simmered in a broth flavored with soy sauce, onions, and fresh ginger. Sometimes served with sautéed spinach, this soup is sure to chase away the blues.

Sourness and tang are an important component to the many-layered complexity of Asian flavor building. Asian countries were producing vinegar long before European cuisine had discovered it. Used as both a condiment and cooking ingredient, there are a huge number of Asian vinegars from which to select. Chinese vinegars, made largely from rice, as used for dipping sauces, marinades and dressings. Shanxi vinegar is the balsamic vinegar of China. It is a black vinegar made from sorghum, barley and dried peas and is popularly used for pot stickers, soups and noodle dishes. Japanese vinegars, also mostly made from rice, are milder than Chinese vinegars. Vinegar trivia: "sushi" translates as "vinegared rice."

Tamarind, a fruit which produces flavorful seed pods, is very widely used in Asian cuisine, as well as Central and Southern American cuisine. If you have enjoyed the soury tang of Chinese, Thai, Indian, and even Cuban, Guatemalan, Mexican, and Salvadoran cuisine, you have experienced the versatility of tamarind. In Asian cuisine, tamarind is used just like lemon in American cuisine, for acid flavoring. Purchase tamarind as an extract, powder, paste or concentrate (it is available fresh, but is too labor intensive to use easily) and include it in hot and sour soups and sauces, curries, marinades and even beverages (think: tamarind-strawberry lemonade).

Ethnic Sweet Endings

Classical and American desserts can be loaded with eggs, butter, cream, sugar, and all those other ingredients that consumers may be trying to avoid. A simple sorbet or fruit ice, a dried fruit compote with ginger or a trio of melons may suffice for a happy meal ending. If you'd like to offer a little more for dessert, think ethnic. Ethnic desserts may not be low in calories, but they can be lower in calories than pie a la mode and can be much lower in fat than traditional American desserts.

Meat can serve as a garnish in Asian dishes.

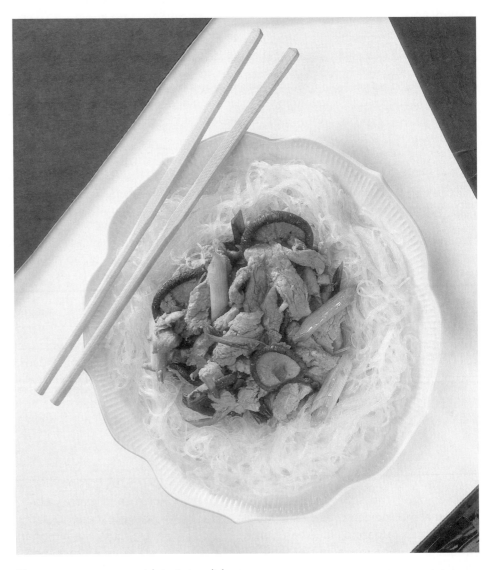

Dessert in the Middle East

Cooking in the Middle East is deeply traditional, with respect for customs and loyalties. Ingredients are selected carefully and may have histories and legends attached to them. For example, milk mixed with honey and cinnamon combined with eggs (you can use vegetarian egg replacer for vegans or egg substitutes for lower cholesterol menus) are said to have awakened thoughts of love in many of the heroes of yesteryear. Spices are particularly valued in Middle Eastern cooking and vary from region to region. Cinnamon, mint, honey, pine nuts, cloves, almonds, dried fruit, such as dates and apricots, coffee, sesame, and yogurt (use low-fat or non-fat or soy yogurt!) are found in some combination in most countries and are used to flavor both sweet and savory dishes.

Yogurt is used both as an ingredient and as a beverage in Middle Eastern cooking. Soy yogurt can be used in place of dairy yogurt. Choose unflavored yogurt if you want to give your menus a Middle Eastern flair. Thin yogurt with a small amount of ice water and flavor with peach or apricot nectar, crushed strawberries or raspberry syrups; serve over ice as a refreshing drink. It is believed that yogurt is a health food in many Middle Eastern countries, capable of prolonging youth and fortifying the soul; it is recommended there for relief of ulcers, sunburn, and to prevent hangovers. You can use it as a dessert sauce, flavored with liqueurs, syrups or pureed fruit or use it to replace some or all of the liquid in baking recipes, to give a pleasant "tang." Try a combination of yogurt, low-fat sour cream, brown sugar, orange zest and orange juice for a modern take-off on *Mandalina*, a traditional Egyptian sweet. A similar combination, flavored with nutmeg and dried apricots is a traditional Lebanese dessert. Use either as a dessert sauce, served over fresh melon or berries, or served over phyllo. You can find vegetarian phyllo in the frozen section of many markets.

The current trend towards flakier and lighter-appearing desserts fits a major ingredient of Middle Eastern desserts to a "t." **Phyllo** dough originated in the Middle East and is lightly textured pastry dough, perfect to show off seasonal or frozen fruit, sorbets, dried fruit, nuts and dessert sauces.

Phyllo (also spelled "filo" or "fillo") is a paper-thin dough or pastry sheet used to make Middle Eastern and Greek desserts. European bakers adapted this delicate dough for their own purposes, using it to enrobe apples, raisins and sweet spices—the apple strudel was born! Purists would tell you that there is a difference between strudel and phyllo, but for our purposes, they are interchangeable. Phyllo is delicate, sweet and flavorful and can be relatively low in fat.

Phyllo dough can, of course, be made from scratch. If you have ever seen puff pastry dough made, you know that it has over 1,000 layers by the time it is completed; phyllo has even more! For our money (and sanity), we work with frozen phyllo dough, which is available in eleven- by seventeen-inch sheets. A one-pound box usually has about twenty-five sheets. Frozen phyllo dough is very delicate and requires a delicate touch. After much pain and aggravation we can give you the two most important points for handling frozen phyllo: be sure to allow phyllo to thoroughly thaw (in the plastic sleeve it comes in) before handling and after opening the package, be sure to keep the sheets covered with a damp towel to avoid drying. Work with one sheet at a time, keeping the remainder covered. If you follow these points and have a little patience, you can create some wonderful phyllo desserts.

If you don't have the time to prepare your own baklava, you can still work with phyllo to prepare desserts. Shred or slice thawed phyllo and bake on a lined baking sheet until golden brown. Serve hot, topped with vanilla, peach or pistachio sorbet, frozen yogurt or orange or lemon sorbet; garnish with a sprinkle of cinnamon or chopped nuts or dried fruit. Thawed phyllo can be shredded and molded into individual containers and baked or deep-fried, to form dessert nests. Fill with sweetened yogurt; make your own by combining unflavored yogurt with chopped nuts, chopped dates, and fresh berries.

Every country has its version of petits four, or small dessert delicacies. To create a Middle Eastern dessert table, create platters with many varieties of dried fruit, especially dates, raisins, figs and apricots. Prepare a yogurt-cream dip for them, flavored with orange and lemon zest, cinnamon, and sweetener. Nuts, especially almonds and pistachios are traditional. Order frozen baklava and serve warm, with clove and cinnamon flavored syrups. Prepare or purchase macaroons and serve garnished with chopped nuts. Halavah, a dry candy made from crushed sesame seeds, comes in a long bar and can be sliced and served with chopped nuts.

Hot coffee or tea is an important part of the Middle Eastern dessert course. In Morocco you will find sweetened mint tea, served piping hot, almost as thick as syrup. Turkish coffee, which can be found all over the Middle East, is brewed to varying degrees of strength and sweetness. With the current popularity of coffee drinks, you might want to invest in several French presses and have a tableside presentation of brewed Turkish coffee. Serve Turkish coffee in espresso or demitasse cups, accompanied by sugar cubes and plates of dried fruit and nuts.

On to India

There are hundreds of Indian cuisines, each with its own range of spices. Largely vegetarian, Indian cuisine can make vegetable and bean stews seem lush and decadent. If you're going to serve it, you have to name it!

Culinary India is a world of spices and teas. Chefs not only need to be versed in cooking techniques, but in the art of spice balance. Every meal must be the correct mixture of "hot" and "cool" spices to please the palate and both stimulate and soothe the soul. Let's take the world's fastest culinary India tour.

Eastern Indian cuisine, with influences from the Bengal region and from Calcutta, is largely a coastal cuisine, with rice as a staple. Curries are thin and sometimes sweet, served with vegetables. Eastern Indian cuisine is not elaborate, taking advantage of the fresh ingredients from coastal growing. The most popular bread is puri (see side bar), fried into puffs. Desserts rely on thickened milk puddings and even a pudding of white potatoes, yogurt, almonds and raisins, called **dum aloo.**

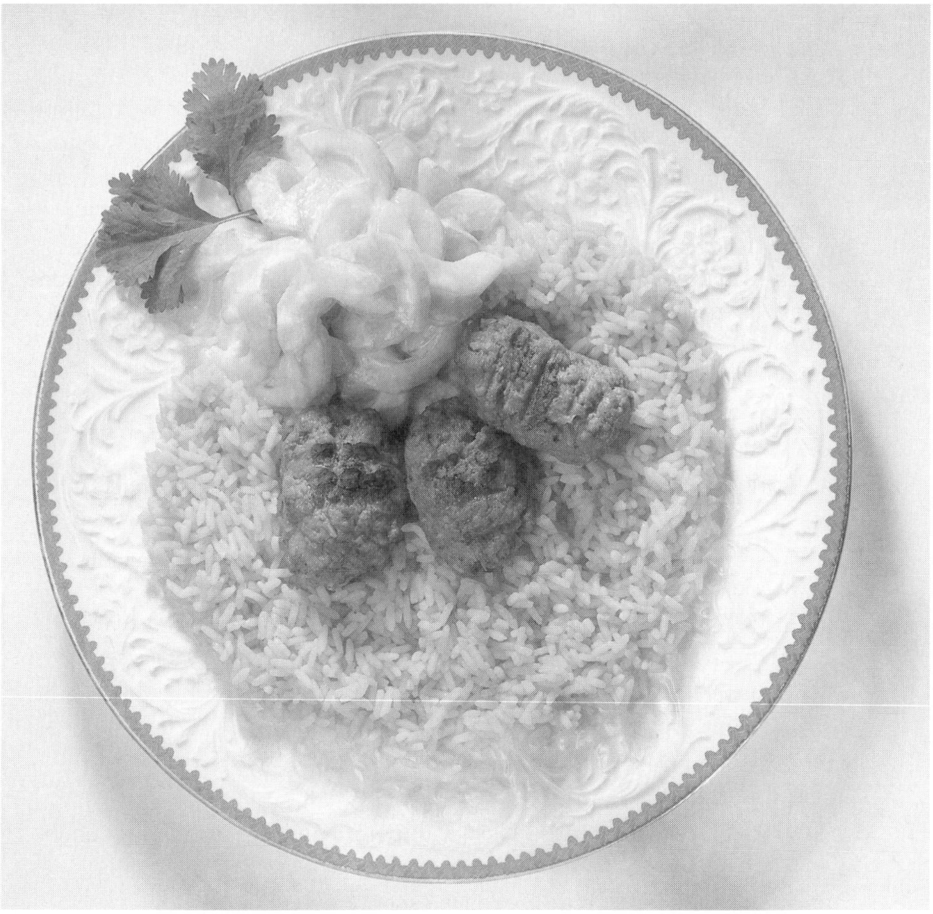

Follow a traditional Middle Eastern entrée with honey-scented, traditional desserts.

Northern Indian cuisine reflects the many visitors who conquered the area. Greek, Persian, Chinese and even Turkish kings left their mark on North India, the center of which is Delhi. From Persia came pomegranates, dates, melons, and figs; the Persians even imported ice from the Himalayas to cool their drinks and summer dishes. Delhi's cuisine is considered the epitome of Indian cuisine, with many elaborate dishes. **Tandoor** ovens are used to barbecue meat and vegetables and bake bread. Pilafs and biranyi are rice dishes prepared with dried fruit and nuts and can be sweet or savory. This is a very fertile growing region, and there are many types of bread prepared from whole and processed grain. Naan is a yogurt-marinated bread baked in a tandoor, chapatis are whole grain flat breads that can be grilled or baked and paratha are similar to whole grain pancakes.

Southern Indian cuisine is largely vegetarian and could be considered the most aromatic of India's cuisines. Curries (dishes with spiced sauces) are popular, served with **raita,** a cooling yogurt sauce made with thinned yogurt and chopped vegetables and fruit, depending on the season. A favorite snack food is **idli,** a crunchy treat of dried beans, Rice Krispie-like grains and chutney or

1. Asafetida: a very powerfully flavored spice blend that takes some getting used to. It is sold in solid form and is used sparingly in vegan dishes.
2. Biryani: a very elaborate rice dish. Usually basmanti rice, layered with raisins, nuts, and seasoned bits of meat, garnished with edible flowers.
3. Chapatis: a flat bread made of whole wheat flour, cooked on grills or directly in the fire. When fried in oil, made to resemble a puff, it is called a **puris.**
4. Curry: not a single spice, but a combination of spices. In India, spice mixes are called **masalas.** In India, curry refers more to a dish served with a sauce. There are as many masalas (what we would call curry mixtures) in India as there are cooks. Masalas are mixed by the individual; there are no commercial mixtures available.
5. Dahl: lentils or split peas cooked, with masala, into a thick sauce.
6. Ghee: clarified butter, used for cooking.
7. Halwah: thick dessert puddings, made from semolina flour or shredded carrots.
8. Idli: a crunchy, savory snack mix sold on the street. Often served with chutneys and other condiments.
9. Kheer: milk cooked until thickened and mixed with sugar, cardamom and cooked rice. Served as a soupy, rice pudding dessert. Try this with rice milk.
10. Lasi: yogurt drink, flavored with mango or rose (sweet) or with cucumber or salt. Try this with soy yogurt.
11. Masala: a blend of freshly ground herbs and spices. Always toasted before being used in dishes.
12. Masala Dosa: Thick, stiff crepes filled with potato and seasoned with cumin, coriander, chili, onion and mustard seeds.
13. Naan: yogurt-thickened bread, baked in tandoor ovens.
14. Papadum: dahl is dried and rolled into small balls and then fried; served as an appetizer.
15. Raita: yogurt mixed with finely chopped cucumber, tomato and onion. Served as a condiment and a side dish.
16. Sambar: a stew of vegetable and beans, served with richly spiced sauces (curries).
17. Samosa: dough stuffed with savory fillings and fried; served as an appetizer or snack.
18. Tandoori: yogurt marinated chicken, seafood or lamb baked in clay (tandoor) ovens. Try this with carrots, sweet potatoes, and white potatoes instead of meat.

Figure 10–1 South Indian Savory

other condiments. **Dosas** are thick crepes that can be stuffed with cooked potato and sweet or savory seasonings.

Western Indian cuisine has Bombay as its base. **Puri,** fried bread puffs are popular, as is **paneer.** Paneer is a dense yogurt cheese that is cut into small squares and used in curries, vegetable dishes and sweet desserts. **Palek paneer** is an Indian version of creamed spinach and is very popular as an entrée or a side dish. **Shrikhand** is a sinfully sweet sweetened, thickened yogurt dessert, flavored with cardamom or mango. It is very high in calories from fat and sugar, but is so rich it is used very sparingly. Two ounces per serving would be more than enough.

Now that we've listed the exotic, let's talk about what you can do. First thing is to visit an Indian restaurant and grocery store, so you can be immersed in the aura of an Indian spice cloud. The next is to procure spices.

Indian chefs do not purchase spice mixes, as combinations vary from place to place. You can purchase separate spices and prepare your own mixtures or you can purchase some of the blends that are available as a convenience items in many Indian groceries. Remember to look for **masala,** as this is the Indian word for "spice." **Garam masala** is a general term for a spice mix, and many types are sold, some sweet and some savory. Spices are toasted dry or with a bit of ghee (clarified butter) before being tossed into dishes. The toasting develops the flavor and color of the spices. Experiment with **tea masala,** a blend for flavoring hot or cold tea, using it in custards, dessert sauces and to flavor melon or orange sorbets.

Pilafs can be Indian-influenced. Use basmanti or jasmine rice as a base. Sauté a spice mix, such as cumin, coriander, turmeric, cinnamon, and cloves, quickly in butter or oil. Add uncooked rice and cook until rice is golden. Add stock and allow rice to simmer until liquid is absorbed. Garnish with chopped pistachios or almonds, chopped raisins or dates and green peas. Saffron can be used to color and flavor the stock, if you have the budget for it. Turmeric is called "poor man's saffron" because it gives the same yellow color to foods as saffron. Just be careful with turmeric, as it can give a bitter flavor if used in excess.

Simple steamed rice or steamed or grilled vegetables can be "India-ized" by the condiments served with them. Chutneys are the Indian version of salsa, served with every meal. Chutneys are available commercially or you can make them in your kitchen. Apricot chutney is a combination of fresh apricots (or you can use peaches), vinegar, sugar, onions, garlic, raisins, fresh ginger, and red pepper flakes, simmered together and allowed to marinate. Chutneys can be made with plums, apples, melon, and berries or most seasonal fruit. Serve chutneys with omelets in the morning, roasted, grilled fish or meat, steamed rice and even used in salad dressings. Other Indian condiments include achar, which are pickled fruit and vegetables, such as mango, cucumber, and carrot; raita, a yogurt dressing; and spicy bhurtas (see recipe). Dhal is a thin lentil stew and is served with all savory dishes. Prepare a batch and serve it with your lunch and dinner items, as a dipping sauce for veggies or chips and as a sauce for rice or vegetables.

Indian breads are wonderful in their variety and their texture. It is possible to prepare them yourself, but we suggest purchasing them frozen and reheating, much as many of us purchase frozen croissants or Danish. Hard to dedicate the time and the talent to preparing them from scratch, especially when frozen items are very acceptable. Naan is made in round or oval shapes and is yeast dough enriched with yogurt and butter. Naan can be reheated with roasted garlic or onions, or with fresh ginger and orange peel. Chappatis are whole-wheat flat breads, and can be used as wraps as well as in a breadbasket. Throw chappatis into the deep fryer and they will puff, wonderful when eaten hot, with chutney. Roti are thin, round or oval discs of lentil flour, available with many different seasonings. They are toasted quickly in oil or in dry, very hot skillet and served instead of chips or dinner rolls. Use naans to make stuffed sandwiches, chappatis to make wrap sandwiches and serve roti with hot or cold dips. Or combine all three for a breadbasket, serve with butter and chutney or bhurta.

Indian desserts can be as simple as chilled melons or sliced oranges served with a sweet raita. Indian rice or carrot pudding is thickened with simmered yogurt and sugar and flavored with cardamom. Served warm, these puddings are garnished with pistachios or almonds and raisins. Sirkhand, a thickened sweet yogurt which can be frozen and served like a chilled mousse, is available already prepared and ready to serve. Indian sweet shops have an amazing array of dessert snacks, made from honey, ground nuts and seeds, dried fruit and lentil, and wheat flour. These sweets are served as a variety on a tray, accompanied by chai masala or lasi. Lasi is a yogurt drink, which, when made sweet is flavored with rosewater or mango. Lasi is easy to reproduce in a restaurant, by blending plain yogurt, ripe mango and honey. Serve lasi over ice, in a smoothie, or freeze it for a frozen dessert.

Chai masala (literally "spiced tea") is ubiquitous on the streets in most Indian towns. You can buy it from street vendors, delivery people bring it to shops and businesses and every food establishment offers it. To prepare chai masala, black tea is strongly brewed and then boiled with milk. This makes a creamy, thick beverage. Right before serving, a spice blend is added. One popular blend is cardamom, ground ginger, cinnamon, cloves, and black pepper. Sugar or honey is added by the customer, depending on taste.

From-scratch chai can be made in a microwave, first brewing the tea and then heating the tea and milk together. Try it with soy milk and vegetarian sweetener. We know it can be done. Our local Starbucks does this very successfully for customers.

Chai is a big seller in the United States. Coffee chains are offering hot and iced chai, chai lattes and chai smoothies. Chai mixes are available in powder and concentrate form. You can prepare chai and hold it in the refrigerator or circulate it in a jet spray. There are even chai mix variations, made with green tea, decaffeinated black tea and with herbal tea and soy and rice milk.

Don't think about chai as only a beverage. It can be frozen and served as a sorbet or thickened and used as a dessert sauce for cake and baked goods. We've seen chai-flavored coffeecakes and cake frosting and fillings.

Treat yourself to a cup of fragrant, aromatic chai at your favorite Indian restaurant and then start thinking about chai applications for your menu.

A La Française

Students of French cuisine know that French cooking is as varied as the country. All dishes are not slathered with butter or steeped in cream. Beyond the grand classics are the traditional dishes, the bistro foods, and the seasonal delights of French menus. You can have a lower-fat meal and still call it French.

It's All in a Name: mixed vegetables sound boring? offer a "bouquetiere legumes" (literally a "bouquet of vegetables")!

a la francaise: a garnish of braised, shredded lettuce; shred sturdier greens, such as romaine, braise quickly in vegetable stock and toss into cooked veggies for a hot garnish.

Dubarry: a garnish of cauliflower; certainly makes cream of cauliflower (crème dubarry) sound a lot more glamorous; want to get your customers thinking? Ask them to consider why chefs looking to honor Madame Dubarry (who was thought to be quite a dish herself) chose the humble cauliflower as her namesake. Try "creaming" with root vegetables, such as potatoes or turnips.

Crecy: named after a famous battle said to have taken place near a carrot field, potage crecy sounds so much classier than "puree of carrot" soup.

Raifort: adding horseradish to the sauce? Then you have a sauce Raifort.

a la Flamande: a garnish of green peas, as in carrots a la flamande (peas and carrots never sounded so elegant).

Princesse: no, not a type of telephone, but a garnish of asparagus tips.

Florentine: actually the French name for the Italian city of Florence, and birth city of one of the culinary d'Medicis, a garnish florentine is always one of spinach.

Freunese: the humble turnip sounds much better in French.

Provencale: the flavors of southern France, usually including tomatoes, garlic olive oil and oils, onions and parsley. Offer a hearty vegetable soup provencale or a bell pepper a la provencale. Sounds pretty antioxidant and trendy to us!

Ragout: sounds much better (and seems to taste better) than a "thin vegetable stew."

Duxelle: a finely chopped paste of shallots and mushrooms which can be used as a filling for vegetables pastries, a garnish or a flavoring. Mild flavored onions can be used in place of shallots.

Nicoise: both an olive style and an entrée salad, you can't say "nicoise" without smiling.

Pommes frites: The debate rages if France or Belgium was the birthplace of these batons of fried potato. Americans prefer their pomme frite dry and golden, requiring the right potato and the correct handling of the oil. In the right balance, pommes frites can fit into a healthy diet. Or try that modern abomination, oven frying.

Cassoulet: a comforting, hearty yet delicate long-simmering stew of baby lima beans, tomato, sausage and duck. Serve as an entrée or as an accompaniment, made vegetarian with soy sausage.

Figure 10–2 Yes, French and Healthy Do Mix

Adding a French accent, whether it be the earthy accent of the bistro or the upscale accent of the salle, is easily accomplished by taking advantage of seasonal produce. French cuisine has a healthy respect for produce that is easily translatable to modern menus. Adding these French accents will enliven your traditional offerings and spark interest in your healthy items.

Put It in the Potage

Every time you add carrots, celery, and onions to your soups, stews, and sauces you can thank the French chefs of yore. Called **mirepoix,** this savory mixture of two parts carrots and two parts onions to one part celery forms the flavor base for many, many dishes.

Vegetable purees are also a timely French cooking technique. Today they are easy to do—whirl the food processor for a second and achieve a rainbow of beet red, carrot or pumpkin orange, squash yellow and pepper green. In the bad old days veggies were pushed through a chinois (a fine-mesh sieve) or cranked through a food mill. Vegetable purees can be used in soups to give the taste and appearance of cream or butter without the added fat. Potage Crecy is a "cream" of carrot soup prepared with carrots, potatoes and fresh herbs. Vichyssoises is a puree of potatoes and leeks, traditionally served cold but doing very well when served hot during the winter months.

French onion soup is a bread-thickened soup, a peasant dish elevated to classical heights. Prepare a hearty onion soup as luncheon entrée by sautéing sliced onions until they are golden and covering with stock, allowing to simmer for 15 minutes. Place two slices of croutons (oven-toasted bread) in an oven-proof dish, pour soup over the croutons, top with a thick layer soy cheese, sprinkle with margarine and broil until brown. Don't confine yourself to one type of onion or unflavored croutons; how about sweet onion soup with rosemary-herbed crouton or a red onion and leek soup with a basil and oregano-herbed crouton!

We're not really sure if **ratatouille** is soup or a stew, but we know it is wonderful. A seasonal melange of stewed eggplant, summer squashes, tomatoes, peppers, onions and garlic, ratatouille encompasses all the flavors of Provence in a bowl. Cost effective, using squash in season, and dramatic in presence, use ratatouille as a vegetarian entrée, instead of pasta or grains to carry an entrée or as a colorful side dish.

Life Is but a Pomme

Gratin dauphinoise, Grandmere mashed potatoes with onions and rosemary, crispy potato and mushroom cake, light as a feather pomme souffle or golden gaufrettes, potato, artichoke and cheese gratin and of course the famous pommes frites. When it comes to potatoes, say "mais oui" (oh, yes!).

Potatoes are versatile, inexpensive, and can be oh-so-French. Puree potatoes (mashed so fine that they can be piped through a pastry bag), mix with a bit of egg replacer, margarine and nutmeg, and pipe in rosettes or borders. Bake or broil, make ahead and freeze, your potato duchess add glamour to vegetable dishes. Duchesse can be done with white potatoes, sweet potatoes, turnips and winter squash for different colors and flavors.

Potato au gratin is a classic and much-maligned side dish. Made correctly, it is potato poetry. To "gratiner" means to bake with a cheese topping. Gratins (which can be made with any sliced, cooked vegetable, such as carrots, zucchini or winter squash) are made by coating cooked vegetables with a cheese or béchamel (cream) sauce, sprinkling with grated cheese, chopped nuts and/or bread crumbs and browned in an oven or broiler. A gratin dauphinois (made in the style of royalty) is a combination of cooked potatoes, cream, garlic and cheese. Try these with soy milk and soy cheeses.

Pommes anna is another simple but elegant potato dish. Thinly sliced peeled potatoes are layered in a circular style in a buttered casserole dish, firmly packed. The potatoes can be covered with stock, melted butter or bouillon and are baked until bubbly. Pommes anna is served in thick slices as an accompaniment to an entrée.

Legumes are about as French as they come; ragouts, cassoulets, confit all rely on dried peas and beans for their texture and flavor. **Cassoulet,** originally from the bean-growing region of Toulouse, is a homey, savory, sophisticated slow-simmered stew of baby lima beans (also called butter beans), tomatoes, onions, garlicky sausage, and duck. There are as many versions of cassoulet as there are kitchens in France. Executive Chef Bob Okura, of the Cheesecake Factory, has an updated cassoulet that he serves over pasta. Cassoulet is low maintenance to prepare and will hold for several days in the refrigerator (it actually seems to get better in flavor over several days). You can try cassoulet with various types of veggie sausage or fake meats. Very little meat is used, in any case, just for flavor.

White, red, or black beans can be made into a ragout (a thin vegetable stew) by simmering with mirepoix, bacon or sausage, peppers, garlic until tender and served as an accompaniment to an entree. Or beans can be simmered until soft and dressed with olive oil and lemon juice or a splash of soy cream for a flavorful side dish. Here are some classic "bean dishes" with a French accent:

Garbure bearnaise: red beans with sausage (use soy) root vegetables and margarine
Cassoulet: white beans with garlic sausage and tomato
White beans with port wine
Baked kidney beans with red wine
Chickpea fritters
Lentils with mirepoix and smoked tofu
Puree of lima bean with onion

Salades, Too

Until modern times, the people of many countries felt that eating raw produce was dangerous, or was, at the least, meant only for the lower classes. The French vacillated between considering raw tomatoes as poisonous or as an aphrodisiac. It was only a matter of time before the French got over their fear of fresh produce. Who could resist the fifty varieties of "butter fruit" (fresh pears) that Louis XII grew in his gardens, the fraise boises (wild strawberries) found in the springtime woods, and yes, the truffles! Cold vegetable terrines and confits made use of cooked vegetables served cold, as did fruit coulis (pureed fruit) for dessert sauces.

Salade Nicoise is a cold entree salad, probably a precursor of our chef salad. Cold new potatoes, tomato wedges, **haricot vert** (tender, slender new green beans), hard-cooked egg slices and poached tuna are shown off on baby greens and garnished with Nicoise olives, concentrated black pearls of the olive family. Dressed simply with olive oil and high quality vinegar, a salade Nicoise makes an excellent pairing with hot soup (try a Crecy!) and freshly baked bread. Make this vegetarian with chilled tofu slices to replace the egg and tuna.

Whether serving peas "a la champignon" (with mushrooms) or "amandine" (with almonds), offering a "macedoine" (mixture) of seasonal fruit or garnishing your red snapper "pamplemousse" (with grapefruit), you can "Frenchify" your menu with seasonal and local produce. Bon temp rollez (let the good times roll)!

Salsa Rules

A little closer to home is the cuisine of the American Southwest. Southwestern Cuisine is a spicy, fragrant combination of Central American and Native American ingredients with a hint of Spanish influence. Today, Arizona farmers raise wheat, greens and citrus fruit. In the past, the Hohokam and Pimas irrigated the desert and grew corn, squash, beans and cotton. The Aztecs contributed jicama, a juicy, mild root vegetable that can be eaten raw or cooked, tomatillos, lemon-flavored, tough vegetables that resemble small green tomatoes with a papery covering, and prickly pear cactus. New Mexico is known for its over two hundred varieties of chili peppers as well as for its state tree, the pinon tree. From the pinon tree comes pine nuts that are used in hot and cold salads, soups, pozoles (stews) and cookies and cakes. Fishing boats along the Gulf Coast of Texas bring in shrimp, crab and red fish, among other sea delicacies. Further inland, rice, pecans, blue corn, grapefruit and oranges are grown. The Texas state food is chili followed by spicy hot barbecue. Although not usually thought of as part of the Southwest, Oklahoma was home to many Native Americans. Oklahoma's large crops are wheat, peaches, and peanuts. The durum wheat grown in Oklahoma is purchased by top level pasta companies. An Oklahoman specialty crop is mung beans. Mung beans can be eaten whole or used for sprouting and are used in many Asian cuisines.

When you think of southwestern holiday food, you can think of color, heat, and an avalanche of tastes. Holiday foods are served on large beautifully decorated platters, heaped with main dishes and garnishes. No food stands alone. There are salsas and pickled chilies, chopped cilantro, epazote (a spiky-leafed herb that has a faint resemblance to bay leaf) and fresh onions and peppers.

In New Mexico, you have your choice of green or red chili sauce, an influence of the states of Sonora and Chihuhua, made with fresh and dried green and red chilies and paste that spark the palate. Green chili sauce is associated with summer, as the chilies are picked while they are young (and green) during the summer months. Green chili sauce is prepared when the green chili is in season and frozen or canned. It is an uncooked sauce, good for dips, used as a salad dressing, or served over tortillas or enchiladas. Ingredients can include fresh green chilies or bell peppers, chopped onions, tomatoes, and cilantro.

Red chili sauce is associated more with winter time and winter holidays. Red chili sauce is made with chilies that have been allowed to ripen to redness and dried. The dried red chilies are ground into flakes or powders. Spices for the sauce include jalapeno chili, garlic, cumin, cinnamon, black pepper and cloves. The chilies are usually sautéed briefly in fat, seasonings are added and then pureed. Red chili sauce is served with tamales, poultry or fish or can be used as a flavoring for soups or stews and is seen in many households on Christmas morning.

Pepitas (pumpkinseeds) and pinones (pine nuts) are harvested from pumpkin patches and pine forests in the autumn and used for holiday treats. The pine forests near Taos and the Rio Grande are a popular place for entire families to go camping in the fall and early winter, gathering pinecones. Pine nuts must be picked from the pinecones by hand, which is what makes them so expensive for culinarians.

Pepitas and pinones are shelled, toasted and salted and served as snack to holiday visitors. You can toast shelled pine nuts by heating them in an ungreased, preheated sauté pan for five to ten minutes, stirring constantly so they don't burn. Or you can toast in a little oil with some chili flakes. You can also roast in a 375° F oven for fifteen minutes, stirring them to prevent burning. Offer your customers pumpkinseeds and pine nuts with their bebidas (drinks), whether it be strong hot coffee, hot Mexican chocolate, rompope (Southwestern eggnog, flavored with brandy and cinnamon) or margaritas.

Holidays and feast days in the Southwest means tamales. Taken from the Aztec word "tamalli," tamales are a mixture of meat, chilies, cheese, and masa that is wrapped in a dried cornhusk and steamed. Fresh green corn tamales is made in the spring with fresh husks and green corn mass, but are rarely eaten out of season.

Masa, the largest ingredient in a tamale, is a mixture of dried corn that has been reconstituted with water and fat. The making of the masa is critical to the success of the tamale. Experiment with a lower-fat masa, using vegetable oils and stocks to substitute for the traditional lard or beef fat.

Actually, tamale making is an art and science onto itself. Tamale making is not a solitary activity. Several families may get together to make large batches of holiday tamales, starting in the early afternoon and proceeding long into the night. The meat must be cooked and spiced correctly, the masa prepared with precision, the husks soak and the prepared tamale wrapped and steamed properly.

If you haven't got a family tamale connection, you'll find many "cottage" tamale industries or small restaurants that take orders for holiday tamales. They are a beehive of activity leading up to Christmas Eve, as everyone wants their Christmas breakfast of tamales with red chilies.

Tamales can be flavored with many different ingredients. A sweet tamale, flavored with bits of pineapple, raisins, coconut and cinnamon is a seasonal holiday treat, served as a breakfast item or a dessert. Tamales may also

FOOD FOR THE MIND

For an amazing number of salsa recipes, check out *The Great Salsa Book* (Mark Miller, Ten Speed Press, 1994, ISBN 0-89815-517-7). To explore American cuisine, go to *American Regional Cuisine: A Coast to Coast Celebration of the Nation's Culinary Diversity* (The Art Institutes of America, 2002, John Wiley and Sons, ISBN 0-471-40544-2).

be flavored with chicken, carnitas (tender, seasoned pork), turkey, potatoes, and squash.

Breakfast tamales can be accompanied by coffee or hot chocolate, but may also be served with atole or champurrado. Atole is a hot beverage brewed with cornstarch, sweetened with sugar and flavored with cinnamon and vanilla. White rice may be cooked in with the atole, making a soupy, warm rice pudding type of beverage. Champurrado is atole flavored with chocolate. Either hot beverage may be served as a fast breakfast during the regular calendar, and supplemented with bunuelos or sopaipillas during the holidays. Look in Central American stores for atole mix and disks of Mexican chocolate.

You need something to drink with this spicy, flavorful fare. Southwestern bebidas (beverages) can include sangria, a wine punch that received its name from missionary priests who saw it "as dark as blood," or beer. Germans and Czechs who settled in the Southwest brewed dark beer that goes well with chili-spiked dishes. Margaritas and other tequila-based drinks are popular if the weather is warm, and rompope (hot eggnog) is served when the weather is cold. Freshly squeezed juices and herb teas are colorful and healthy bebidas. For example, jamaica (pronounced ha-mi-ca) is the dried flower of the hibiscus tree. It makes a deep crimson flavorful tea that is high in Vitamin C.

Christmas is not the only southwestern holiday celebrated in December. Native American Hopis observe the Soyal ceremony in December during the winter solstice. Many dishes that feature corn are served, as the corn plant is revered in Hopi tradition.

Pumpkins abound in the Southwest and are used as both a vegetable, in soups and stews, and as a sweet ingredient in candy and cookies. Pumpkin candy, made with pumpkin meat, sugar and lemon juice and rind takes patience. Uncooked pumpkin meat is cut into strips, sprinkled with sugar, and soaked in lemon juice and rind and allowed to stands for at least twelve hours. It is then cooked until the pumpkin is clear and firm, about ninety minutes. The cooked pumpkin is removed from the sauce, allowed to dry at least twelve hours, rolled in sugar or covered in syrup and stored.

Salsa can be fresh or cooked, fire-hot or cool. Salsa can be used as a low fat dipping sauce, as an entrée accompaniment or as a dessert sauce. Traditionally, red salsa was a combination of fresh tomatoes, onions, cilantro and chilies. Green salsa's base was boiled and mashed tomatilloes. With salsa's growing popularity comes many variations. Vegetables are grilled or smoked before chopping, seafood is added, beans are mashed and fruit is incorporated.

Chef Mark Miller's book, *The Great Salsa Book* (Ten Speed Press, 1994) offers a collection of salsas from all over Central and South America. There are fusion salsas with Mediterranean and Asian ingredients. Here are just some of the salsas Chef Miller offers for your imagination: mint and carmelized shallot salsa, seaweed and red chile salsa, kim chee salsa, carrot and black olive salsa, Aztec white bean, leek and mushroom salsa and lemon fig salsa. As people become more aware of the nutritional value of foods and seek out lower fat options for sauces and gravies, the popularity of salsa will continue to rise.

PUTTING IT ALL TOGETHER

After reading this chapter you should have a good insight into the healthy aspects of ethnic cuisines. Many ethnic cuisines are traditionally lower in animal products and fats, making them lower in cholesterol and saturated fats.

Ethnic cuisines take advantage of regional and seasonal ingredients. Cooking methods are used that enhance the nutrient values of foods. The accent is on flavor and taste. Spices, herbs, fruits, vegetables, and nuts are used for flavoring. Meat and fat are often used more as a condiment or flavoring agent rather than a main ingredient.

Asian and Indian dishes can be used as accents or served as main meals. The balance of produce, meat or fish and herbs and spices make these cuisines interesting and healthy. When designing menus or creating recipes, consider reducing the portion size of the solid meat entrée and increase the vegetables, rice and noodles. Rethink cooking techniques that require large amounts of fat; consider tandoori, clay pot cooking, one pot cooking and hot pots.

French cuisine can be a lower-fat, higher-fiber cuisine, depending on the ingredients chosen. French menus can include dishes whose main ingredients are beans, legumes, potatoes, vegetables and salad items.

The culinary nutrition student would be wise to learn how to incorporate ethnic dishes into menus. According to a National Restaurant Association survey (National Restaurant Association, 5), the American taste for ethnic cuisines is on the rise. Over 45 percent of the people surveyed said they chose ethnic restaurants when they eat out. Italian, Chinese, Japanese, Mexican and Indian dishes are becoming more popular. Ethnic cuisines will "sell the plate" and add healthy choices to the bottom line.

FYI: VARIETY IN A BOWL

One-pot meals are a hallmark of many Asian cuisines. Cooking all ingredients in one container allows the flavors to concentrate and captures many of the nutrients. One-pot meals are one-pot wonders of taste, health, and interest.

Clay pot chicken and vegetables incorporate sautéing and stewing in one pot. Chicken thigh pieces are marinated in soy sauce and sherry and sautéed with thin slices of sweet potato, onions and mushrooms. Ingredients are sautéed until soft, mixed with a small amount of flour and simmered in chicken stock until tender. Served with steamed brown or white rice, the flavor of this dish improves if made a day or two ahead of service.

Coconut vegetable curry is one of Indonesia's answers to one-pot cooking. Onions, garlic and fresh chilies are sautéed with fish sauce in a large pot until soft. Coconut milk, bay leaves and tamarind are added and allowed to simmer to combine flavors. Diced carrot, potato and pumpkin (winter squash can be used) are added and simmered until soft and then green beans and zucchini are added. Cooked fish or shrimp (presumably left over from a previous meal) are added before service.

Coconut milk has great flavor and great texture, but unfortunately, also has a great amount of saturated fat. You can create the illusion of coconut flavor by using rice milk with a splash of coconut milk. You will obtain the creaminess with a minimum of fat.

A vegetarian one-dish from Indonesia combines seasonal vegetables, such as cabbage, spinach, onions, corn, potatoes and squash with a vegetable stock and is flavored with tamarind, cinnamon, bay leaf, garlic, and ginger. This is allowed to simmer until all the vegetables are tender and the flavors combined.

Shrimp and rice noodle one-pot hails from Malaysia. Peeled shrimp is simmered in a broth flavored with soy sauce, onions and brown sugar. When tender, noodles are added and allowed to cook. Fresh spinach is added just before service to hold its color and texture. This dish is served with a condiment plate of chopped garlic, chopped green onions, bean sprouts, and fresh chives.

From the Philippines comes oxtail and vegetable stew. With the resurgence in "comfort" or diner-style foods, this dish could score well with your customers. Oxtail pieces (stew beef or pork could be used if oxtail is not available) are heated in a large pot until brown. The browned meat is tossed with garlic, onions, soy sauce and fish sauce. Broth is added and the mixture is brought to a simmer. Peeled, cubed eggplant, diced turnips, and sweet potatoes are added and allow to simmer until soft. Paprika and chopped peanuts are used as a garnish.

Tom Kha Gai is Thai heavenly smoothness in a one-pot. Coconut milk and ginger are brought to a boil and then allowed to simmer until slightly reduced. Chicken stock is added, as are chicken pieces, red chili, fish sauce, and a touch of brown sugar. The mixture is allowed to stew until the chicken is tender. Fresh cilantro is used as a garnish.

A cousin of Tom Kha Gai, green chicken curry follows the general directions of Tom Kha Gai, adding green beans as a vegetable, and excluding the green chili and brown sugar. Flavoring for this powerful curry is limejuice and green curry paste (available commercially). In place of chicken, fish fillets are sometimes steamed with the coconut milk. A vegetarian version of green curry is red vegetable curry. Coconut milk and red curry paste are simmered together; when slightly reduced, diced potatoes, cauliflower, green beans, red bell pepper, and baby corn are added and allowed to simmer until tender. Additional seasonings are green peppercorns and limejuice.

Chicken and pumpkin stew, from Laos, requires some additional ingredients. Fresh turmeric, which resembles miniature ginger and gives a slightly bitter flavor and bright orange color to dishes, is used, as is green papaya (a sour cousin of the usual orange papaya) and galangal, a cousin to ginger. This is an oven-cooked dish, unusual for a one-pot. Uncooked rice is spread in the bottom of a heavy pot and allowed to toast in a hot oven. This toasted rice is ground and mixed with a small amount of oil (you could take a short cut and use Cream of Rice cereal). The rice mixture is combined with garlic, turmeric, galangal, and onions. Chicken pieces are coated with the rice mixture, stock is added, as is pumpkin and papaya, the pot is returned to the oven and allowed to simmer until everything is tender. Something quite different!

Sukiyaki is the traditional Japanese beef and vegetable hot pot. Served in a miniature cauldron to the table, this hearty dish is a four-course meal in one dish. Thin slices of beef are simmered with onions, carrots, mushrooms, cabbage, bamboo shoots, bean sprouts and tofu. Sliced hard-cooked eggs and surimi (imitation crab) are sometimes used as additional ingredients. Additional flavor comes from a sauce added to the broth made of Japanese soy sauce, beef stock, sake and sugar. Note that in traditional sukiyaki, the eggs are not hard cooked. The sukiyaki is brought to the table boiling hot, and raw eggs are cracked into the pot by the customer.

A cousin to Japanese sukiyaki is Korean tofu soup. Customers can choose from beef, chicken, or vegetarian broth that is spiced to the degree of heat desired by the customer. The broth, with small bits of meat and vegetables and a large serving of firm tofu, is brought to the table bubbling and boiling and an egg is cracked into the broth, whisked to perfection by the customer. Condiments for tofu soup include at least four or five different types of kim chi, preserved and pickled vegetables (not just cabbage, kim chi can be made from radish, summer squash, peppers, and greens).

Burma's national dish is *Moh Hin Gha* or spicy fish soup with noodles. Fish fillets are sprinkled with salt and turmeric and allowed to marinate. Peanut oil is used to sauté onions, garlic and ginger, the heat is lowered, and the fish, along with coconut milk and fish sauce are allowed to simmer. Noodles are added and allowed to cook until tender. This is served piping hot with fresh chili.

Pho Is Fine

Pho restaurants are found throughout Vietnam and are becoming quite popular in the United States. Pho, or soup, is eaten as a hearty breakfast, as a light lunch or dinner, as a "chicken soup" cure for anything from the common cold to hangovers or as a midnight snack. Phos have got to be the trendiest one-pot on today's restaurant scene.

Variety in one bowl is hard to do, but phos succeed. The customer has a choice of several broths, usually chicken or beef, but we've seen duck and seafood as well. Chopped veggies, such as green and white onions and slivered carrots flavor the broth, which will be served containing rice or rice noodles, depending on customer preference. Beef is the most popular ingredient, which can be selected from lean to fat and rare to well-done. Chicken, duck, shrimp, and eggs can also be ordered. Many pho restaurants even have different-size bowls and different-size meat orders; the customer is really king. Pho condiment plates include large servings of bean sprouts, lime slices, Asian basil, fresh chilies and shredded lettuce. On the table is generally fish sauce, soy sauce and chili paste.

Phos are something that you can easily do. Chicken or beef broths can be served with noodles or rice and lightly sautéed onions. To make an authentically flavored pho broth, add black peppercorns, cinnamon stick, whole cloves, coriander seeds, and fresh ginger to simmering beef broth. Add green peas or snow peas, minced ginger and garlic and shaved carrots for flavor and color. Thinly sliced beef or chicken can be added to the hot broth, as can cooked shrimp, crab or lobster. Assemble a condiments plate which will please your customers palate, including sprouts, fresh bell pepper and chili, lemon or lime slices and soy sauce.

Breakfast or Dinner

One pots are a sure hit for lunch and dinner menus. If you're up to it, have hot pots at breakfast. For the morning bunch, offer a Vietnamese pho, a Korean sizzling tofu soup, or a Japanese miso (served with hard-cooked eggs and pickled vegetables). Breakfast hot pots appeal to health-conscious consumers as well as those looking for a new morning thrill. Be sure to include fresh fruit, such as honeydew melon, watermelon, pineapple, oranges, and grapes as a counterpoint to the saltiness of the soup. Hot or cold black, green, or herb teas are beverages as choice for a breakfast hot pot.

Lunch or dinner hot pots can be accompanied by fresh fruit or vegetable salads, pickled vegetables and candied fruit (such as ginger, kumquats, or pineapple). Beer, sparkling waters, and freshly squeezed fruit juices offer a refreshing accompaniment to hot pots.

Nutri-Words

Asian cuisine: cuisine typical of the span of Asian countries, such as Thailand, Burma, Vietnam, Japan, and China. Emphasis is on fresh ingredients and lower-fat cooking techniques.

Bok choy: member of the cabbage family, grows in a bunch with long, pale green and white stems and dark green leaves. Baby bok choy is served whole, steamed or braised. Boy choy leaves are as an ingredient in soups and hot pots.

Cassoulet: a regional dish of Toulose, France, made as a thick stew of fresh baby lima beans, duck or veal sausage and tomatoes.

Chai: the Indian or Asian term for "tea."

Chinese five-spice: a powdered blend of star anise, fennel, black pepper, cloves and cinnamon. Used to flavor sauces, fake meat dishes and noodle dishes.

Cilantro: also called Spanish parsley. Used as a flavoring agent in Spanish and Asian cuisine. The dried seeds of cilantro are sold as the seasoning coriander.

Gai lan: member of the spinach family, can be steamed, braised or stir-fried to add a spicy note to dishes.

Garam masala: an Indian spice mixture which varies according to region. "Masala" means "spice." Garam masala can be used in soups, stews, vegetable, rice and grain dishes.

Ghee: the Indian term for clarified butter or butter oil.

Haricot vert: literally, "beans, green." Generally understood to be a very slender, long, delicate green bean.

Jackfruit: the closest a fruit comes to resembling a porcupine. Jackfruit is used in juices, fruit purees and desserts, in baked goods and rice.
Lemon grass: is a long-stemmed herb that has a citrus flavor. Fresh lemon grass has the most flavor, and is used in Thai, Vietnamese and Chinese dishes, such as Thai coconut soup. If fresh lemon grass is not available, use lemon zest instead.
Mediterranean cuisine: cuisine typical of the Mediterranean countries, such as Spain, Portugal, Italy, southern France, Turkey, etc. Menu selection is low in red meat and dairy and high in fresh produce, whole grains, and olive oil. Considered to be low in saturated fats
Mirepoix: a 2:1:1 ratio mixture of onions to carrots to celery. Used as a flavoring in stocks, soups and sauces.
Miso: a seasoning used in Japanese cuisine, made from fermented soy, available in different flavors and strengths.
Paneer: a soft white cheese, often cut into small squares and used as an ingredient in Indian tomato or spinach stews.
Phyllo: a delicate, many-layered dough. Used to prepare baklava and many Greek, Mediterrean and Middle Eastern desserts.
Pummelo: also called a "shaddock." Thought to be the original grapefruit, originated in South East Asia. Pummelos can weigh up to three pounds, with a deep pink interior.
Raita: an Indian condiment with a base of yogurt, usually flavored with minced cucumber, tomato, and onion.
Ratatouille: a regional dish of Provence, France, made as an eggplant stew with tomatoes, olive oil, garlic, parsley, carrots, onions and other summer squash.
Seitan: the "meat of the wheat." Seitan is gluten, protein extracted from wheat flour. Seitan is chewy and can be used as a vegetarian alternate to meats.
Starfruit: also called "carambola." A citrus fruit that resembles a yellow or green five-pointed star. Sliced and used as a garnish or as a flavoring for sorbets and sauces.
Tandoor: a clay cooking implement, resembling a small oven, used to slow-roast vegetables, potatoes, breads, meat and seafood.
Tempeh: tofu that has been allowed to ferment to develop flavor, color, and texture. Can be sliced and roasted, grilled, steamed, or baked.
Wasabi: a small, green-leafed plant growing in river beds in Japan. In appearance, wasabi looks similar to watercress. Often dried and sold as a paste. Nicknamed "Japanese horseradish" for its flavor resemblance to European or North American horseradish.

Whaddaya Think?

1. What are some of the health and economic advantages of ethnic cuisines?
2. Is traditional Italian cuisine a lower-fat, lower cholesterol cuisine?

3. Can you think of ways to incorporate Asian cooking techniques and ingredients into American cuisine (and sneak some nutrition in there as well?)
4. How about some Middle Eastern desserts that are lower in cholesterol and sodium than ice cream and cake?
5. List all the ways low fat yogurt can replace butter and sour cream in American recipes.
6. Do you think Indian cuisine can be incorporated into some American dishes?
7. Design a four-cuisine French dinner that is lower in fat and sodium (and still interesting and flavorful).
8. Create a cassoulet of the future, low fat and full of flavor.

Critical Application Exercises

1. Review the Mediterranean and the Asian Food Guide Pyramids (Chapter 2):
   a. Design a three-day, Mediterranean healthy menu for a summer promotion in your restaurant.
   b. Design a three-day, Asian healthy menu for a winter promotion in your menu.
2. Obtain regular sour cream, nonfat sour cream and soy or imitation sour cream and low-fat (unflavored) yogurt:
   a. Have a taste testing. Do some cooking with each product to see how it responds to heating and chilling.
   b. Compare fat and calories for each product. Do you think you might be able to use low fat yogurt where some recipes call for sour cream? Record your observations.
3. Visit several ethnic restaurants of your choice:
   a. Did you notice any cuisines which were inherently healthy?
   b. How would you incorporate these cuisines into an American menu?
   c. Comment on interesting flavors or ingredients you encountered.

References

Barer-Stein, Thelma (1999). *You Eat What You Are*. Buffalo, NY: Firefly Books.

Batra, Neelam (1998). *Chilis to Chutneys: American Cooking with the Flavors of India*. NY: William Morrow and Company.

Kaplan, Karen (2000). *The Purple Kiwi Cookbook*. Nashville: FRP Press.

Kittler, P. G., & Sucher, K. P. (1998). *Food and Culture in America*. Belmont, CA: Wadsworth Publishing.

National Restaurant Association (1999). *Ethnic Cuisines II*, Survey 1999. Chicago, Illinois.

Rozin, Elisabeth (1992). *Ethnic Cuisine*. NY: Penguin Books.

PLATE I

Knife Skills

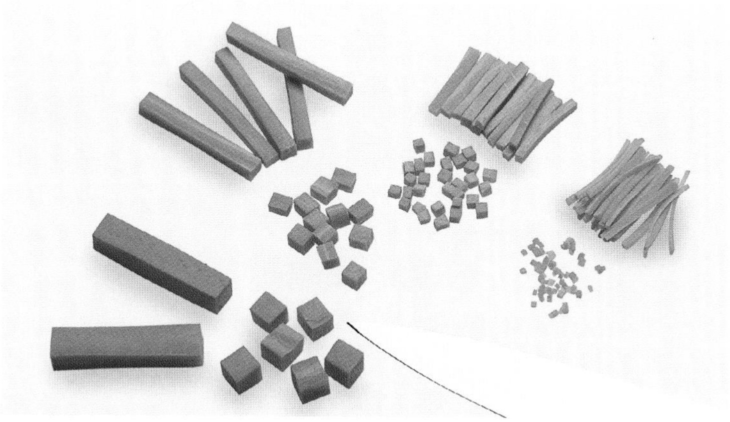

Batonnet and julienne sticks and the large, medium, small and brunoise

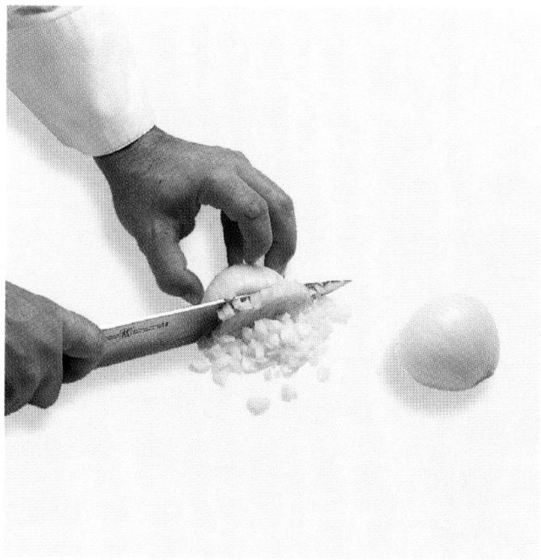

Dicing onions

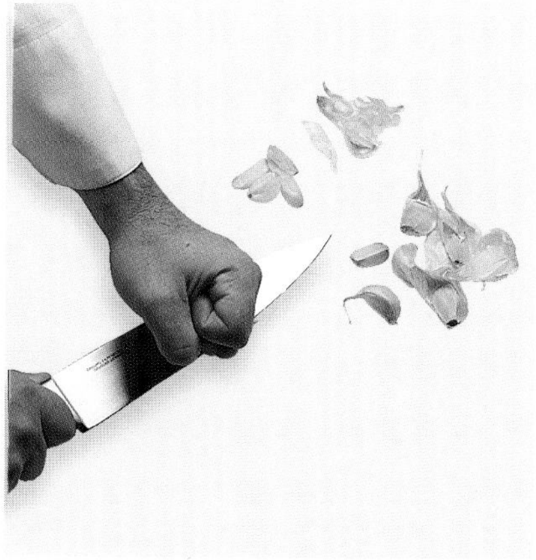

Mincing garlic

PLATE II

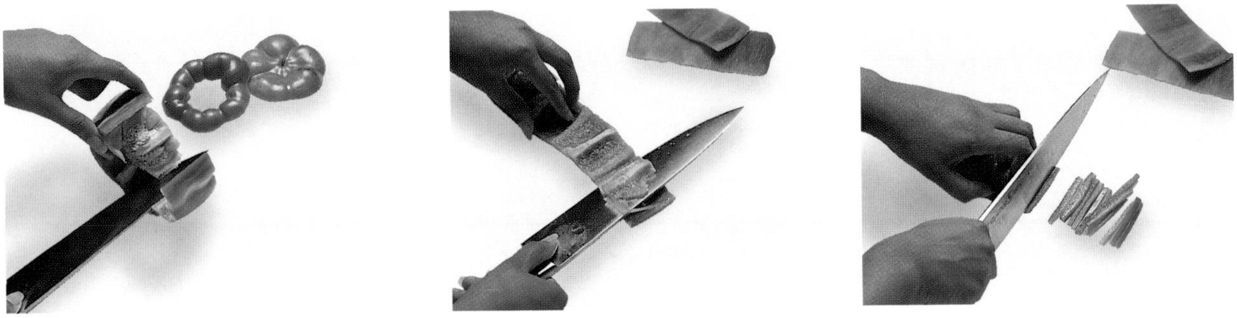

Julienne Peppers

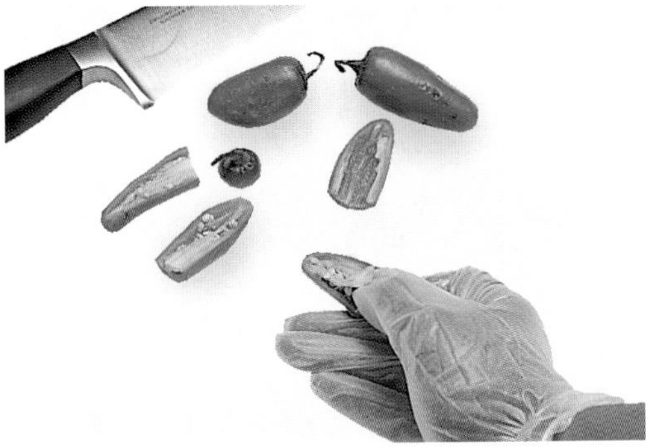

Deseed & chop chili

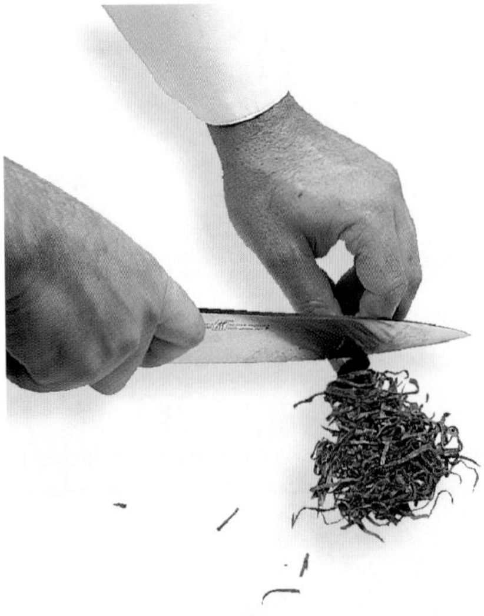

Shred fresh herbs
and baby greens

PLATE III

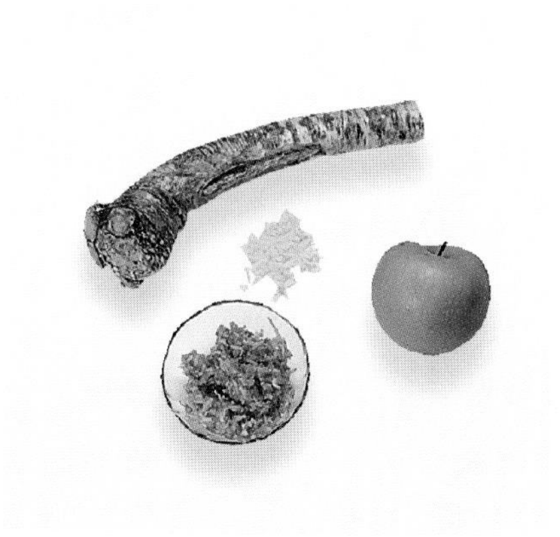

grate fresh horseradish

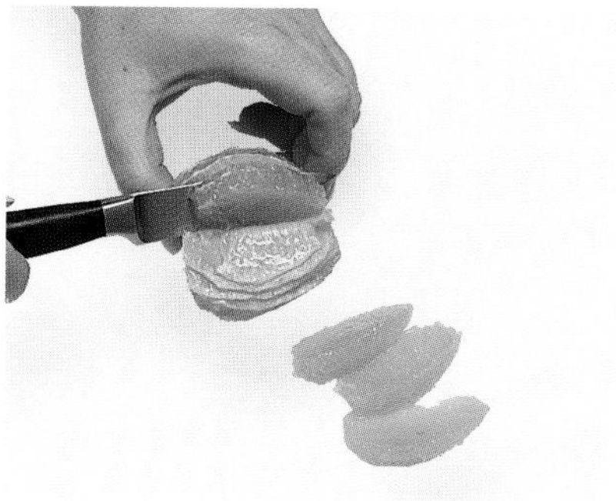

Citrus Fruits

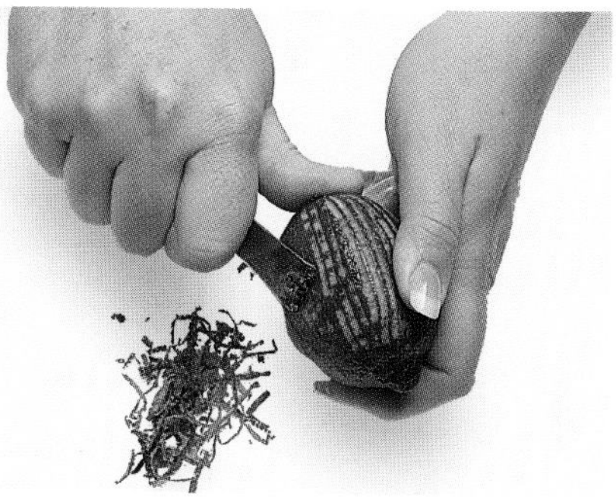

Zest Citrus Fruits

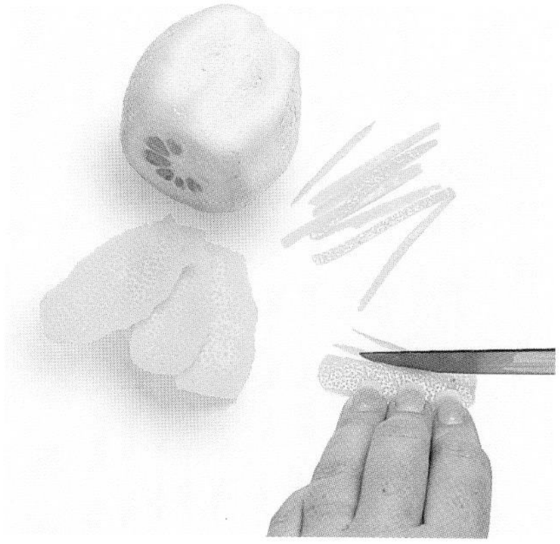

Cut Citrus Peels

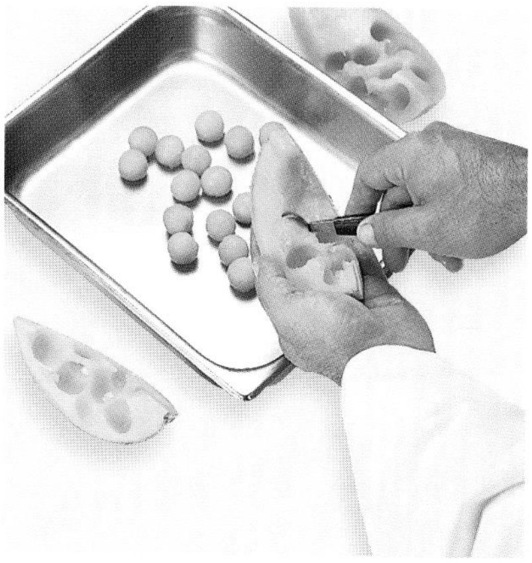

Parisional fruit & vegetables

PLATE IV

Several Cold Techniques

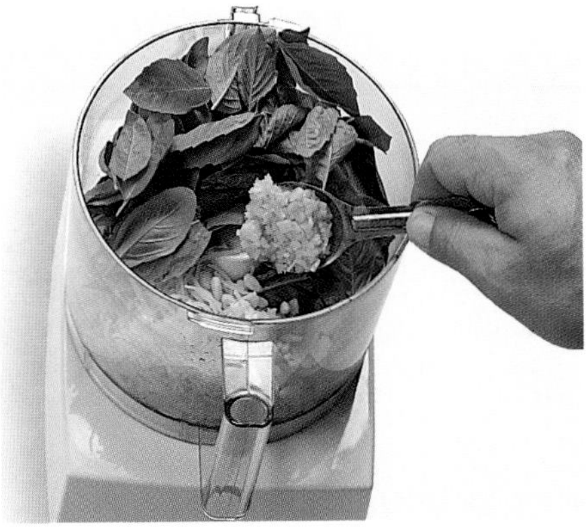

Pureeing pesto sauce

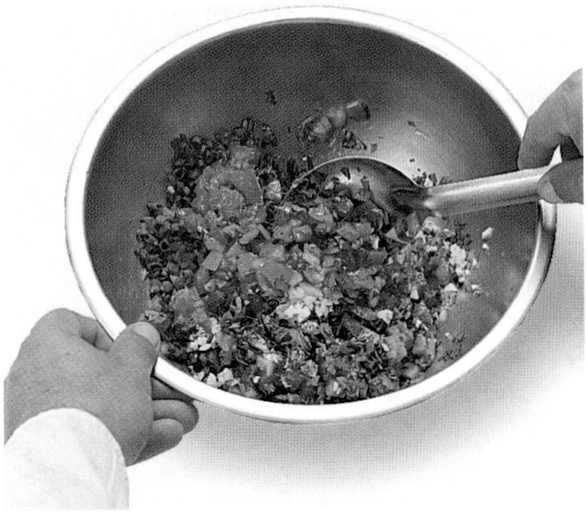

Chopping & mixing salsa

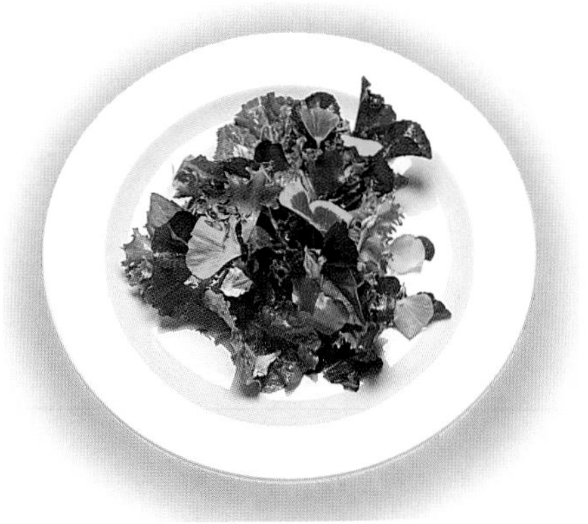

Composing fresh salads

PLATE V

Cooking Techniques

Preparing Ratatouille (Provençal-Style Eggplant Stew)

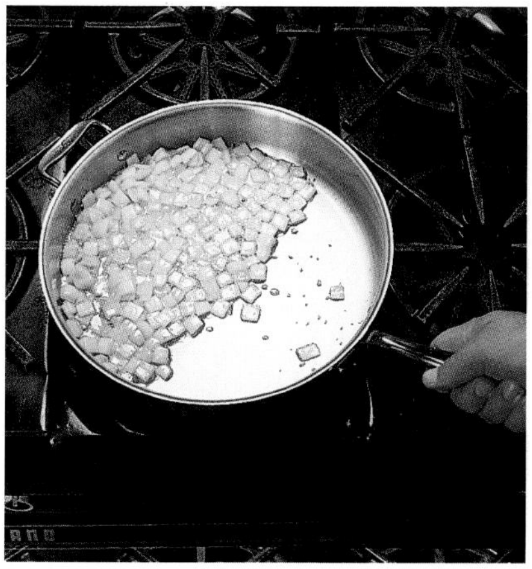

Sauté onions and garlic.

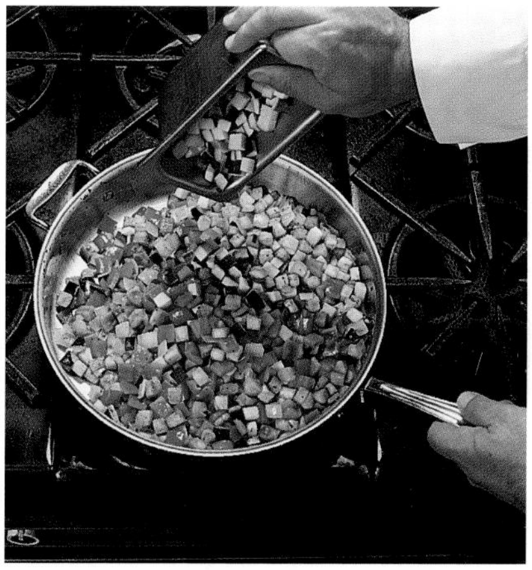

Add peppers, eggplant and zucchini.

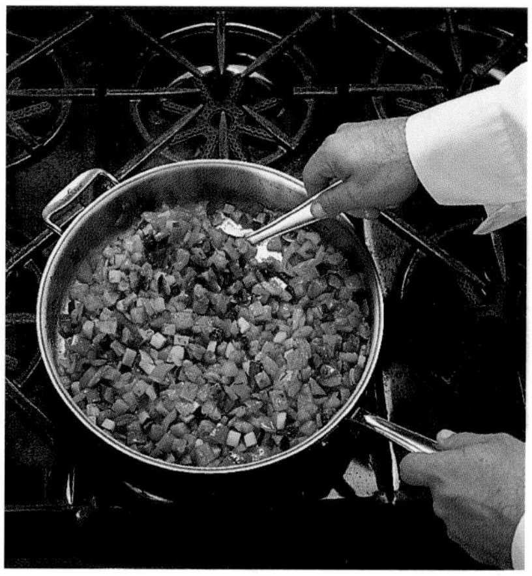

The finished ratatouille.

PLATE VI

Steaming Vegetables

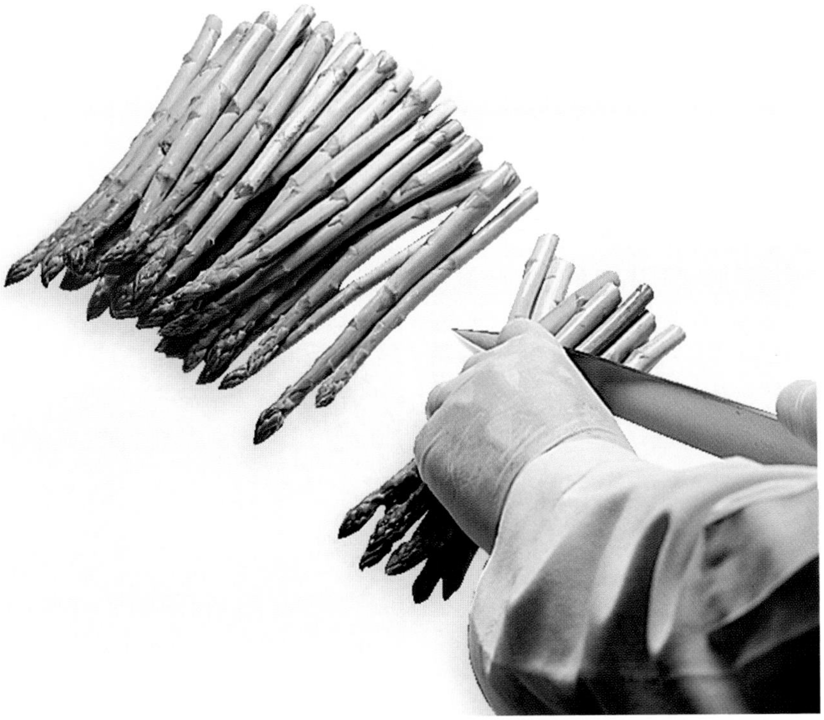

Cut items to fit steaming pan

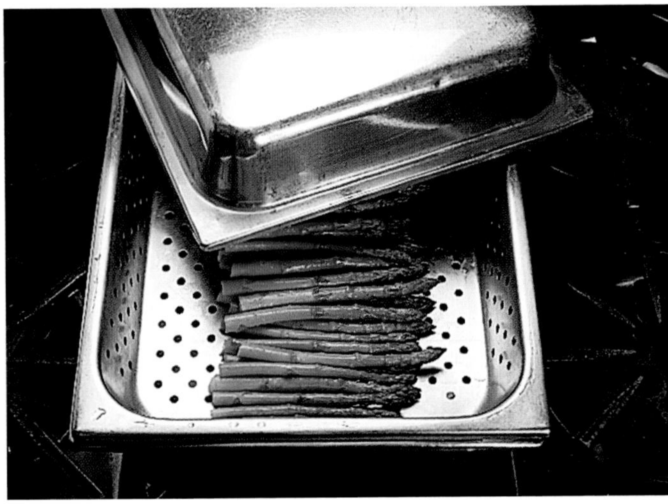

Steam for as little time as possible

PLATE VII

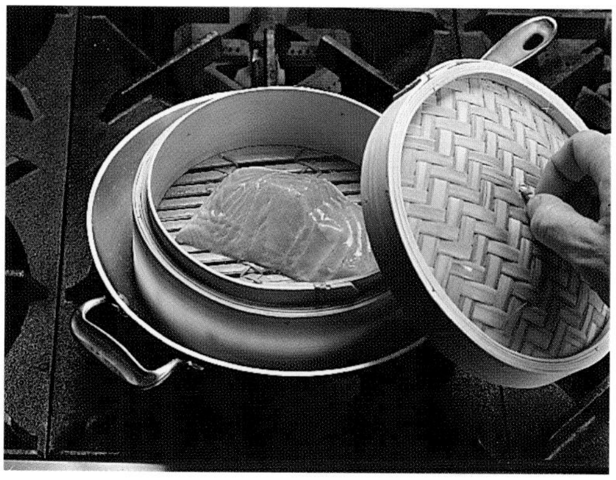

Steaming fish

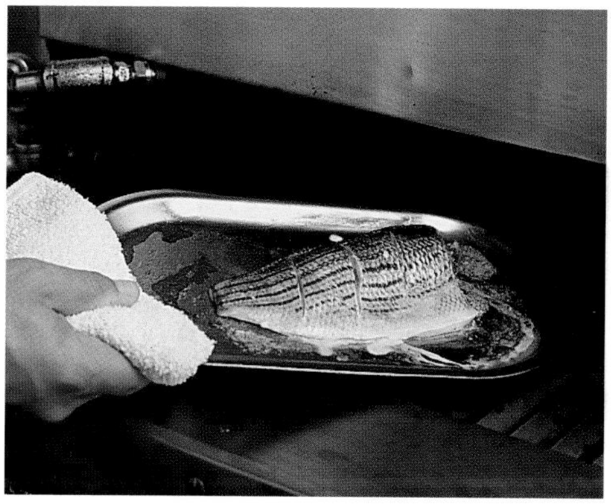

Broil

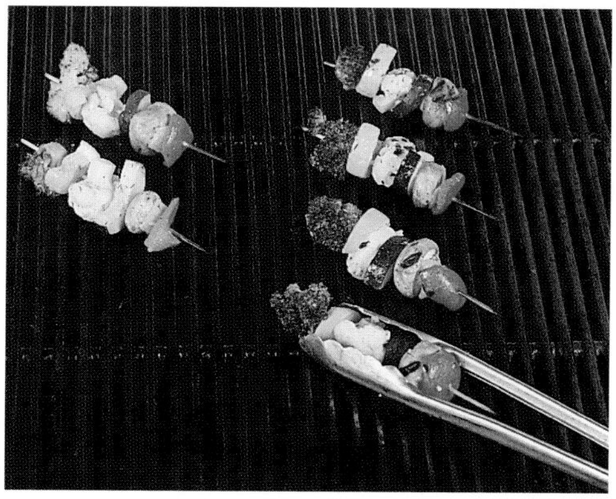

grill

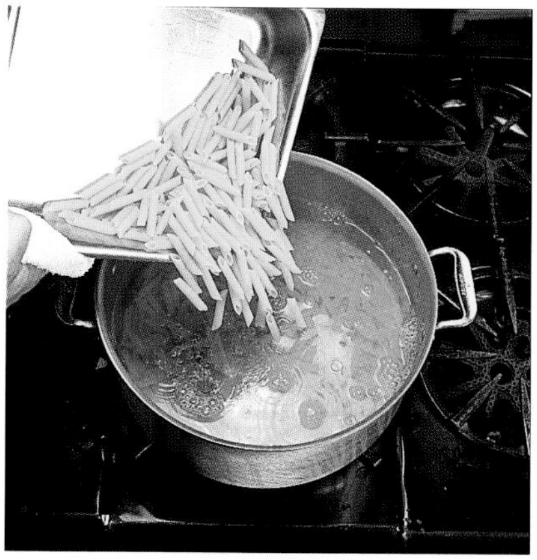

Boil

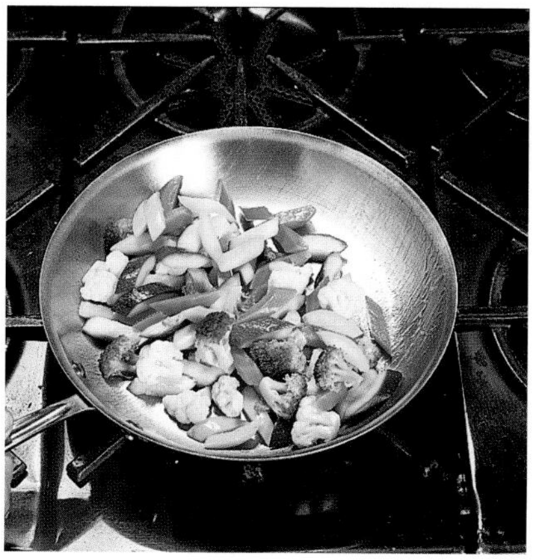

Sauté

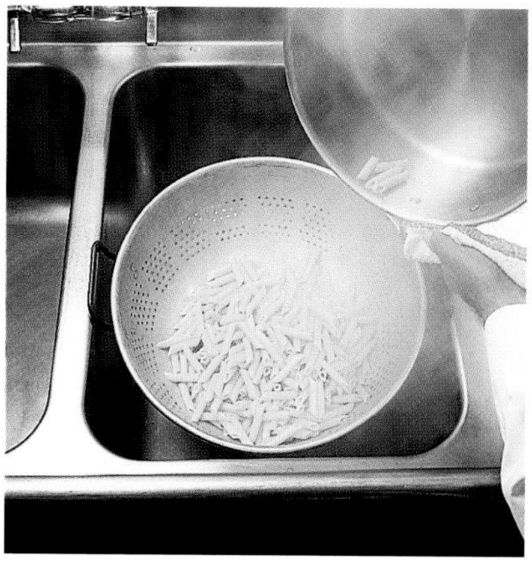

Strain

PLATE VIII

Preparing a Coulis (Puréed Sauce)— Fruit (Such as Strawberries) and Vegetables Can Be Used to Prepare a Coulis

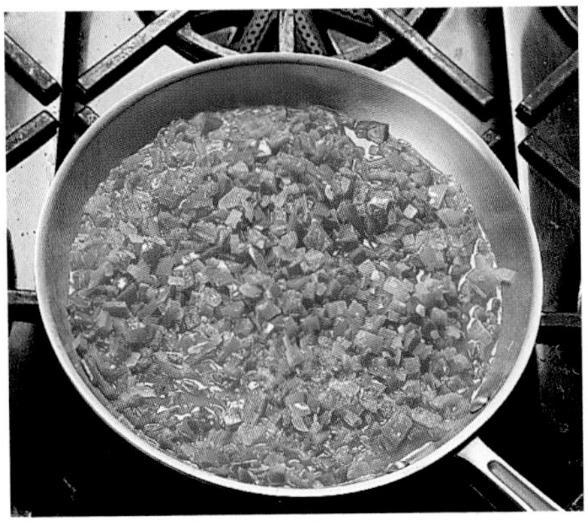

Sauté red peppers.

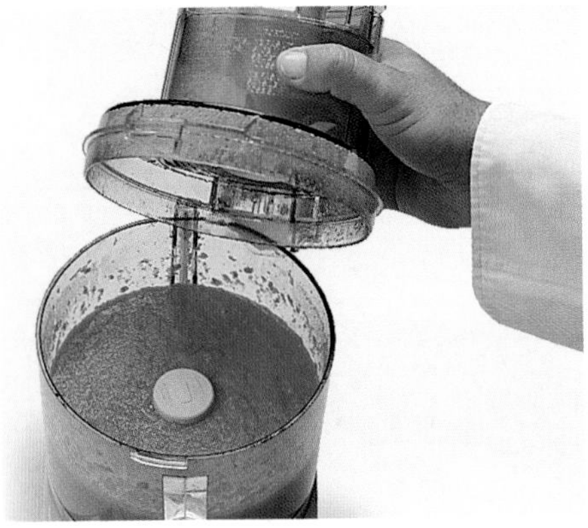

Purée the cooked peppers.

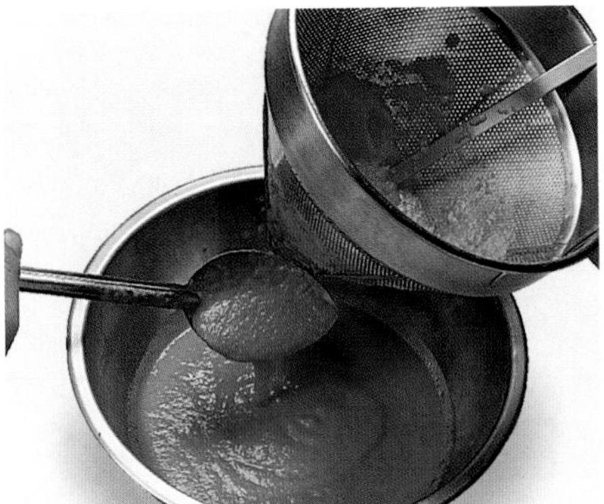

Straining the coulis.

PLATE IX

Poaching

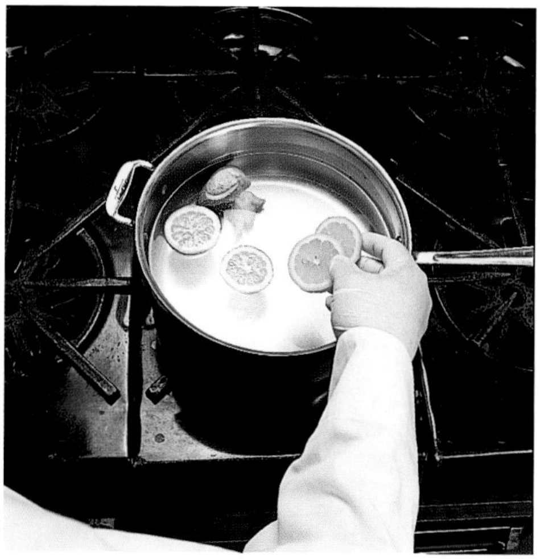

Season liquid

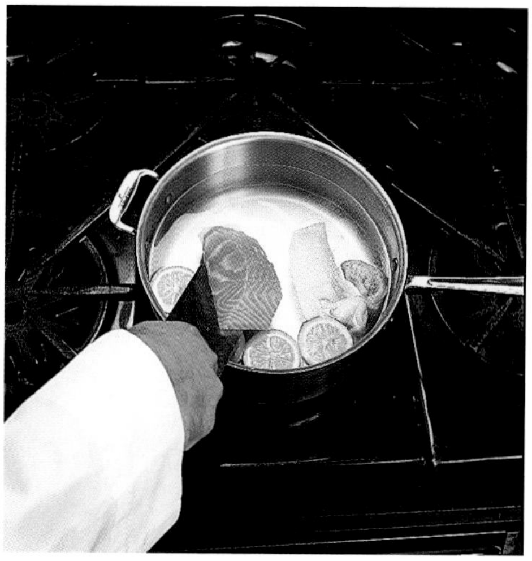

Place items in liquid

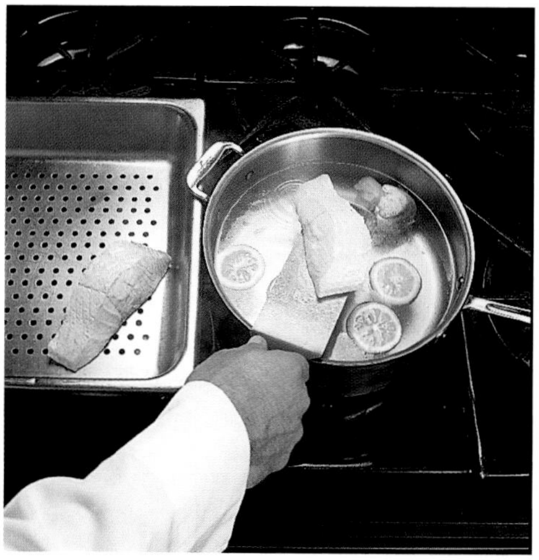

Remove & drain items

PLATE X

En Papillote *(Oven Steaming in Parchments)*

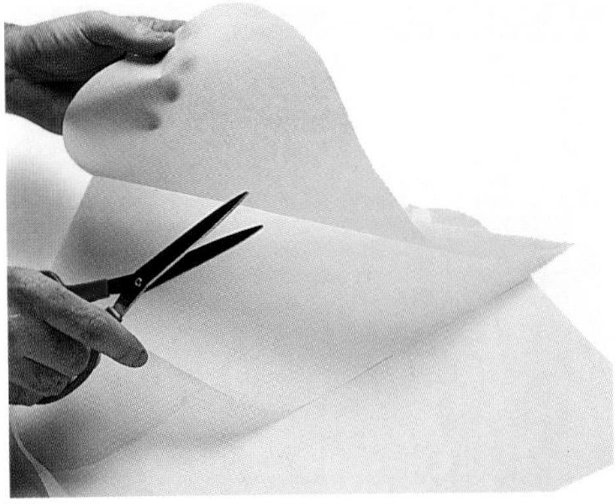

Cut heart-shaped pieces of parchment paper.

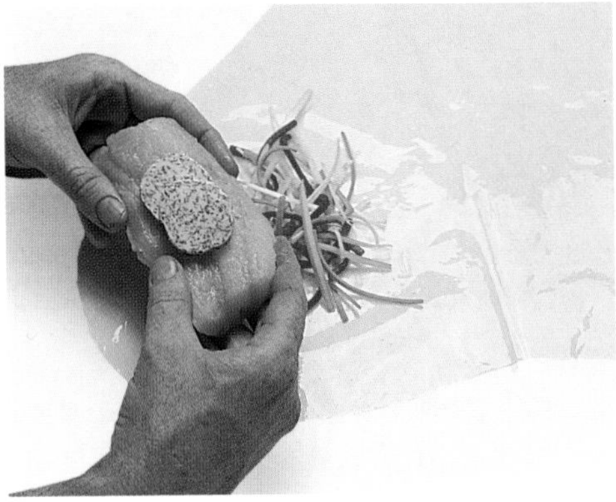

Place items on parchment

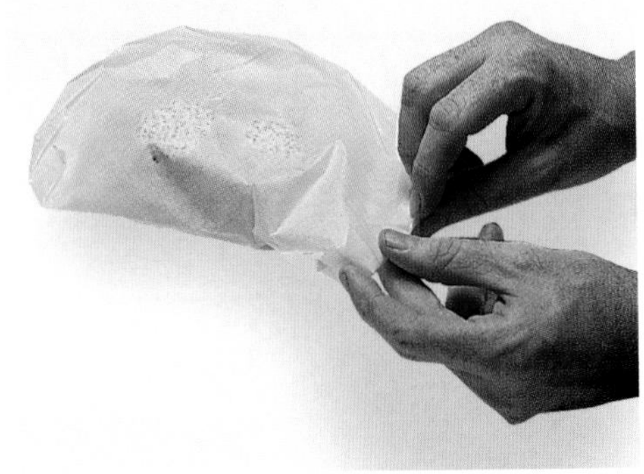

Crimp edges

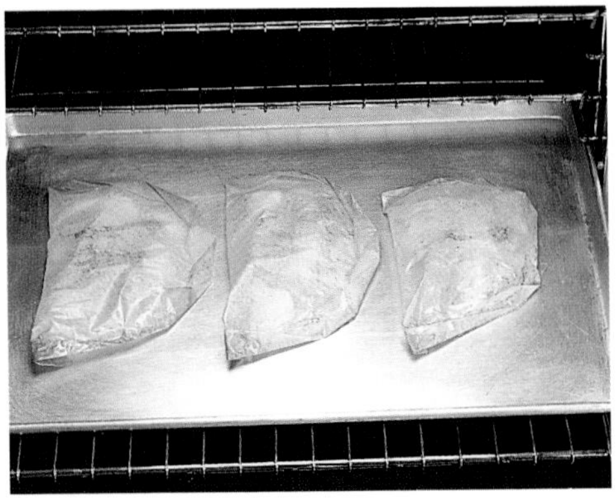

Finished product

PLATE XI

Preparing a Cold Fruit Soup

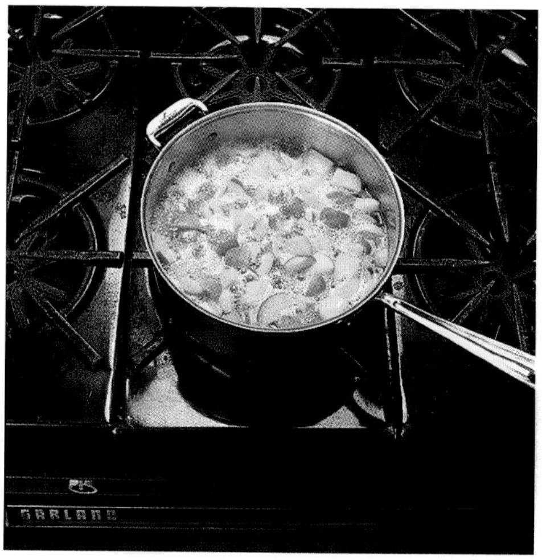

Simmer fruit

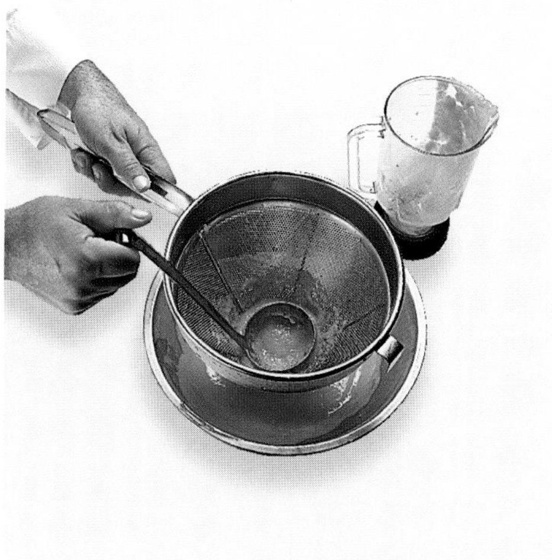

Strain the pureé.

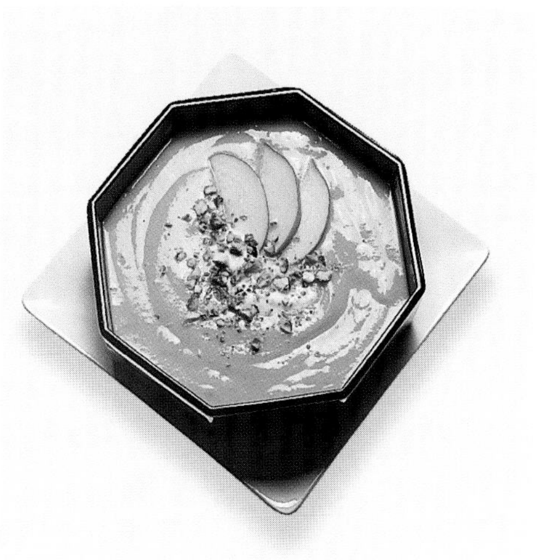

The finished soup.

PLATE XII

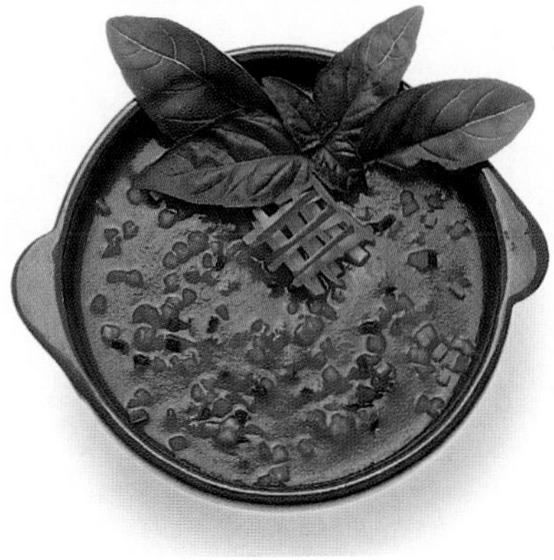

Gazpacho

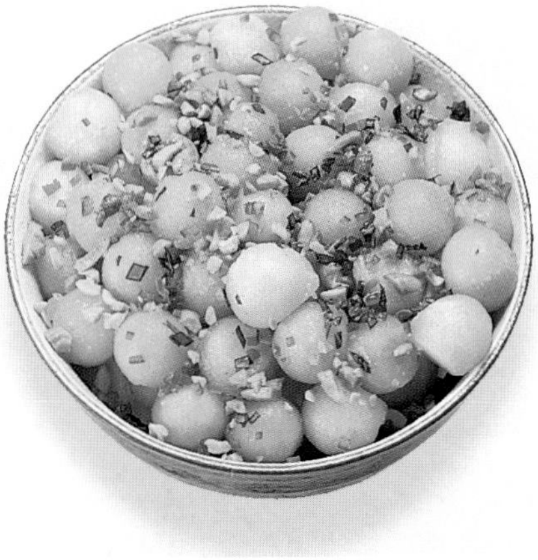

Thai Melon Salsa

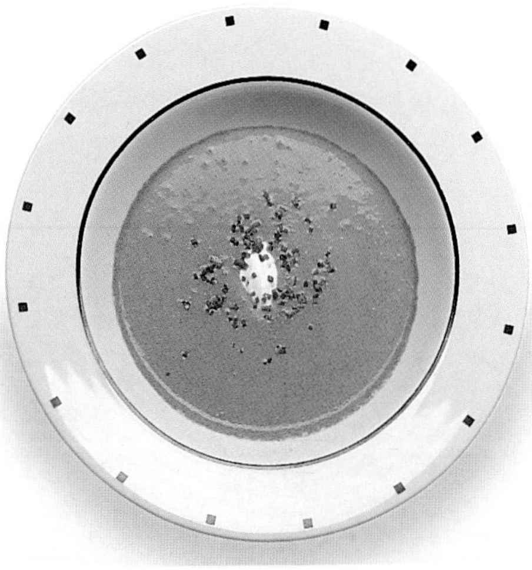

Chilled Beet & Buttermilk Soup

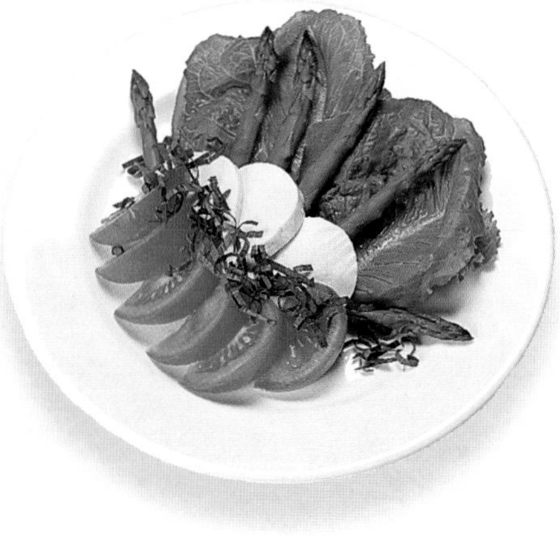

Salad caprese and part-skim mozzarella

Chapter 11

Putting It All Together: Healthy Menu Planning

Chapter Overview

Healthy Menus and the Bottom Line
Nutrition and the Culinarian
Corporate Nutrition
Healthy Menu Construction Methods
Individual Ingredients
- *Pork as a Lean and Low-Salt Item*
- *Winter Vegetables in Soups and Sauces*
- *Beans in Soups, Sauces, and Dips*
- *Fruit as a Savory Accompaniment*
- *Salsa Instead of High-Fat Sauces*

Healthy Segments of the Menu
- *Breakfast*
- *Seasonal*
  - *Grill On!*
- *Desserts*
- *Fast Food*
- *Catering*

Equipping the Nutrition Kitchen
Evaluating Web Sites for Nutrition Information
Swapping Ingredients
FYI: Soy Speak
- *Beyond Tofu*
- *Care and Feeding*
- *The Meat of the Wheat*

Chapter Objectives

After reading this chapter, the student should be able to:

1. *List the reasons why nutrition makes good monetary sense for a food operation.*
2. *Name some of the chefs and corporations who include nutrition in their repertoire.*
3. *Suggest some programs to use for healthy menu construction.*
4. *Explain how alternate meats, such as pork or buffalo, can be included on healthy menus.*
5. *Replace fat and salt with healthy, satisfying ingredients, such as root vegetables and beans.*
6. *Use fruit and salsa in place of some of the fat on a menu.*
7. *Construct a low-fat breakfast menu.*

8. *Demonstrate how fast food can be healthy.*
9. *Write a healthy catering menu.*
10. *Evaluate Web sites for nutritional information.*
11. *Suggest food preparation equipment that can assist in the preparation of healthy menus.*
12. *Explain how to exchange ingredients in menu items.*

Introduction

When we started this book, we discussed all the reasons food professionals needed to know about nutrition. We mentioned personal health, helping the world, understanding how the ingredients you work with can improve your life and the life of your customers. The best, though, is . . . the MONEY.

Good nutrition is a good business practice for food service companies. Good nutrition means good health for employees. Healthy employees are able to work effectively and bring a vibrancy to the workplace. It's hard to bring passion to the menu when you don't feel well.

In this chapter, we will examine how nutrition can affect the bottom line of food service operations, making suggestions on how to play the nutrition card in various types of operations. We'll look at individual ingredients to see how they fit in the health portion of the menu.

We'll discuss using the Web as a tool for nutrition information, including how to assess if the information you are getting is valid and current. Finally, we'll look at a typical food-service operation and make suggestions for equipment purchasing and ingredient selection so you can offer the maximum amount of healthy items with a minimum of labor and expense.

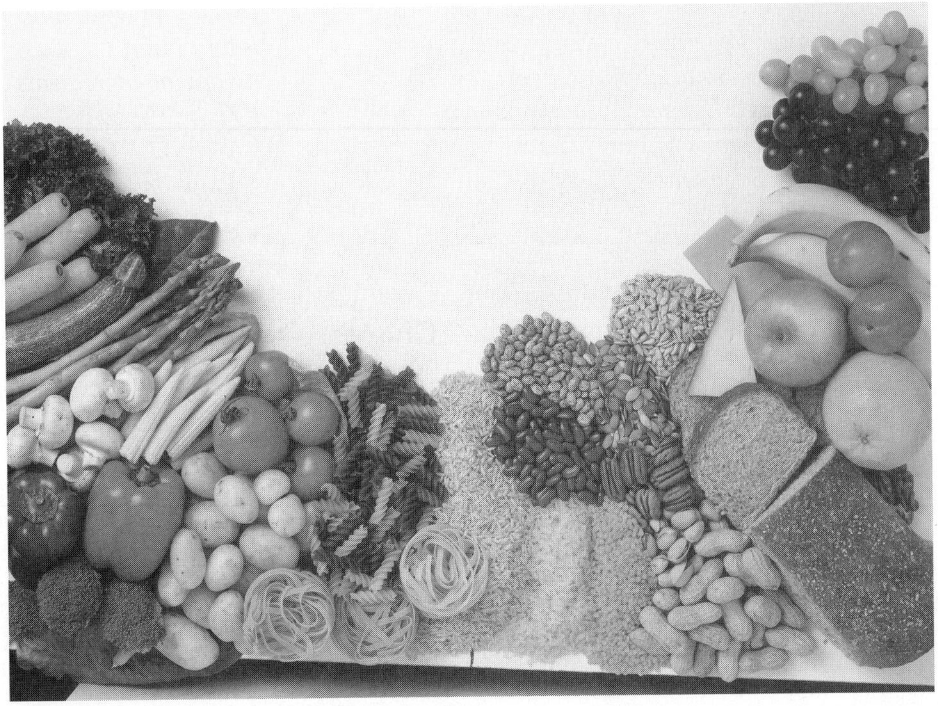

HEALTHY MENUS AND THE BOTTOM LINE

Many customers are looking for good nutrition on the menu. Since many people eat out more than they eat in, restaurant food is no longer an indulgence that can be high in fat and salt and lacking in nutrients. If you offer good nutrition along with good value, you'll have happy customers that come back often, probably bringing their friends, family, and co-workers. If you offer good nutrition on your menu, you can attract more people. With a varied menu, one member of a dinner party can have steak and potatoes au gratin, another can have a grilled salmon Caesar salad and another can have a mixed meal, with poached chicken breast tarragon and French fries. Don't be surprised if breakfast customers order "schizophrenic" meals, such as egg-white omelets with shredded cheddar cheese or hollandaise sauce or French toast made with egg substitute. The idea is that you are satisfying the customers needs or ideas about nutrition, and bringing in a profit at the same time.

NUTRITION AND THE CULINARIAN

Famous chef and food personalities have certainly acknowledged the idea that "nutrition sells." Some culinarians responded to their customers' health issues. Some had family member with medical problems that required nutritional intervention. And some recognized the benefits of a healthy diet for a long and happy life.

We've mentioned Master Chef Victor Gielisse in previous chapters. His "cuisine actuelle" was just the beginning of the association between good nutrition and luxurious cuisine. Food personality Graham Kerr (known as the "Galloping Gourmet") had taught millions of television viewers the techniques of classical cuisine. After he and his wife overcame some health issues, Chef Kerr devoted his food instruction and writing to sumptuous foods that were low in fat and salt. He has had great national and international success with his healthy cooking techniques.

Chef Paul Prudhomme is known as "Chef Paul" to the thousands of people who have visited his world-renown restaurant, K-Paul's, in New Orleans, used his spice blends, or read his cookbooks. Chef Paul has published a collection of lower-fat, lower-salt recipes, using the intrigue of Cajun seasoning to replace the need for some of the fat and salt in selected recipes. On a different nutrition note, Chef Paul wrote a series of highly nutritious recipes based on USDA **commodity foods** for use by homeless shelters feeding families with children. These recipes have been distributed by the American Culinary Federation to food banks across the country, to ensure that children are receiving the nutritious foods they need. Food service people can help to provide good nutrition for the diverse needs of the American population.

CORPORATE NUTRITION

In previous chapters, we've discussed some of the healthy food programs that hotels and restaurants have put into effect in response to customer interest. The Omni Hotel chain launched an "Ideal Nourishment" menu, to accommodate travelers who want to eat healthy on the road. The menus offer health-conscious meals that are either heart-healthy, high-protein/low-carbohydrate (a la Atkins), low-sodium, sugar-free, and/or vegetarian.

The chain had a competition among all their corporate chefs. Recipes had to be designed for gourmet cuisine that fit at least one of the categories listed above. Here are just some of the winners selected to be offered on chain-wide menus:

Cardamon-encrusted Atlantic salmon, apple/fennel slaw and vegetable nage (heart healthy), rosemary lamb chops (low sodium), black-bean enchiladas and grits and vegetables (veggie), chocolate/strawberry cheesecake (sugar-free). To continue the healthy theme throughout the property, most hotels have in-house health clubs or swimming pools. In-room mini-bars were stocked with healthy snacks.

Some operations construct their own elaborate nutrition programs. Others simply offer a variety of menu items prepared to the customer's request. For example, fish or poultry can be fried, grilled, sautéed, broiled, poached or roasted. Potatoes are available in low fat options. Salad dressings, sauces and gravies can be served on the side. Burger selections can include beef, turkey, chicken and vegetarian. We've even seen salmon, buffalo, and ostrich (both very lean), and **portobello** mushroom burgers.

Sorbet, sherbets, and fruit ices are lower-fat alternatives to ice cream on the dessert menu. You don't have to spend a lot of time and money to offer menus with healthy food options. In fact, you don't want to order a lot of "special" ingredients, as you will just have to carry them on an inventory and find alternate uses for them. The wise chef knows how to use the ingredients already in the kitchen to prepare healthy foods.

HEALTHY MENU CONSTRUCTION METHODS

Organizations such as the American Heart Association or the American Cancer Society have packaged nutrition programs that can be easily adapted to a restaurant's menu. These programs generally have guidelines for healthy eating along with recipes that have been nutritionally analyzed. A food establishment can submit their recipes and menus to these organizations to obtain approval. For example, the American Heart Association has a "heart healthy" ❤ ™ symbol that signifies menus or recipes that meet the American Heart Association's guidelines. For a fee, a recipe, menu or food product can carry this symbol, letting customers know that they are ordering or purchasing a bona fide healthy food.

Review the designations for label claims if you want to add "salt free," "low-fat," "low-cholesterol," or other claims to your menu items, you must be able to prove that they meet the USDA standards for these designations. You can prove that a menu item is low-salt by analyzing the recipe with a computer program, hiring a dietitian to analyze it for you or by preparing the menu item from a recipe that has already been analyzed.

INDIVIDUAL INGREDIENTS

Let's spend the rest of the chapter talking about how to offer menus and recipes that meet particular nutritional needs. We've included some recipes at the end of the chapter for you to sample and convert to your own needs.

Pork as a Lean and Low-Salt Item

Some ingredients are perceived as being high in fat. Pork is a product rarely associated with "lean." The following information will give you something to communicate to customers when they ask "How can you have savory herbed pork chops with caramelized onions on the heart-healthy menu?" Do your own nutritional investigation of particular ingredients that you would like to offer on your healthy menus.

Modern pork production is geared to reduce the fat content of pork. For example, three ounces of skinless chicken breast has about 140 calories and 73 milligrams of cholesterol. Three ounces of pork tenderloin also has 140 calories and 67 milligrams of cholesterol. Three ounces of beef tenderloin has 175 calories and 71 milligrams of cholesterol. Lean cuts can be found in pork as well as poultry and beef.

In addition to being fairly lean, pork has some extra-added nutrient values. Three ounces of cooked pork shoulder (good for braising, stewing, and barbecuing) has about 180 calories, 319 milligrams of potassium, 3 milligrams of zinc, 22 milligrams of magnesium, and about a milligram of B_{12}. Fresh pork is very low in sodium, with about 50 milligrams per three-ounce serving.

Recognizing that pork can be both healthy and economical, you'll have to make some decisions on the pork cuts to order. If you have limited oven or stove space and need to cook quickly, order smaller cuts of pork, such as stir-fry strips, or end-to-end chops (which are less expensive than center cuts). If you have more time, order fresh pork roasts, such as rolled top loin, shoulder, or boneless blade.

Optimize the leanness of pork by cutting fat from kitchen techniques and recipes. Trim any visible fat before cooking and prior to service. Plan your preparation and cook pork several hours to a day ahead of time. This will allow you to skim fat from surfaces of stews and to more easily trim fat from solid cuts, such as roasts. Use minimal amounts of oil, or even better yet, vegetable oil spray when cooking. Put roasts and other baked pork cuts on a rack, so any fat drips away from the meat.

Lean pork cuts give you the opportunity to work with marinades, rubs and seasoning blends. Anyone can slap a chop or steak on the grill. You'll impress them with your flavorful, savory offerings. When using lean cuts of any type of meat, you need to replace the flavor and the juiciness with alternate ingredients.

Select pork stew cubes, shoulder butt or tenderloin medallions for braising, short ribs, and cubes for stewing, ground pork and strips for sautéing and shoulder butt and tenderloin for roasting. Remember that most cuts of pork are lean and shouldn't be overdone. You're looking for an internal temperature

Here are lots of Web sites that can assist you in healthy menu planning.

Web Site	*Info*
www.diabetic-recipes.com	Search for recipes by ingredient or category, holiday, party and kids menus and recipes, links to *Diabetic Lifestyle* magazine
www.chef2chef.net	Food news, recipes, wines, chefs forum, chef rankings, and background
www.foodsubs.com	The *Cook's Thesaurus* has suggestions for ingredient substitutes and lots of photos
www.epicurious.com	Over 12,000 recipes, prep methods, cuisines
www.globalgourmet.com	Food and wine info, culinary tips from thirty-six countries
www.orst.edu/food-resource/food.html	This Oregon State University site has food links and resources for every type of food
http://soar.berkeley.edu/recipes	Searchable archive of 70,000 recipes organized into cuisine and country
www.foodtv.com	Thousands of recipes and a full culinary encyclopedia
www.chowbaby.com	International recipes, cooking and purchasing types, restaurant menus, cooks' dictionary
www.foodallergy.org	The Food Allergy Network has ideas for designing recipes and menus for people with food allergies
www.talksoy.com	The United Soy Board's Web site has soy-based quantity recipes
www.winetoday.com	A database of 7,000 wines with suggestions for pairing

Figure 11–1 Savor the Web

of 160 degrees; measure the temperature in several places to ensure doneness.

Trichinosis is virtually nonexistent in the United States because of controlled production conditions. So there is no longer the need of "incinerating" pork to ensure safety. Just to make you feel better, if there were any trichinosis lurking about, it would be destroyed with the 160-degree temperature.

Stewing pork can be "down home," comfort food. Order pork shoulder, cut into one-inch or one-half inch cubes, smoked shoulder roll, or even hocks or neck bones (if your clientele are familiar with them) for stewing. To seal in flavor and develop a golden brown color, lightly coat pork with flour, breadcrumbs or seasoned bread crumbs. Spray vegetable oil or heat a small amount of stock in a stockpot or tilting skillet and brown pork on all sides. When pork is browned, add cooking liquid, such as mushroom broth or chicken stock, cover and simmer (on top of the stove or in the oven) for one to three hours.

Web Site	*Info*
www.vrg.com	The Vegetarian Resource Group's Web site with vegan quantity recipes, vegan kitchen set up and ingredient purchasing, on-line vegan nutrition courses
www.aeb.org	The American Egg Board's site with recipes and encyclopedia
www.alaskaseafood.org	Ideas for ordering and preparing fresh and frozen seafood
www.avocado.org/foodservice	Everything you need to know and how to use avocado
www.beeffoodservice.org	Everything you need to know about beef
www.otherwhitemeat.org	Pork recipes, cooking ideas, menu ideas
www.eatturkey.com	Virtual chef demos, purchasing and preparing turkey ideas
www.fcso.org	Foodservice Consultants Society International—how to find consulting services
www.kelloggsfoodservice.com	Info on Kellogg's cereal products
www.tetleyusa.com	Tips on brewing and cooking with tea
www.oceanspray.com	Product info and recipes for cranberry dressings, entrees, beverages, and desserts
www.conagra.com	Foodservice information on Conagra's "healthy" products, including egg substitutes, Healthy Choice items, etc.
www.chickenofthesea.com	Recipes, nutritional information and kids' menus ideas for tuna
www.ent.iastate.edu/Misc/InsectsAsFood.html	Need a recipe for banana worm bread or Root beetle dip? Go to Iowa State University's Web site. Even has ordering info for edible bugs (ick!)

Figure 11–1 Savor the Web *(cont'd)*

You can tell pork is tender when it is soft to the touch of a fork. Add vegetables and cooked potatoes towards the end of cooking, about the last twenty to forty minutes; this will ensure plenty of moisture.

Stewing pork can transform a less-than-tender cut into a soft-as-butter cut. Just be certain to allow enough time for cooking and to add enough liquid. For a German-style pork stew, use beer as part of the simmering liquid and season with onions, caraway and thyme. For a continental stew, add white wine, tarragon, fennel, pearl onions, and green peas. For a Mediterranean melange, use a hearty red wine, tomato puree, olives, and garlic. All lower fat, all tasty.

Braising is a close cousin to stewing. Stewing usually involves simmering less-tender cuts for several hours in a liberal amount of liquid. Braising requires liquid only to cover and can be done in as little as twenty minutes. To obtain the full flavor of braised pork, season pork, sear meat on all sides to

Got Ambition? Want to analyze your wonderful new recipes and menus? Here's some resources:

Free for the Asking:

Resource	*Contents*
www.internets.com/sfood.htm	Nutritional Food Database Index Site: searchable database of over 4,000 food items
www.nal.usda.gov	USDA Food Values Data Base: searchable database of over 10,000 food items
www.heartinfo.org	Heart Information Network: Restaurant Nutrition Claims: definitions of health claims, nationwide listing of restaurants and their health claims
www.chowbaby.com	Food Web site including analyzed recipes and ingredient information
It'll Cost Ya	
www.nraef.org	National Restaurant Association's Web site includes information about recipes analysis software
www. computrition.com	Computrition has many types of nutritional analysis software for recipes and menus
www.culinarysoftware.com	Chef Tec Software has intregrated software that can link recipe analyses with inventory and purchasing information
www.firstdatabank.com	Nutritionist Pro™ will plan and analyze menus and has food labeling options

Figure 11–2 Analyze This!

brown, just cover with liquid, cover tightly and simmer on the stove top or in the oven until meat is tender. Braising liquid can include chicken, mushroom or vegetable stocks, tomato sauce, wine or beer, vegetable juice cocktail, or prepared gravies. Use the braising liquid as a sauce for the cooked meat.

Both stewed and braised pork dishes benefit from marinades or rubs. To make a marinade, combine an acid ingredient, such as citrus juice or vinegar, with a small amount of oil and seasonings. Allow the meat to soak in the marinade for at least thirty minutes. Marinades also help to tenderize. Less-tender cuts, such as pork stew or shoulder, can marinate for up to twelve hours. Try a marinade combination of orange juice, cloves and a small amount of canola oil or tomato juice, Italian seasoning blend (basil, oregano, black pepper), and olive oil.

Rubs are mixtures of herbs and spices that are rubbed directly into meat before it's cooked. Rubs impart flavor and color to meat, combining with the natural juices of the pork to accent flavor. Try a rub of coarsely ground black pepper, granulated garlic and dried parsley or mild chili powder, thyme and onion powder. This adds flavor without fat or salt.

Whichever cooking method you choose for pork be sure to be safe. Avoid cross contamination by having separate cutting boards for pork. Be sure kitchen knives are sharpened regularly; nothing is more dangerous in a kitchen than a dull knife. Be sure to defrost frozen pork in the refrigerator, allow about three to five hours per pound of pork. Thin cuts of pork such as strip or thin patties can be defrosted as they are cooked.

When you think pork, think creative. Think country-stuffed pork roast (order a boned and rolled shoulder), stuffed with a bread dressing aromatic with sage, thyme, dried cranberries, and garlic, and serve with an orange cranberry sauce. Think pork leg, marinated in lemon juice, vegetable stock, ginger, curry powder, rosemary, and lemon zest and serve with a brown sauce made from mushroom stock seasoned with red wine, tomatoes, parsley and garlic. Think savory pork and vegetable pie, made with pork shoulder cubes, onions, peas, carrots, thyme, and rosemary, baked into a fresh crust. Try tossing pork strips with soy sauce, Worcestershire sauce and curry powder, quickly stir-frying and add broccoli, tomatoes and cooked pasta. Steam smoked pork picnic shoulder with cabbage, carrots, turnips and potatoes, season with pickling spice and serve with a low fat sour cream, mustard, onion and honey sauce. Just start thinking pork, and start adding flavorful, fun for the palate and fun for the pocketbook menu items.

Winter Vegetables in Soups and Sauce

When people reduce calories, they don't necessarily want to reduce mouthfeel or the amount of food on their plate. The secret is to select ingredients that have lots of "chew" without lots of calories.

Winter vegetables are sturdier in structure which means they'll stand up to lots of preparation. They are high in fiber, which means they are lower in calories. Fairly large servings can be eaten without excess calories. Winter vegetables give a pleasant, "full" sensation without a lot of fat or salt. Hearty greens, such as cabbage, kale, mustard and turnip greens, a variety of onions, such as leeks, white, yellow, and red onions and shallots and root vegetables are high in vitamins and minerals with little fat or salt. They have lots of texture, flavor, and color. Presented in a creative way, customers will forget that they are "eating their vegetables" without benefit of lots of butter or cream. Winter vegetables are economical as well, usually less expensive than dairy or meat ingredients. Combine good nutrition with good business.

Delicate greens are for the summer months, but sturdy greens, such as collards, kale and chard are available fresh and reasonably priced throughout the winter. Store fresh greens in a closed container to keep them from drying out and keep them cool. Shred greens finely and use, uncooked, as a garnish for salads. Lightly steam shredded greens and use them to garnish soups and stews. Or chop and steam, mix with egg whites or silken tofu and breadcrumbs and fry or bake as a green pancake to accompany entrees.

Greens have a reputation for being difficult to clean and being overly strong in flavor. Solve the cleaning issue by purchasing already-cleaned greens (and already chopped, to save labor). Forget the notion of simmering greens for hours. Most greens can be quickly steamed or lightly sautéed for a holiday-colored, fresh-tasting side dish.

Greens can be used as a side dish, tossed into other side dishes, such as pasta or rice and even used as part of a stuffing mixture for poultry and seafood. When fresh greens aren't available or convenient, purchase frozen. Be sure to allow them to thaw and to squeeze excess water from them to ensure a non-soggy finished product.

Onions are available fresh in the spring and summer and then are available as storage veggies the rest of the year. We all know onions to be great ingredients, but think of them also as a vegetable that can stand alone as an accompaniment dish.

Leeks, resembling overgrown green onions are mild in flavor, can be sliced and stewed, sautéed or steamed, and served with a light, creamy sauce. Leeks have a delicate onion flavor and a moist, tender mouthfeel. Use leeks in stuffings and in soups when you want an insinuation of onion flavor.

Yellow (or white onions) can get a bit powerful in the winter months. Knock off some of that power by baking or broiling. The heat releases some of the acid and caramelizes some of the onion's natural sugar, resulting in a soft-but-crunchy, slightly sweet new side dish. Leeks and onions add lots of flavor without any fat or salt.

Winter squash are not grown or harvested in the winter, but got that name for their ability to be stored throughout the long winter months. Winter squash are allowed to mature more than their cousins, the summer squash (zucchini, crookneck, pittypan, etc.) and have a tougher and darker skin. Butternut, hubbards, acorn, and banana squash are popular varieties.

Winter squash can be sweet or savory, used in a dessert pie or in savory soup. Purchase fresh winter squash, cut it in squares and bake (cut-side down) on a baking sheet with a little water on it (about ½-inch). For a sweet squash, sprinkle with cinnamon, nutmeg, ginger, mace, cloves, and orange zest. For a savory squash, sprinkle with garlic and onion powder, white or black pepper, red pepper flakes, thyme, or rosemary.

Squash side dishes can be simply cubed baked or steamed, seasoned squash or use pureed winter squash as a sauce for poultry or green vegetables or as a base for a hearty winter soup (think winter squash, carrots, potatoes and celery soup). Mashed winter squash can be an ingredient in soups or pasta fillings. When fresh squash is not available or convenient, explore your frozen options. Frozen winter squash is very easy to handle, as it is already cut up and cooked—you just have to decide how to season it and heat it.

Potatoes—sweet or savory are wintertime favorites. Baked, boiled, steamed, sautéed or fried, potato dishes can warm the cockles of the coldest customer's heart. White potatoes can be baked and heaped with toppings (try a stuffed baked potato paired with a vegetable or bean soup for a wintry evening meal), mashed with fresh herbs and other veggies (mash in some carrots for sweetness and color or turnips for some "snap"), roasted with dried herbs and sautéed with peppers, onions, and herbs. Used leftover mashed potatoes in potato pancakes or as a topping for baked casseroles. Roesti potatoes resemble potato pancakes made with hash browns, and can be served with sautéed onions and cracked black pepper.

Fresh sweet potatoes can be simply baked or roasted. Their natural color and flavor require little assistance. If you have the urge to create, mash sweet potatoes with pineapple juice and minced oranges and create a sweet potato pancake. Pureed sweet potato makes a great base for soup and for the famous sweet potato pie. Mashed sweet potatoes can be mixed with mashed white potatoes to create a new dish (with a lovely color).

Carrots, beets, turnips, celery root, and parsnips are reliable winter vegetables. They are colorful, flavorful, full of texture, and best of all, relatively inexpensive. You can steam carrots, celery root, or beets until they are soft enough to puree. Add herbs, onions, and garlic to pureed root vegetables for "creamy" soup with no fat calories. Use the same puree as the base for a sinless sauce or gravy.

Potage Crecy (puree of carrot soup) is classical and colorful. Cook carrots and potatoes together until they are tender enough to puree. Puree until creamy, season with garlic, white pepper, and parsley and you have a silky soup that gives the impression of being creamy and buttery. The same soup routine can be done with winter squash (try banana or butternut), sweet potatoes or any root vegetable. Season squash or sweet potato soups with white pepper, cumin and thyme (savory) or ginger, mace, and nutmeg (holiday flavors). If you have the time, create a compound butter or margarine by softening the fat, mixing in herbs and spices. Serve the otherwise low-fat soup with a small dollop of savory compound butter. This adds texture and eye appeal.

With the miracle of Mr. Birdseye's process, many veggies are available at a reasonable price year-round. If you are using frozen veggies in the wintertime, consider using the heartier veggies to fit the season, leave the zucchini for the warmer months.

Frozen vegetables are blanched, so they require very little cooking time. Take advantage of their just-harvested flavor and color and create your own blends. Add a sauce (use some of the pureed winter squash), another vegetable (mushrooms and onions are always a welcome addition) or some dried herbs (dill, tarragon, mint, and rosemary spice up green veggies, such as peas or green beans) to complete the flavor.

Remember not to thaw frozen vegetables, as this will make them soggy. Right from the freezer to the frying pan (or steamer or oven) is the correct technique. Brightly prepared vegetables can be served in larger portions on an entrée plate, adding flavor and color without cholesterol or sodium.

Beans in Soups, Sauces, and Dips

Cold months are the right months for hand- and tummy-warming bean soups and side dishes. Purchase beans dried or canned, depending on time and labor. Dried beans do take more preparation time and are low in salt; canned beans are quick to use but can be high in salt.

Think of the colors and flavors that beans can add to your menu: green, yellow, pink and red lentils, white, yellow and green limas, black beans, cranberry beans, Christmas beans (yes, Virginia, they are red and green), pink and red pinto beans, white navy beans, beige and white garbanzo beans, and white or green soy beans.

Fresh, frozen or canned, wintertime is the perfect time to offer comforting, hearty, warmly spiced produce; here are some ideas:

Swiss chard sautéed with garlic

Steamed Swiss chard topped with seasoned bread crumbs and Parmesan cheese

Steamed spinach tossed with spicy tomato sauce

Steamed greens tossed with salsa (this can be served hot or cold)

White potatoes mashed with steamed parsnips

White potatoes mashed with rosemary and garlic

Veggies

Fresh or canned mushrooms sautéed with onions and peppers

Frozen peas with fresh or frozen pearl onions and chopped red pepper

Peas, pearl onions and mushrooms served with a creamy celery sauce

Winter squash baked with sautéed onions

Winter squash baked with cinnamon, nutmeg and ginger

Winter squash mashed with chicken or vegetable stock, margarine and garlic and onion powder

Acorn squash filled with stuffing or rice pilaf

Sweet potatoes oven-roasted with a teriyaki sauce

Sweet potato pancakes served with hot apple slices

Sweet potatoes mashed with margarine, cinnamon, nutmeg and ginger

Sautéed red or green cabbage

Sweet and sour red cabbage (made with vinegar and apples)

Cabbage rolls (stuffed with rice or barley)

Beets with orange sauce

Fruit

Dried apricots, apples, raisins and prunes stewed with apple juice, ginger, mace and cloves

Apple and pear sauce (cook apples and pears together)

Baked apples and pears (bake with raisins, apple juice concentrate, and cinnamon, ginger)

Poached apples and pears (poach in water and wine combo, simple syrup spiked with cinnamon sticks or apple juice)

Apple or pear brown Betty

Canned or frozen peach, berry or pineapple cobbler

Apple or berry bread pudding

Apple or banana fritters

Apple or pear dumplings

Pink grapefruit broiled with honey or orange juice concentrate

Citrus ambrosia

Orange and grapefruit tart

Cranberry and orange relish

Baked pumpkin custard

Apple and pear pie with raisins and walnuts

Figure 11–3 Winter Wonderland

Some cooks will tell you that the more you soak and rinse beans, the less likely they are to cause socially inappropriate flatulence. We can tell you that you can produce a successful bean dish without soaking, if time is constrained. Cooking time and liquid content should be increased if beans are not soaked.

Cook several types of beans together for a flavorful side dish. Smoked turkey wings and tofu hot dogs can be used to get that smoky flavor without the fat and salt of bacon. Salsa chopped peppers, tomatoes and onions and dried herbs and spices (red pepper flakes, tarragon, white and black pepper, garlic, oregano, curry, and chili powder, etc.) can be added during cooking to give even more flavor.

Cooked beans can be pureed to form the base for soups and dips. Thin pureed beans with tomato juice or vegetable stock to make a vegetable-based sauce for entrees and other vegetables. Cooked beans can be used as ingredients in stews, casseroles and in stuffings and hot sandwich wraps. Be sure you stock up on a variety so you can add them as needed.

If you go overboard on bean preparation, puree them for low-fat, savory dips. Bean dips can be served hot or cold to accompany crudite (crunchy vegetables), bread sticks, hot breads, baked vegetable chips, and roasted vegetables or potatoes.

Fruit as a Savory Accompaniment

Regional fresh fruit may not be available in large varieties in the winter months. However, you can do a lot with traditional winter standbys, apples, pears, and citrus fruit.

In many cases, apples and pears can be used interchangeably for sweet and savory dishes. Bake and stew both apples and pears and serve hot with roasts and desserts alike. Apple or pear sauce can be used as an accompaniment to an entrée, rather than a fat-based sauce. Add apples or pears to stuffings and breads for a hint of sweetness and crunch. Finely diced apples can "smooth" out heavily flavored soups and stews.

Citrus is readily available throughout the winter. Follow the citrus season, as different types of oranges, tangerines, grapefruit, and lemons become available. Fresh citrus sections are always a welcome addition to salads (green, pasta, seafood, etc.) but also consider cooking them with poultry, green vegetables, rice, and even chicken soup (the famous Greek soup, Avgolomono, is a chicken-rice-lemon soup). Think about scattering tangerine sections on poultry or using pink grapefruit segments as a garnish for poultry. Fresh citrus can be used as a garnish for hot entrées and side dishes and for dessert items, such as fruit tarts, custards and puddings.

Dried fruit is popular during the winter. The captured summer sunshine is reflected in the sweetness of black and golden raisins, dried peaches, apricots, apples, pears, cranberries, cherries, figs, and dates. Add dried fruit to pie fillings and muffin batters, to poultry, pork and beef dishes, stuffings, sauces, and as a garnish for desserts. In addition to sweetness, dried fruit is a concentrated source of many nutrients.

Even when the wind is blowing and the snow is piling, fruits and veggies are an important component of your menu, adding color, variety, flavor and nutrition. Remember, five a day is what the USDA says and what menu planners need to offer.

Salsa Instead of High-Fat Sauces

Salsa is a low-fat, high-flavor alternate to gravies and sauces. If made with fresh vegetables, salsa is low-fat and low-sodium, not to mention high in vitamin C and several minerals. No longer just for chips, use salsa as a condiment for meats, fish, salads, soups, casseroles and vegetables. Red tomatoes were the traditional base for salsas, but with popularity comes variety! Now when you think salsa, think mango, papaya, pineapple, orange, summer squash and roasted vegetables. The term "salsa" has come to mean just about any combination of chopped fruit or vegetables with hot or mild spicing.

Although most salsa ingredients are used uncooked, chilies can be roasted and nuts can be toasted for more flavor and a variety in texture. For the uninitiated, peppers are roasted directly on a stove flame (right in the burner or under a broiler) and allowed to cook, turning, until the skin has blistered. If no direct flame is available, peppers can be roasted on a baking sheet, in the oven, on high heat (400° F or higher). Place the roasted peppers in a plastic bag and allow to "rest" for several minutes. This makes the peppers easier to peel. Remove from bag and peel, and peel off the blistered skin and remove the seeds. *Do not* touch your eyes after you've touched peppers, as the capsaicin contained in the peppers will burn any sensitive skin.

Take a salsa-building tour of a local grocery store or farmers' market. You'll see that chilies can be purchased fresh, canned or dried, selecting them on the basis of the heat desired. Bell peppers are extremely mild. Anaheim chilies are fairly mild. Moving up the scale, jalapenos and serranos are hot and habanero (also called Scotch bonnets) and Thai chilies are very hot. Removing the seeds removes some, but not all, of the heat.

Salsas can be sweet or savory. Try sweet combinations, such as strawberries, vinegar, sugar and black pepper or navel oranges, mango, chopped chili, chopped cilantro and limejuice. To a basic blend of chopped onions and chopped chilies, add a combination of several ingredients such as cooked beans, olives, parsley, cut corn, minced garlic, chopped pimentos (roasted red peppers), chopped fresh pineapple or canned, drained pineapple tidbits, mango, papaya, kiwi or banana, zucchini, crookneck squash or apples, avocado, grapefruit, oranges, or berries. For extra flavor, grill fruit or veggies, allow them to cool and then chop them and add them to the salsa.

Salsas can be made ahead of time and stored in the refrigerator for up to two days. Think salsa instead of sauce or gravy for poultry, fish, seafood, beef, pork, vegetable, and grain side dishes, chips or raw vegetables and dessert. Salsa can also be used instead of salad dressing and is a way to sneak yet another serving of vegetables into the meal.

HEALTHY SEGMENTS OF THE MENU

Breakfast

Fried eggs, pancakes, and sausage are not the only items customers are looking for on the breakfast buffet. In the winter, offer assorted hot cereals, baked hash browns or baked white or sweet potatoes, steamed or grilled tofu, steamed or stir-fried white or brown rice, hot baked apples or pears, warm apple sauce, assorted breads for toasting and fresh fruit. Condiments should include margarine (nondairy if possible to meet the needs of vegetarian and lactose-intolerant customers), low-fat cream cheese, nut butters (peanut, almond, pistachio, etc.), fruit preserves (some made without sugar, if possible), ground cinnamon, nutmeg and ginger, dried fruit, wheat germ and chopped nuts. Beverages could include non- and low-fat dairy milks, **veggie milks** (soy, rice, grain, etc.), hot tea and coffee, coffee beverages, such as lattes, hot cocoa, and fruit juices. To heat up the morning, include a veggie chili (with steamed tortillas and fresh salsa).

For the warmer weather, replace hot cereal with cold (have several made without sugar), chilled, cubed tofu, assorted bagels, fresh fruit salad, whole fruit, melon slices, assorted mini-muffins, and cold breakfast burritos (filled with mashed pinto beans, chopped chilies, chopped tomatoes, and chopped cilantro).

If you want to offer tofu on your buffet, purchase firm tofu and let it drain overnight in a colander (this will firm it up even more, so it retains its shape during service). Marinate tofu in a seasoning blend (think: Southwestern, Asian, Mediterranean) of your choice for at least thirty minutes before steaming or grilling. Leftover tofu can be chopped and used in pasta or rice salads, tossed with vegetarian mayo to make an "egg-less" salad, added to stirfries or used in soups.

Grab-and-go beverages are a hot (pun intended) morning item. To ensure you are attracting your health-minded customers, add the following ingredients to your coffee bar: non- and low-fat dairy milks, assorted veggie milks (rice, soy, grain, available in regular and low-fat, vanilla, and chocolate), nutritional yeast (Red Star has a yeast that meets the nutritional needs of vegans), peanut butter, applesauce, dried fruit, bananas, flavor extracts and (if available) soy yogurt. Here are some low fat, high energy beverage ideas: latte with muscle (latte blended with bananas, raisins and dates), chocolate-covered capp (cappuccino blended with cocoa powder, fresh berries and a shot of vanilla extract), banana split (steamed milk blended with banana, strawberry preserves, crushed pineapple and cocoa powder), nutrition 'r'us (steamed milk blended with nutritional yeast, orange juice concentrate, banana and raisins).

One dish (for the customer, not for the cook) morning meals can be served as grab-and-goes or teamed with accompaniments for a larger meal. Scramble firm tofu (just like you would do eggs, on the griddle, in a sauté pan or in the oven) with sautéed veggies and serve on it's own or over steamed rice or hash browns. Breakfast burritos are a good way to utilize leftover beans, potatoes and chopped veggies (even spinach). Wrap them up (check flour tortilla labels to be sure there's no lard around) and steam a bunch off or microwave them individually, as your customer flow dictates. Have salsa, chopped cilantro, chopped tomatoes, chopped chilies and hot sauce available as condiments. Breakfast parfaits can be made a day ahead of time and displayed in a refrigerated area. Using glass or plastic large cups and alternate layers of "creamy," crunchy and soft ingredients. "Creamy" could be soft, mashed tofu (flavor with a little almond extract), soy yogurt, cottage cheese

Slice brown bread (see page 338) or zucchini bread and keep moist on steam table; as accompaniments, have heated, spiced applesauce (think: ginger, cinnamon, nutmeg, mace, clove), heated apple or peach slices, fruit compote (dried fruit that has been stewed with cinnamon sticks and ginger and sweetened with apple juice concentrate).

Offer condiments such as peanut butter, apple butter, flavored margarine (whip-softened margarine with fruit preserves and spices), fruit jams, and marmalades.

Offer fruited yogurt to which people can add wheat germ, chopped nuts or granola. Low-fat cottage or ricotta cheese to which people can add chopped fresh or frozen fruit.

Offer fresh Waldorf salad (try adding chopped dates or pineapple for sweetness).

Figure 11–4 Serving Ideas for Lower-fat Breakfasts

or fruited yogurt. Crunchy could be granola, crushed cold cereal, chopped nuts, trail mix, fruit chips (like apple or banana chips) or wheat germ. Soft ingredients could include fresh seasonal fruit, stewed fruit, and thawed frozen fruit, leftover bread pudding, or leftover fruit cobblers.

Potatoes make a good base for healthy breakfast. Bake off russets and offer topped with sautéed onions, peppers and tomatoes or chopped fresh vegetables and salsa. Use the same toppings for baked hash browns. Steam some new or red-rose potatoes and season with fresh, chopped herbs or roast off some yams, sprinkle with cinnamon and nutmeg and add some margarine. Mashed potatoes can be made with soymilk, topped with salt and pepper and served as a warm morning comfort food. Leftover mashed potatoes can be mixed with breadcrumbs, a little milk, salt and pepper, formed into patties and become morning potato pancakes.

If your healthy morning audience is too small to add many extra items, look at what you already have. You most probably have peanut butter, nuts, dried fruit, fresh, canned and frozen fruit, fruit and vegetable juice, margarine, breads and crackers, tortillas, potatoes and beans. Don't relegate your healthy breakfast customers to dry toast and black coffee in the morning. Capitalize on their needs and increase your breakfast count. You've probably got the makings for a great healthy breakfast staring right at you.

Seasonal

Hot weather dictates refreshing menus. People are trying to slim down or stay that way when it's bathing suit weather. When it's hot and humid, nobody's in the mood for heavy, fatty meals. Eliminating fatty meat and whole-fat dairy products means eliminating fat and heavy-on-the palate menu items.

Grill On!

Nice greasy burgers are good for some customers, but you want to capture the whole audience. You can offer lower fat grilled items that are tempting for everyone. Purchase frozen **veggie burgers** and throw them on the grill. Read the label for fat and salt content before you buy. All veggie burgers are not necessarily made of air! Purchase turkey burgers, boneless chicken fillet, and even buffalo burgers for low-fat burger options. Got some time? Marinate portobello caps in a small amount of oil, minced garlic, chopped onions and cracked pepper and grill until just tender. Prepare your own veggie burgers from combinations of cooked rice or barley, chopped fresh and cooked vegetables, tomato or vegetable juice and spices, bake, cool, and freeze.

Firm tofu can be marinated overnight in Italian dressing, grilled and served hot or cold. For a fat-free marinade try a combination of vinegar, lemon juice, ground oregano, cracked pepper, minced garlic and chopped mushrooms. Try smoked or flavored tofu and seitan served as a grilled vegetarian "steak," paired with corn on the cob, baked beans and a fresh green salad. Make the most of your grill time and toss some vegetable kebobs (button mushrooms, cherry tomatoes, pearl onions, garlic cloves and radishes work well) on the coals to serve with the "steak."

A veggie "steak" sandwich is a new offering at Los Angeles City College. Firm tofu is marinated overnight in barbecue sauce and then marked off on a grill. Served on a cracked wheat burger bun and topped with seasonal salad greens, sliced cucumber and fresh sweet corn (cut, uncooked, from the cob) this sandwich is a top seller for outdoor-catered events and at the student cafeteria. This summer selection is crunchy, tasty and flavorful; customers do not miss the fat and cholesterol.

What's a burger without the sides? Wedge or dice tomatoes, slice onions and cucumbers, shred carrots and beets, chop bell peppers and fresh basil, cilantro and shred green and red cabbage, romaine, and spinach as toppings. Offer tomato or fruit salsa, spiced tomato puree, hot sauce, Tabasco sauce, plain and flavored mustards, and soy sauce as condiments. Soy sauce and chutneys make good veggie burger seasonings, as do barbecue sauce and Worcestershire sauce.

Picnic or box lunches, sandwiches are summer fare. Not too many people want heavy, fatty and salty foods in the hot weather. While the barbecue or grill is hot, toss thinly sliced, marinated eggplant, carrots and summer squash (sliced lengthwise), sliced bell peppers, wedged red and white onions and mushrooms and cook until tender. Chill until ready to use. Marinate tomatoes, cucumbers, green and wax beans, and mushrooms in vinegar, dried herbs and chopped onions. Chop lettuce, radishes, green and black olives and pickles, rinse alfalfa and soy bean sprouts, drain and rinse canned black, kidney, red, and garbanzo beans; open some salsa and mix up some **humus** and you're ready to assemble cool sandwiches.

Stuff whole-wheat and plain pita with grilled veggies, radishes, humus, olives and sprouts. Wrap flour, tomato and blue corn tortillas with marinated veggies, beans, lettuce and salsa. Try wrapping with cracker bread, spring roll wrappers, and soft pizza crust. Instead of a veggie burger, top a burger bun with grilled veggies, pickles, and salsa. Create a summer sub with grilled and marinated vegetables, dried herbs and salad greens on a crusty baguette or in a demi-loaf of walnut–green onion or black olive–sun dried tomato.

Green salads are cool, crisp and receptive to change! Build a basic salad with head and leaf lettuce, baby greens, endive, radicchio, and cabbage, and then go beyond.

As an Entrée, Add:

Cold black, white, kidney, lentil and red beans
Smoked, barbecued or grilled tofu
Sliced fake deli meats
Grilled Eggplant
Bean and salsa combinations
Humus and olive combinations
Grilled or marinated mushrooms
Cold ravioli, tortellini and gnocchi
Chopped walnuts, pistachios, pinenuts and cashews
Cold lentils tossed with mushrooms and tomatoes
Baked or grilled tofu

As Side Dish:

Green and wax beans
Cut corn
Chopped onions, radishes, tomatoes, garlic, olives
Shredded carrots, beets, zucchini, crookneck squash
Chopped pickled vegetables
Sliced marinated or fresh mushrooms
Chopped nuts, such as walnuts, peanuts, cashews, pumpkin and sesame seeds

Figure 11–5 Dress Up That Green Salad

Some people order entrée salads because they truly like them and some order them to be virtuous. You offer entrée salads because they're good for the customer and good for sales. Entrée salads can start with cold rice, pasta and grains (such as barley or kasha). Prepare and set aside cold ingredients to have available for assembly. Toss cold rice or pasta with chopped olives, celery, green onions, tomatoes, minced carrot and garbanzo or black beans, top with chopped nuts (think pine nuts, almonds and pumpkin seeds), croutons, and shredded herbs (think basil, oregano and rosemary) and dress with oil and vinegar or a tomato and herb dressing.

Couscous can be served cold, tossed with basil, chopped mushrooms and tomatoes or with chopped green, red and yellow peppers, minced garlic, and onions. Try a sweet, cold couscous, tossing it with fresh blueberries, shredded fresh mint, and pinenuts. These combinations also work well with cold, cooked barley and with small pasta, such as **orzo** or pastina.

Utilize extra portions of cold spaghetti, pasta sauce, black olives, sliced mushrooms, oregano and chopped canned tomatoes. Pair with a green salad and sliced baguette. **Tortellini** or ravioli work well with this combination.

Desserts

Everyone likes to end even a quick meal with something sweet. You can bring in the bucks if everyone orders dessert to complete their meal. Along with the ooey-gooey double chocolate creations, offer lower calorie selections. Then no one will have an excuse to skip dessert.

Fresh berries, served chilled on their own or with sorbets are easy and fast to assemble. Pair strawberries with orange sorbet, blueberries or raspberries with lemon or strawberry sorbet. If you have extra berries, puree them with a small amount of orange juice or apple juice concentrate and use as a dessert sauce.

Melon can be sliced, wedged or balled, served chilled on its own, soaked in white wine or sprinkled with fresh orange or lemon zest. Serve a trio of melon slices studded with a chiffonade of fresh mint or sprinkled with berries. Create your own honeydew or watermelon sorbet by pureeing melon with a small amount of fruit juice concentrate or fruit liqueur and freezing in individual serving dishes.

Frost grapes, strawberries or melon balls. Moisten grapes with water or apple juice before freezing; berries and melons have sufficient natural moisture. Simply place fruit, single layer on a baking sheet (use parchment paper), and allow to cool in the freezer until frosty but not frozen. Serve as soon as removed from the freezer.

Fresh peaches, plums and apricots can be cut and sprinkled with orange zest and orange juice concentrate and allowed to marinate overnight in the refrigerator. Serve garnished with raisins and nuts or use as part of a sorbet sundae. If there's room on the grill, wrap peach or apricot halves seasoned with cinnamon and ginger in foil, and allow to cook until just tender. Use as a "fire and ice" dessert with sorbet or soy ice cream.

Take advantage of the great flavors and appearance of summer ingredients to create lighter menus.

Fast Food

Fast food is a way of life. Every age group seems to have bought into the idea of food prepared and served quickly, and if it can be consumed while driving a car and speaking on a cell-phone, even better! Lower in fat and calories, even better yet!

If you are serving fast food, you'll have to make a decision whether to make the products from scratch or to purchase them already made. Making items from scratch will involve more labor, but will give more control over the product design; **Ready-to-use (RTU) products** require less labor and have a consistent quality, but are more expensive to purchase. You may decide to go one way or another or use a combination of both types.

Even if you prefer to make everything you serve from scratch, some products are simply easier to purchase. Soy or tofu hot dogs come to mind. While it certainly is possible to make your own vegan sausage, it is a time-consuming process and requires a certain amount of skill and equipment. Depending on the volume you sell, marinated or spicy "fake meats," usually seitan or tempeh, may also be easier to purchase than to prepare yourself. For example, Nasoya, a division of Vitasoy, has recently released a chilled baked tofu product, available in Tex Mex, mesquite, Thai peanut, and teriyaki flavors. Just slice them to use as the filling in a cold sandwich or grill them for a hot one. Visit *www.vitasoy-usa.com* for information. Read the labels to guarantee that your vegetarian fast-food items are low in fat and salt.

As we've mentioned, the ever-popular vegetarian burger is always a good sell. We have seen RTU burgers made from every conceivable ingredient—textured soy, seitan, okara (a soy byproduct of tofu production that resembles cottage cheese), beans, corn, mushrooms, grains, potatoes, and whole-grain flour. You will need to do some tastings to see which product your customers will best accept. Many of the RTU veggie burgers must be fried for an acceptable texture so take this into consideration when choosing. Other points to consider are: Do the burgers hold up when held in heating equipment of any length of time, will the supplier be able to fill orders in the amounts needed, and are the salt and/or spices at a level acceptable to the customer?

Ethnic foods are quite popular as fast food items. Pizza and pasta, **falafel** and stir-fries are easily made lower fat. Fresh or frozen pizza shells can be made into a quick meal. Top shells with tomato sauce (straight from the can or seasoned with tomato puree, fresh or dried basil and oregano, chopped tomatoes, onions and peppers, etc.) and offer ingredients such as sliced mushrooms, peppers, onions and garlic, spicy sprouts (try radish or broccoli sprouts), broccoli or cauliflower florets, shredded carrots, capers (the pickled plant, not the fish), artichoke hearts, chopped tomatoes, seasoned tofu, veggie crumbles, and for the more adventurous—diced pineapple. For variety, make individual calzone (stuffed pizza crust resembling a pizza crust turnover) with the same ingredients; an advantage of a calzone is that it can be premade, frozen (uncooked or cooked) and then heated as needed.

Pasta can be a fast meal that is easy to grab and eat on the go. Offer pasta with several types of sauce or offer combination pasta platters, with bread sticks and tossed salads as side dishes. If you have the time, prepare your own pasta dishes (lasagna, stuffed shells filled with seasoned tofu or mashed beans, veggie balls), freeze and heat as needed. Tomato and pesto sauce can be made without too much fat. Several types of cheese are available in skim-milk versions. You can use whole fat cheeses, just keep the amount limited.

Falafel (ground chickpea patties) can be purchased frozen and ready to cook, as a dry mix or can be made from scratch. Depending on the product, falafel can be fried or baked- test before deciding on a purchase. Offer falafel in pita bread, as a sandwich or as a combination platter, with tabbouli (a sprouted wheat and parsley salad, available as a mix or made from scratch), chopped fresh and pickled salad and hummus. Hummus is a pureed chickpea, garlic and lemon juice spread, which can be spiced with cumin, pepper, and turmeric—or experiment! We've seen Southwestern hummus (with jalapenos and cilantro) and Asian hummus (with soy sauce and sesame seeds). Hummus can be purchased RTU (ready to use) or can be made from scratch.

If you would like to do fast food stir-fries, you will have to consider the equipment necessary to do it. Electric woks can be used without making any modifications, but gas-fired woks benefit from specialty gas fittings which bring in more heat (use your local utility companies as resources when researching this). If equipment is an issue, consider offering steamed noodle or rice bowls, rather than stir-frys. Stir-fries are quick to make, but, depending on the style of ingredients purchased, the pre-preparation can take a lot of time. Consider your costs to see if you can purchase precut vegetables, marinated tofu, etc.

When designing Asian fast-food menus, take some time to educate yourself about the wide variety of noodles available, both dry and RTU. Exclude the products made with eggs and include wheat, rice, lentil, and bean noodles in every width and length. Noodles topped with steamed, seasoned veggies and tofu or seitan strips makes a great fast food. Rice (try brown, jasmine, wild, basmanti, glutinous) can be topped in the same way.

A discussion of fast food would not be complete without mentioning French fries. Once again, you can buy them frozen, RTU in many shapes, sizes and flavors. Be sure to read labels, as some commercial fries use animal fat, which translates into cholesterol, as an ingredient in the coating. We have seen skin-on, skin-off, wedges, rippled, basket weave, thin- and thick-cut with a variety of seasonings. We have seen sweet potato and eggplant fries and, that cousin to French fries, tempura-style veggies. Tempura batter mix can be purchased or you can make your own with rice flour, spices and water. Select the type of French fry that can be baked rather than deep-fried. While you've got the oven on, throw in some baker potatoes and offer hot baked potatoes for a fast meal.

Depending on the season and on your clientele, you may want to offer soups-to-go and other easily packaged and eaten foods, such as baked beans or cold salads (think potato or pasta). Remember, with fast food, think about eating your menu items while driving in the car or perched on a park bench—a fact of life in our society.

What's life without dessert? Fast-food desserts can be convenience items, such as rice or soy ice cream novelties (we've seen sundaes and sandwiches), scooped sorbet, fruit ices, popsicles, and whole fruit or fruit salad.

Fries, veggie burgers, and soy dogs do not stand on their own. They need condiments! Depending on your property, these may be single-serve or large dispensers of ketchup, mustard and pickle relish (you can purchase or make veggie mayo) or you may offer more exotic flavors. Add some salsa (available RTU or made from scratch), gardiniera (pickled vegetables), chutneys, flavored mustards, satay (Thai peanut sauce), kimchi (marinated, aged, spicy cabbage, available commercially or you can make your own), sauerkraut, soy sauce, tapenade (olive spread), hummus and sliced veggies if your cost will support it and your customers will use it. Sliced tomatoes, shredded carrots, sliced cucumbers and different types of lettuce add color and crunch to the grab-and-go meal. Accessories sometimes perfect the dish!

Catering

Culinary elegance is universal and healthy and vegetarian catering is becoming more and more popular. Leaving out the meat and the fat doesn't mean leaving out the finesse.

Catering for elegant occasions requires the correct ambiance. Go for simplicity with a grilled portobello fillet or for bounty with a grand grain-tasting menu.

Vegetarian entrees can include a center-of-the-plate attraction, such as a seared tofu steak in a cabernet au jus or a vegetable cutlet with a lemon-caper sauce. If dairy products are acceptable, fettucini Alfredo or a four-fromage quiche are simple to prepare and gorgeous when served.

If several small items are preferable to the traditional entrée and two sides, try a spicy vegetable, a more subtle vegetable, a crunchy grain and a soft finish. Spicy Moroccan eggplant or chicken with roasted herbed carrots, couscous with onions and garlic and sautéed mushrooms come together for visual and palate appeal. More ideas: ratatouille (eggplant and summer squash stew with tomatoes, olive oil, olives, parsley, and garlic); rosemary mashed potatoes; spicy green beans and roasted corn; mushroom and barley pilaf; sautéed bell peppers (try at least three different colors); jasmine rice and petite pois (baby green peas); spinach fettucini (served as individual baskets) topped with fresh tomato sauce and basil; wilted greens with garlic and crisp carrot and cabbage sauté.

For make-ahead elegance, prepare crepe skins or purchase premade crepes. Stuff with chopped, grilled seasoned vegetables and freeze, unsauced. When ready to use, place frozen on a baking sheet, sauce and reheat and serve. Lasagna, stuffed shells, and manicotti made with low-fat cheeses or tofu can make a beautiful plate and hold up well to freezing. Stuff tomatoes or sweet onions with herbed grains, smoked fish turkey or tofu, sautéed mushrooms and nuts, such as almonds or pistachios. Cook them off and freeze until ready to use. For vegans, use soy-based cheese or pureed tofu in place of sliced cheese or soft cheese (such as ricotta).

Accompaniment dishes add the color and texture to the plate as well as complimenting the entrée. Fresh seasonal vegetables, such as asparagus, broccoli florets, baby carrots and summer squash, lightly steamed and herbed require little handling while offering lots of class to the plate. Grains and rice can be steamed into pilafs, shaped into timbales (small drum shapes) or sautéed with fresh or dried herbs. Potatoes, white or sweet, can be pureed or whipped with complementary seasonings, piped as a Duchesse, browned as an au gratin or oven-roasted. Rice, brown, jasmine, basmanti or wild, can be used as a bed for an entrée or tossed with herbs or nuts to stand on their own. Pasta can be sauced, tossed with sautéed vegetables or also used as a bed to carry an entrée.

Accompaniment dishes don't always have to be hot. Chill and toss wilted spinach or kale with chopped onions, olive oil and vinegar; grill root vegetables with an Asian marinade and chill for a crunchy side dish. Fresh fruit medleys are a complement to every type of entrée, especially when the textures are assorted, as in a pineapple-mango-orange-apple medley.

Continue the healthy black-tie affair with dessert. Offer a trio of sorbets garnished with fresh berries or topped with a simple tuile cookie. Bread pudding can put on a tuxedo with specialty sauces, such as a brandy-ginger sauce or a fresh apricot and strawberry coulis. Poach pears in wine or syrup and serve with a sorbet, chocolate sauce, or with a sprig of fresh mint. Tropical sundaes can be made with sorbet or frozen soy or rice dessert topped with chopped papaya, mango, and shredded coconut create a cool ending.

Although not a culinary topic, edible centerpieces are dramatic and aromatic ways to decorate tables. Try bouquets of herbs (think of the aroma of fresh basil, lavender and rosemary) carved fruit and vegetable arrangements and edible flower bowls. This style of centerpiece will add a simple elegance to your table and will prime your customers for dinner!

Here are some suggestions for elegant and healthy dinner menus:

Chilled gazpacho with fresh breadsticks
Grilled portobello steak with rosemary jus lie
Garlic mashed potatoes
Asparagus spears with balsamic glaze
Poached Bosc pear with ginger sorbet

or

Baby greens salad with pine nut vinaigrette
Baked tofu steak with mango chutney and tomato accents
Basmanti rice pilaf
Baby carrots and baby beets with lemon sauce
Citrus sorbet with fresh berries

or

Puree of black bean soup, Cuban style
Grilled ahi with risotto with trio of mushrooms
Ratatouille
Wilted Swiss chard with sesame dressing
Lemon tart with raspberry coulis

EQUIPPING THE NUTRITION KITCHEN

We've talked a lot about individual fresh ingredient selection and preparing healthy foods from scratch. Very few kitchens today have the luxury of preparing every item from scratch. Labor costs, seasonality, time, and the need for larger menus with more selections force food service managers to choose which items will be made from scratch and which will be purchased ready-to-use.

There are no absolutes when it comes to making the from-scratch or convenience decision. You have to take a look at your budget, your food preparation and storage space and the skill of your staff; in addition, you'll want to make a quality comparison to make your decision.

For example, you need several low-fat salad dressings. You don't have much call for them, but would like to have them available for the customers that request them. Your food purveyor has several very good-tasting, low-fat salad dressings that come packed in one-gallon jars. Your chef can whip up several different types of low-fat salad dressing, such as a balsamic-garlic and yogurt-cucumber, in the quantities needed when they are needed. The commercial salad dressing is cheaper per ounce, but comes packed in such a large size, it will have to be discarded before it can be used. Your chef's dressing is a little bit more costly per ounce, but it can be made in useable quantities with no waste.

What's your decision? We would suggest the chef-made dressing. In the long run, the cost will be less. In addition to eliminating waste, a "homemade" salad dressing will have customer appeal.

You decide to use tofu as a base for nondairy smoothies and cheesecakes, frozen desserts, and salad dressings. Your chef tells you that you can

A NUTRI-BAR

The Girl Scouts Do Sushi

When you are thinking about "going healthy" you need to get everyone into the act. The more ownership there is, the more people will buy into new menu items. Sodhexo Marriott is a contract food service company with many school accounts. The company food service directors and chefs look to provide interesting and nutritious menus for the student population. Students in the Palo Alto (California) School District asked Sodhexo to offer more vegetarian options and healthier options. A local Girl Scout troop was asked to survey students to find out the types of foods that would be appealing. One of the most popular requests was for vegetarian sushi.

The District's food-service director located a supplier and set up a tasting. The Girl Scouts loved the sushi and took responsibility for publicizing it in the schools. They made banners and signs, started a phone campaign and made announcements over the schools' PA systems.

The following items were introduced and accepted: vegetarian avocado rolls, cucumber rolls, carrot rolls and pickled radish rolls. California rolls, with imitation crab, were the only non-vegetarian item. To comply with HACCP regulations, no raw protein ingredients were used. Sushi has become so successful in the primary, junior, and senior high schools that a separate "sushi line" has had to be added to most cafeteria serveries. At the college level, Sohexo Marriott has introduced an entirely vegan menu. Boston College and the University of Vermont tested menu items such as mushroom risotto cakes, Turkish grilled eggplant sandwiches, mushroom walnut tofu burgers, and grilled herbed polenta. The menu has been a big success with both vegetarian and non-vegetarian students.

purchase equipment to make your own tofu. You know that you can easily purchase tofu.

After tasting a sample of "homemade" tofu versus commercial tofu, you can't tell the difference. The homemade tofu will require the purchase of equipment, additional labor hours, time and food safety concerns. Commercial tofu is readily available, inexpensive, and has a good flavor and texture. What would you do?

There are many healthy items that can be prepared or purchased. Salad dressings, sauces, stocks, gravies, condiments like low-salt soy sauce or no-sugar ketchup, dessert items, dairy products, and cereals are available in low-fat, low-salt, no-sugar and no-cholesterol variations. Low-fat mayonnaise might be hard to quickly whip up, but low-salt stock might be easy to make and inexpensive. Veggie burgers might be more convenient to purchase, and frozen and low fat marinara sauce very easy to prepare.

Make decisions about healthy items just as you would any food item. Can I make a profit after purchasing this product? Can the kitchen make a

Topic	*Information*
Contributors/credentials	Are there health-care professionals, registered dietitians, chefs, or recognized authorities contributing to the site?
Claims	Are claims based on scientific findings, such as found in respected journals? What guidelines are used to analyze menus or recipes?
Promises	Is the site promoting healthy eating or "lose bazillion pounds by eating carrots"? Does the site explain how to incorporate all types of food into a healthy diet?
Cost	If a fee is charged, what is covered? Do free sites provide the same type of information. How commercial is the site?
Contact	Is there a customer service e-mail address or phone number if you have further questions?
Links	Are there links to reputable sites, such as the USDA databank?
Updates	Are there regular updates and postings?
Options	Is there versatility in menu and recipe planning?

Phrases that do not lend credibility: "Outstanding," "Named best of . . . .," "In the top ten," "Nine out of ten doctors, nurses, etc." given by non-nutrition or nonscientific organization.

Backing that does not lend credibility: free offers, celebrity endorsements, number of users (or hits) or endorsement by users, company endorsements, flashy graphics, streaming videos, music, etc.

Figure 11–6 Evaluating Web Sites

quality product or will the quality be more consistent if I purchase the item? Does my staff have the time and the equipment. And, most importantly, which one will the customer enjoy the most?

EVALUATING WEB SITES FOR NUTRITION INFORMATION

In this plugged in age, you may want to use the Web to assist you with menu planning. You'll need to evaluate sites to be sure they are credible and convey reliable information. The Web can be a font of information or misinformation, depending on the sites you choose. We'll run you through an analysis of two Web sites to show you what we mean.

Web site 1: www.diets.com Developed by registered dietitians and an eating disorder specialist. It costs $25 to 30 for a three-month membership and a $15 registration fee. Nutrition information is based on the U.S. Food Guide Pyramid. The site has assessment, links, resources, and chat rooms. Menus are calculated by a computerized program, so there is not a great deal opportunity to customize your menus. There is a customer service line, but you are not speaking with nutritionists. Very commercial site, promoting lots of products.

Web site 2: www.dietsite.com Also developed by registered dietitians, this site is free. Menu and recipe analysis is based on the Food Guide Pyramid. Access to information is easy. There is information on regular nutrition, sports nutrition and nutrition for people with medical conditions. There are links and chat rooms. The site is geared to adult nutrition for healthy menu planning. Sources have credible references. Pages are hard to print.

Looking at nutrition or health-based Web sites in this way will help you in selecting material from people who are committed to communicating reasonable information.

SWAPPING INGREDIENTS

If you want to cook healthy, you need the tools. You'll have to write a menu first and then you can decide on what you need. Of course, a good chef can do anything with a knife and cutting board, a stove top and an oven. If you'd like to have all the toys, you can purchase some kitchen equipment that will make life easier and healthy cooking a fast deal. We asked some chefs who were into healthy cooking what they would stock their dream nutrition kitchen with. Here are several of their answers:

Steamers: come in all shapes and sizes, from a pot with a rack and a tightly fitting lid to a $10,000 pressure-less model, steamers run the gamut of bells and whistles. Decide on what you'll be cooking in it and what type of capacity you'll need. Beyond veggies, you can steam potatoes, fish, poultry, rice, eggs and pasta in a steamer.

Instead of:	*Try:*
Mayonnaise	Yogurt, blended tofu
Whole eggs	Egg whites, vegan egg replacer, fruit purees
Frying	Sauteeting, braising, stewing, poaching, grilling
Bacon	Ham, Canadian bacon, smoked turkey
Cream	Yogurt, whipped low-fat milk
Butter (for baking)	Cream cheese, peanut butter
White sugar	Fruit-juice concentrates, pureed dried fruit

Figure 11–7 This Instead of That

Instead of:	*Try:*
8 ounces ricotta cheese	8 ounces mashed firm tofu or 5 ounces okara
8 ounces milk	8 ounces soy or rice milk
8 ounces yogurt	8 ounces blended silken tofu or soy yogurt
1 large egg	2 Tablespoons blended firm tofu
1 ounce baking chocolate (has dairy)	3 ounces unsweetened cocoa powder and 1 Tablespoon soy oil
1 pound ground beef (for burritos, meat sauce, etc.)	1 pound diced firm tofu, 12 ounces crumbled seitan or tempeh (marinate for extra flavor before cooking)

Tempeh: marinate in Italian dressing or barbecue sauce and grill or dice and mix into soups or chilies, slice and grill and serve as a "tempeh"dip sandwich

Soy milk: use in place of regular milk in puddings, custards and sauces, make hot chocolate or coffee beverages, use in soups

Soy crumbles: sauté, bake or grill with fresh or dry herbs and use as pizza toppings, in chili, in ""beef" and mac casseroles or "meat" sauces, in tacos, with tofu as a "morning scramble"

Soft tofu: use instead of ricotta cheese in stuffed shells and lasagna, make fruit smoothies, use in salad dressings, scramble instead of eggs (remember to season with pepper, hot sauce sautéed veggies, etc.)

Silken tofu: use instead of mayo or sour cream in recipes, use to make pudding, pie fillings or custard, smooth out sauces (tofu Alfredo or primavera) or soups and make a frosting by blending a small amount of tofu with instant pudding mix

Firm tofu: add to brochettes instead of meat, use in stir fries, cut in cubes to make an egg-less or chicken-less salad (toss with celery, onions, pickles, regular, or vegetarian mayo), grill, roast (use the same seasonings as you do for meat) or bake with bread stuffing

Figure 11–8 Soy Instead

Blender and/or food professor: in the good old days, chefs pureed foods by cooking them until they were soft and then forcing them through a chinois or cranking them through a hand-held food mill. Blenders or food processors allow today's chef to preserve some of the nutrients in foods, as you don't have to cook them down to a pulp before processing them. They certainly save time and work. You can whip nonfat milk, blend veggies or berries for sauces, chop nuts and grate cheese (so you use less) with blenders and food processors, along with pureeing soups for "creamier" textures.

Cheesecloth: to get a firm texture from yogurt or tofu, you need to drain them. This is best done through cheesecloth. In both the nutrition and the culinary kitchen, cheesecloth is used to tie up herbs and spices to flavor stocks, stews, soups and broths (no one want to bite down on a whole peppercorn) and to strain liquids to remove fat.

Salad spinner: crisp is good. If you're going to eat a salad, you want the veggies to be crisp and dry.

Smoker: although the American Cancer Society frowns on smoked foods, smoking is a way to cut down on fats while adding flavor and texture to foods.

Grill or barbecue: If you want the fat to drip away in a flavorful way, then grilling or barbecuing could be a good choice. In addition to meat, poultry and fish, vegetables, potatoes, and fruit can be grilled for extra flavor and texture.

Everybody would like to eat whatever they want without suffering any health consequences. It would be nice if food professionals had magic wands and could take all the sugar out of chocolate cake and all the fat out of prime rib.

We may not be able to do that, but we can offer many menu items that taste good without so much of the "bad stuff." For example, you can replace some of the fat in baking recipes with fruit purees. The cakes and muffins come out moist, tender and fluffy. An acceptable swap.

A portobello mushroom cap can be marinated and grilled and slapped on a bun. Customers looking to reduce their fat or animal product intake will enjoy the swap. Salsa can be served as an alternate to some sauces, gravies or salad dressings. Foods can be stir fried or sautéed rather than deep-fried. There are many times when health and taste can get along very well.

There are sometimes when substitutes or swaps will not produce a desirable outcome. As a food professional, you need to be knowledgeable enough to know where to draw the line. Customers will not thank you for preparing a low fat or low salt dish if it is tasteless and colorless. Be prepared to offer alternates, rather than substitutes.

For example, a customer pleads with you to prepare a low-fat, low-salt eggs Benedict. As you know, eggs Benedict is a poached egg served on a toasted English muffin with a slice of Canadian bacon, topped with Hollandaise sauce (made with egg yolks and butter).

So, what have you got to work with? The English muffin is both low-fat and low-salt. The poached egg has some fat, but should be allowable. The Canadian bacon is lower in fat than bacon, but it is not exactly lean. The salt content is really up there. The Hollandaise sauce is a cardiologist's delight. Could you create a Hollandaise with margarine or oil and egg substitute? You could probably make something that looked like Hollandaise but tasted like *Blecch!* So, what are your options?

If the customer wants something like an eggs Benedict with no fat and no salt, that would be very difficult to do. If the customer is willing to work with you, you could offer an eggs Florentine, which is a poached egg served on a bed of savory spinach, topped with Hollandaise. This would be very low salt.

If you just tickled the egg with the Hollandaise, then you would be appreciably cutting back on the fat. To cut back on the salt, you could remove the Canadian bacon from a traditional eggs Benedict and replace it with a very small piece of grilled salmon. There'd still be lots of fat, but very little salt. Or you could scrap the whole eggs Benedict idea and offer the customer something special, something tasty and good looking, like an eggs Florentine (if you really wanted to get crazy, you could poach just the egg whites) with a grilled salmon fillet, served with roasted mango salsa. See how you have to play with your food to get that correct combination of health and good food?

When you are looking on your menu to see which items you can modify as healthy options, keep in mind that the customers want to enjoy their meal. Even though they say that they want fewer calories, less fat, less salt or less cholesterol, they still want to eat. They want to see a plate with a reasonable amount of food on it, want to bite into a big sandwich. Some foods can be modified and still be interesting, and some cannot.

For example, take a club sandwich. Three slices of bread, bacon, turkey, tomato, lettuce, mayonnaise. The fat in the sandwich comes from the bacon and the mayo. You could offer an avocado club, switching the bacon and the avocado. You'd have the same amount of fat calories, but they'd come from unsaturated fat rather than saturated fat (translation: try our "no cholesterol" club) and would be lower in salt. Or you could swap bacon for sliced ham, which is lower in fat.

Eggs are easy. When you are baking, experiment to see if you can leave out some egg yolks and use fruit purees or concentrates, vegetable oils or mashed bananas. This will work in items like chocolate cake, brownies, carrot cake and less delicate baked goods. Won't work for angel food cake. Of course, you could do angel food cake or meringues for low-fat bakery items, since they only use egg whites. Low-fat, not low-calorie. Egg white omelets are gaining in popularity, as is baked French toast. A little less fat and still enjoyable.

Two very easy ways to cut down on calories work well for the kitchen budget. Pare down portions and serve gravies, sauces and salad dressings on the side. Offer "petit" steaks so those people who would like a little red meat still have an option. Price your "petit" to include labor, service, etc. You can make a decent profit on smaller items. When you serve sauce on the side, both the kitchen and the customer tend to use less.

Chefs are not the only ones "swapping" ingredients. Food scientists and technologists have been thinking up ways for years to make foods taste creamier or sweeter without the calories. We've discussed sugar and fat substitutes in Chapters 3 and 4. If you'd like to delve more deeply into the world of food additives, you might want to research the Institute of Food Technologists Web site, *www.ift.org* or the Research Chefs Association, *www.rca.org*. There you can find out about using mannitol or maltodextrins to give baked goods the mouthfeel of butter and fat without the butter and fat. Or how about a little agar gum or carageenan to smooth out a sauce without any fat? Hydrolyzed yeast can replace some of the salt in food products and powdered whey can give a creamy taste without the cream.

Healthy menus are easy to do, with a little addition here, a little cut there. Take a reasonable approach, remembering that you don't want to purchase a lot of fancy ingredients. And remember, if you wouldn't eat it yourself, don't serve it to your customers.

FYI: SOY SPEAK

Soy is in, it's hot, it's healthy and your customers want it *now!* At a recent seminar, sponsored by Protein Technologies International, over five-hundred nutritionists, food service people, chefs and health professionals sampled such soy items as Texas barbecue soy nuggets, soy-fortified pancakes, and tofu smoothies. Dubbed the "human bean," soy is appearing on more and more menus as a meat and dairy alternate.

What's the buzz? Although still high in fat (unless you select a low fat soymilk or tofu), soy products are very low in saturated fats. Soy's proteins and isoflavones (natural plant estrogens) are thought to reduce cholesterol, reduce the risk of heart disease and ease symptoms of menopause. Conveniently, The United States is one of the world's largest growers of soybeans (although close to 75 percent of the crop is exported or used for animal feed).

Tofu is probably the most familiar soy product. Nothing more than coagulated soymilk (think: cheese making), tofu is available in different firmness and flavors. Silken tofu is custard-like and can be the "cream" in pies, soups, custards and sauces. Soft tofu blends well and can be used instead of dairy in smoothies, salad dressings and dips. Firm and extra firm tofu are toughies and can be marinated, chopped, diced sautéed, baked. . . you get the idea.

Tofu has a neutral flavor so it will take on whatever personality you give it. Marinate tofu in fresh or dried herbs, salad dressings, vinegars, barbecue sauce, chili sauce, etc. If you need a really firm tofu, such as for grilling or roasting, you can drain blocks of tofu. Place tofu between weights, like several china dinner plates, and allow to drain for several hours. This will condense and compress the tofu and works well for tofu "steaks," fajita strips, and barbecued tofu sandwiches.

There are commercially available flavored tofus, both sweet and savory. Try almond-flavored tofu for dessert items, and barbecue, Southwestern, Mediterranean and Asian flavored for entrées.

Freezing is okay for tofu and makes it chewier in texture. Drain tofu and slice before freezing. To use frozen tofu, let it thaw in the refrigerator, squeeze out excess fluid and marinate or cook.

Soymilk is available in several flavors and fat levels. Soymilk is naturally high in protein but low in calcium, vitamins A, D, and B_{12}. If nutrition is a concern, look for fortified brands. We have seen vanilla, almond, mocha, and chocolate soymilk available in individual and food service packs.

Beyond Tofu

There is life beyond tofu. Tempeh is a firm cake of pressed, fermented soybeans, sometimes mixed with grains, such as rice or wheat. Tempeh's mild, smoky flavor and chewy texture works well in chili, casseroles, stir frys and hot sandwiches. Tempeh is sold in blocks and is usually available in various flavors. In terms of food safety, treat tofu and tempeh like meat.

Soy nuts are roasted soybeans and have a nutty, peanut flavor. Use them in Thai dishes, as salad toppings and as an ingredient in baking and trial mixes. Fresh soy beans, called "edamame," can be quickly steamed and eaten as a bar snack, tossed onto salads or served as a vegetable with an entrée.

Soy cheese and yogurt can be used just like their dairy cousins. Soy cheese is available in various types, such as mozzarella and cheddar. Soy yogurt is generally available as a sweetened, fruit flavored product. Use it as is, in sauces or freeze it for a fast dessert. Frozen soy milk (also rice milk) is the soy equivalent of ice cream and is available in many flavors and forms (sandwiches, popsicles, etc.).

Meat analogs, such as tofu dogs, burgers, crumbles, breakfast strips, and "fake" sandwich meat are generally made from soy protein and are designed to mimic their animal counterparts. Experiment with different brands to find the type that have the flavor and texture acceptable for your customers. For example, several brands of soy burgers must be fried to be palatable, which may defeat the purpose of your healthy offerings.

Care and Feeding

HACCP is in effect for all soy products. Except for aseptically packaged products (tofu and soymilk is available in this), all soy products must be kept refrigerated until used and have use-by dates to which you must adhere. Once opened, all soy products must be handled just like meat or eggs. Avoid time-temperature abuse, cross-contamination, multiple re-heating of left overs, etc.

Tofu, tempeh, soymilk and seitan (a wheat product) can be frozen. They must be thawed in the refrigerator. The tofu, tempeh and seitan will be tougher when thawed and the soymilk will be watery. Plan on using thawed products as ingredients rather than as stand-alone items.

All soy products are available in organic or standard forms and may be fortified or not. The products used to process them may differ. For example, some tofu is processed with calcium, some with nigari (a sea vegetable). Save the labels, as some of your customers may request this information.

The Meat of the Wheat

Although not a soy product, seitan is a popular vegetarian meat substitute. Originally processed by Buddhist monks, seitan is in wide national and international production. Seitan is compressed, fermented gluten (wheat protein). It is available in blocks, strips and crumbles and can be frozen until ready to use. Seitan is perishable, so all the HACCP guidelines apply.

Seitan has a very firm texture and will hold up to poaching, roasting, grilling and baking. Serve it as a "steak" (marinated in lemon or limejuice, garlic, and onions) or add it where you would use beef or chicken strips. There are commercially available meat analogs made with seitan, some in the shape of roasts, which can be flavored and served just like roast beef.

Soy products have been around for the last two thousand years or so—definitely not a fad! Incorporate them into your menus for health and interest.

Nutri-Words

Commodity foods: foods made available through the USDA, obtained from farm surplus crops.
Couscous: pasta that resembles grains of sand, often made from semolina flour.
Falafel: fried or baked patties made from garbanzo beans.
Humus: a Mediterranean-influenced vegetable or bread dip based in garbanzo beans and flavored with sesame paste, lemon and garlic.
Orzo: pasta formed in the shape of large rice kernels.
Portobello: a type of mushroom with a large cap. Can be used to replace meat in some recipes.
Ready to Use (RTU) products: convenience products that are fully or partially prepared, requiring little or no preparation.
Sorbet: a frozen menu item used as an intermezzo or dessert made of fruit pulp or fruit juice.
Tortellini: small pasta pieces stuffed with vegetables, cheese, meat, nuts or grain.
Veggie burgers: RTU products made from non-animal ingredients, served in place of beef, seafood, or poultry burgers.
Veggie milks (soy, rice, oat): milks made from plant, rather than animal, sources.

Whaddaya Think?

1. What's the culinarian's incentive to add nutrition to the menu?
2. What do you think about Chef Gielisse's "cuisine actuelle"? Do you think chefs should get involved in this sort of thing?
3. What type of healthy promotion would you have at your restaurant?
4. If you had sufficient budget, suggest a healthy food product you would market.

PRODUCTS

HINOICHI Foods America Corporation 7351 Orangewood Avenue Garden Grove, CA 92841	(producers of tofu)
TOFUTTI Brands, Inc. 50 Jackson Drive Cranford, NJ 07016 908-272-2400	(producers of soy-based frozen desserts, filled pasta and cookies)
Vegi-D'Lite and hot'n'spicy tofu) 4332 Cadena Circle Yorba Linda, CA 92886 714-996-5889	(manufacturers of tofu specialty products, such as hickory smoke
Vitasoy USA, Inc. 400 Oyster Point Blvd. Ste. 201 So. San Francisco, CA 94080 650-583-9888	(producer of soy milk, Tofu mate and Vegiburgers)
Eden Foods, Inc. 701 Tecumseh Road Clinton, MI 49236 517-456-7424 *edeninfo@eden-foods.com*	(producers of soy milk and drinks, miso, tofu products, soy sauce)
Ener-G Foods, Inc. 5960 First Street, South Seattle, WA 98124 800-331-5222 *www.ener-g.com*	(producers of soy drinks and vegan egg replacer)
Lightlife Foods PO Box 870 Greenfield, MA 10302 413-774-6001 *www.lightlife.com*	(producers of tofu dogs and sausage, tofu meat analogs, tofu burgers, tofu tacos, etc)
White Wave, Inc. beverages) 1990 N. 57th Street Boulder, CO 80301 303-443-3470 *www.whitewave.com*	(producers of soy cheese and yogurt, tempeh, tofu products, soy

Figure 11–9 Soy Resources

5. How about a root vegetable soup that no one can resist? Use at least three vegetables.
6. What do you think about using salsa instead of gravy for some menu items?
7. What would you like to see on a healthy breakfast buffet?

Critical Application Exercises

1. Design your own "cuisine actuelle." Name it and explain what it would cover, including your nutritional philosophy.
2. Now take your cuisine and:
   a. Design a marketing promotion for it.
   b. Create two packaged products for it.
3. Create two new kinds of salsa and suggest at least five food items (each) with which they can be used.
4. Your employee cafeteria wants to have a breakfast and lunch buffet. Some employees are asking for "healthy" items. Using several ethnic items, design your buffets with at least three entrées, ten side dishes and appropriate beverages, condiments, and accompaniments (such as breads and garnishes).

References

United Soybean Board
16305 Swingley Ridge Road Suite 110
Chesterfield, MO 63017
1-800-825-5769
(ask for their *Soy Connection* newsletter, lots of recipes and health info and for *US Soyfoods Directory*, state-by-state listing of soy foods distributors)

Soyfoods Association of America
1723 U Street, NW
Washington, DC 20009
202-986-5600
info@soyfoods.org

Soyfoods Center
PO Box 234
Lafayette, CA 94549
510-283-0234

Melon Salsa

This sweet-but-hot salsa is a good accompaniment to poultry, beef, fish and hot soups, and makes about 2 cups of salsa.

Ingredients

1 cup diced cantaloupe
¾ cup diced honeydew or Persian melon
1 cup diced watermelon
1 teaspoon minced and seeded chili (you choose the heat)
1 teaspoon chopped fresh mint
1 tablespoon fresh lemon or lime juice
1 tablespoon orange juice

Method

1. In a nonreactive bowl, combine all ingredients.
2. Allow to chill for at least 30 minutes before serving.

Nutritional Analysis: 21 calories per serving, 1 gram protein, 0 grams fat, 5 grams carbohydrates, 9 milligram calcium, 3 milligrams sodium.

Olive and Carrot Salsa
(Yields about 2 cups)

This Mediterranean salsa goes well with fish, seafood and poultry.

Ingredients

1½ cups grated carrots
8 large, pitted and chopped green olives
4 large, pitted and chopped black olives
2 teaspoons chopped bell pepper
¼ cup olive oil
1 teaspoon cayenne powder
1 tablespoon fresh lemon juice

Method

1. In a nonreactive bowl, combine all ingredients.
2. Allow to chill for at least 30 minutes before service.

Nutritional Analysis: 82 calories per serving, 1 gram protein, 7 grams fat, 5 grams carbohydrates, 100 milligrams sodium, 1 gram fiber.

Baked Banana Salsa

Use this salsa as a dessert sauce, served over ice milk, sorbet or soy ice cream, fruit salad or sliced angel food cake or as a sauce for savory pork, chicken or duck.

Ingredients

4 ripe unpeeled bananas (about 2 cups)
2 teaspoons vanilla extract
1 teaspoon maple syrup
½ teaspoon brown sugar

½ teaspoon cracked black pepper
2 tablespoons chopped nuts (such as walnuts or almonds)

Method

1. Preheat oven to 375 degrees. Place whole bananas (in their skins) on a baking sheet and allow to roast for 20 minutes; skins will turn brown. Allow to cool.
2. Peel and dice bananas and place in a medium mixing bowl. Add remaining ingredients and toss gently until combined.

Nutritional Analysis: 100 calories per serving, 1 gram protein, 8 grams fat, 8 grams carbohydrates, 8 milligrams sodium, 1 gram dietary fiber.

VEGGIE BREAKFAST IN A SLICE

Boston Brown Bread

(Yield: 60 portions from 8 loaves)

Boston Brown Bread resembles a steamed pudding and is rich, flavorful and chewy. It can be packed with dried fruit or nuts for extra texture, flavor and nutrition. With a few add-ons, this bread is an a.m. meal in itself. It fits the vegetarian bill because it requires no eggs or milk, and molasses is the sweetening agent (some vegans avoid refined sugar) This recipe is healthy for everyone.

Ingredients

1 pound cornmeal
14 oz wholewheat flour
12 oz all-purpose flour
1 oz salt
1 oz baking soda
1 qt 1 pint buttermilk*
2½ cups molasses

*Rice milk may be used if a vegan product is desired

Method

1. Mix all dry ingredients together in bowl of mixer. Mix on low speed, with paddle, until ingredients are blended.
2. In a blender or food processor, blend milk and molasses. Add immediately to dry ingredients and mix on low speed until well-combined.
3. Scale into 8 greased loaf pans (3¼ × 4½″), cover tightly with foil.
4. Steam in commercial steamer for 1½ hours or until knife inserted in middle of loaf comes out clean.

Notes: Loaves may also be baked, using 3 larger loaf pans (5 × 9); bake at 375 degrees for one hour. Dried, chopped fruit, such as raisins, dates, prunes or figs, totaling 14 ounces, may be added when the molasses is added. Garnish with chopped walnuts, almonds, chopped dried apricots or cranberries.

Nutritional Analysis: 154 calories per serving, 3 grams protein, 2 grams fat, 10 milligrams cholesterol, 32 grams carbohydrate, 253 milligrams sodium, 1 gram dietary fiber.

SPLASH ON THAT TOFU

Basic Tofu Salad Dressing

(Yield: 1 pint)

Use this as a "creamy" salad dressing.

Ingredients

10 ounces silken or soft tofu
2 ounces minced onions
1 clove minced garlic
1 ounce chopped fresh parsley
1 tablespoon lemon juice
1 teaspoon white pepper

Method

1. Place all ingredients in a blender and process until smooth.
2. Chill until ready to use.

Variations

Tomato-basil: add 2 ounces tomato puree and 1 tablespoon fresh chopped basil
Mediterranean: add 1 ounce chopped green olives, 2 teaspoons chopped bell pepper, 1 teaspoon oregano, 2 teaspoons chopped tomatoes
Asian: add 1 ounce soy sauce, 2 teaspoons fresh minced ginger
Thousand Island: add 1 ounce tomato puree, 2 teaspoons pickle relish
Tangy Strawberry Orange: add 2 ounces chopped fresh strawberries, 2 teaspoons orange juice concentrate

Nutritional Analysis for basic recipe: 136 calories per serving, 11 grams protein, 6 grams fat, 11 grams carbohydrate, 26 milligrams sodium, 3 grams dietary fiber.

Veggie Mayonnaise

(Yield: 1 pint)

You can purchase vegan mayo or you can whip up this quick recipe—use in salads or, add your favorite herbs and chopped veggies to create a salad dressing.

Ingredients

2 cups silken tofu
1 ounce oil

2 ounces lemon juice
1 teaspoon dry mustard
1 teaspoon ground white pepper
1/2 teaspoon garlic powder

Method

1. Place all ingredients in a blender and process until smooth.
2. Keep refrigerated until service.

Nutritional Analysis: 16 calories per tablespoon, 1 gram protein, 1 gram fat, 1 gram carbohydrates, 1 milligram sodium.

Sweet Potato Burgers
(Yield: 25 burgers)

This slightly sweet and very colorful burger can be made and grilled ahead and then reheated in the oven or microwave. It has a faint taste of India and goes well with eggplant fries or a lentil soup. (Adapted from *Vegan in Volume*, Berkoff, 2000.)

Ingredients

3 pounds raw sweet potatoes
12 ounces quinoa
1 1/2 pints vegetable broth
1 pint water
Vegetable spray
1 pound onions
3 ounces garlic
1/2 ounce ground cumin
1/4 ounce ground turmeric
2 pounds chopped cashews
6 ounces bread crumbs

Method

1. Preheat oven to 375 (convection 350).
2. Steam potatoes until tender. Allow to cool.
3. In small stock pot, bring quinoa, broth and water to boil. Reduce heat, cover, simmer until quinoa is fluffy (about 10 minutes). Allow to cool.
4. Spray sauté pan and heat. Sweat onions and garlic. Add cumin and tumeric and stir to combine. Remove from heat.
5. In food chopper, combine potatoes, quinoa and veggies. Process until well blended. Add cashews and bread crumbs and process again to blend well.
6. Shape into 1/4 inch thick burgers. Put on sprayed baking sheet and bake for approx. 30 minutes, turning once.

Note: additional breadcrumbs can be used if mixture is too loose to form burgers.

Nutritional Analysis: 356 calories per burger, 10 grams protein, 42 grams carbohydrates, 18 grams fat, 74 milligrams sodium, 5 grams dietary fiber.

Cream-less, Creamy Cream of Du Jour Soup
(Yield: 20 eight-ounce servings)

Ingredients

Vegetable oil spray
8 ounces diced onions
18 ounces cooked and chopped veggie of choice (see note)
4 cloves minced garlic
3 teaspoons chopped fresh parsley
2 tablespoons lemon juice
1 tablespoon white pepper
1½ quarts soy milk
2 pounds firm tofu, drained

Method

1. Heat sauté pan, spread with oil and sweat onions, veggies and garlic.
2. Add parsley, lemon juice and pepper and sweat until veggies are tender.
3. Place in small stock pot, stir in soy milk and heat on low flame, stirring for 5 minutes or until mixture is heated. (Using high heat may cause soy milk to curdle.)
4. Remove from heat, stir in tofu. Place mixture in blender and blend until just smooth.
5. Return to stock pot, reheat and serve hot.

Notes

1. This recipe is a way to utilize leftover fresh or frozen veggies. Chop to uniform size. Try combos such as celery-mushroom, carrot-sweet potato, broccoli-corn, cauliflower-tomato, summer squash-sweet onion or broccoli-mushroom.
2. Soup does not have to be blended. For a chunky texture, dice tofu before adding and serve as is. Or blend a portion of the soup, stirring in blended mixture for a semi-smooth, semi-chunky texture.
3. This soup may be made ahead of time and stored, refrigerated, for up to two days.

Nutritional Analysis: 66 calories per serving, 5 grams protein, 2 grams fat, 6 grams carbohydrate, 44 milligrams sodium, 1 gram dietary fiber.

Appendix 1

RDA and RDIs

1989 Recommended Dietary Allowances (RDA)

Age (yr)	Energy (kcal)	Protein (g)	Vitamin A (μg TE)	Vitamin E (mg α-TE)	Vitamin K (μg)	Vitamin C (mg)	Iron (mg)	Zinc (mg)	Iodine (μ grams)	Selenium (μ grams)
Infants										
0.0–0.5	650	13	375	3	5	30	6	5	40	10
0.5–1.0	850	14	375	4	10	35	10	5	50	15
Children										
1–3	1300	16	400	6	15	40	10	10	70	20
4–6	1800	24	500	7	20	45	10	10	90	20
7–10	2000	28	700	7	30	45	10	10	120	30
Males										
11–14	2500	45	1000	10	45	50	12	15	150	40
15–18	3000	59	1000	10	65	60	12	15	150	50
19–24	2900	58	1000	10	70	60	10	15	150	70
25–50	2900	63	1000	10	80	60	10	15	150	70
51 +	2300	63	1000	10	80	60	10	15	150	70
Females										
11–14	2200	46	800	8	45	50	15	12	150	45
15–18	2200	44	800	8	55	60	15	12	150	50
19–24	2200	46	800	8	60	60	15	12	150	55
25–50	2200	50	800	8	65	60	15	12	150	55
51 +	1900	50	800	8	65	60	10	12	150	55
Pregnancy										
Lactation	+300	60	800	10	65	70	30	15	175	65
1st 6 mo.	+500	65	1300	12	65	95	15	19	200	75
2nd 6 mo.	+500	62	1200	11	65	90	15	16	200	75

In addition to the values that serve as goals for nutrient intakes (presented in the adjacent tables), the Dietary Reference Intakes include a set of values called Tolerable Upper Intake Levels—the maximum amount of a nutrient that appears safe for most healthy people to consume on a regular basis.

Tolerable Upper Intake Levels for Selected Nutrients (per day)

Age (yr)	Vitamin D (μg)[a]	Niacin (mg)	Vitamin B_6 (mg)	Folate (μg)	Choline (mg)	Calcium (mg)	Phosphorus (mg)	Magnesium (mg)	Fluoride (mg)
Infants									
0.0–0.5	25	—[b]	—[b]	—[b]	—[b]	—[b]	—[b]	—[b]	0.7
0.5–1.0	25	—[b]	—[b]	—[b]	—[b]	—[b]	—[b]	—[b]	0.9
Children									
1–3	50	10	30	300	1000	2500	3000	65	1.3
4–8	50	15	40	400	1000	2500	3000	110	2.2
9–13	50	20	60	600	2000	2500	4000	350	10.0
14–18	50	30	80	800	3000	2500	4000	350	10.0
Adults									
19–70	50	35	100	1000	3500	2500	4000	350	10.0
>70	50	35	100	1000	3500	2500	3000	350	10.0
Pregnancy	50	35	100	1000	3500	2500	3500	350	10.0
Lactation	50	35	100	1000	3500	2500	4000	350	10.0

Note: An Upper Level was not established for thiamin, riboflavin, vitamin B_{12}, panthothenic acid, and biotin because of a lack of data, not because these nutrients are safe to consume at any level of intake; all nutrients can have adverse effects when intakes are excessive.

[a]To convert μg to IU, multiply by 40. For example, 50 g × 40 = 2000 IU.

[b]Upper Levels were not established for many nutrients in the infant category because of a lack of data.

Source: Adapted from the first two of the *Dietary Reference Intakes Series*, National Academy Press. Copyright 1997 and 1998, by the National Academy of Sciences.

Courtesy of the National Academy Press, Washington, D.C.

DAILY VALUES FOR FOOD LABELS

The Daily Values are standard values developed by the Food and Drug Administration (FDA) for use on food labels. In creating the Daily Values, the FDA first established two sets of reference values. The first set, the Reference Daily Intakes (RDI), are for protein, vitamins, and minerals and reflect average allowances based on the RDA. The second set, the Daily Reference Values (DRV), are for nutrients and food components, such as fat and fiber, that do not have an established RDA but do have important relationships with health. Together, the RDI and DRV make up the Daily Values used on food labels.

Reference Daily Intakes (RDI)

Nutrient	Amount
Protein[a]	50 g
Thiamin	1.5 mg
Riboflavin	1.7 mg
Niacin	20 mg NE
Biotin	300 μg
Pantothenic acid	10 mg
Vitamin B_6	2 mg
Folate	400 μg
Vitamin B_{12}	6 μg
Vitamin C	60 mg
Vitamin A[b]	5000 IU
Vitamin D[b]	400 IU
Vitamin E[b]	30 IU
Calcium	1000 mg
Iron	18 mg
Zinc	15 mg
Iodine	150 μg
Copper	2 mg

[a]The RDI for protein varies for different groups of people: pregnant women, 60 g; nursing mothers, 65 g; infants under 1 year, 14 g; children 1 to 4 years, 16 g.

[b]The RDI for fat-soluble vitamins are expressed in International Units (IU), an old system of measurement. The current RDA and tables of food composition use a more accurate system of measurement. Equivalent values are as follows: for vitamin A, 875 μg RE: for vitamin D, 6.5 μg: for vitamin E, 9 mg α-TE.

Source: Adapted from the first two of the *Dietary Reference Intakes Series*, National Academy Press. Copyright 1997 and 1998, by the National Academy of Sciences.
Courtesy of the National Academy Press, Washington, D.C.

Daily Reference Values (DRV)

Food Component	DRV	Calculation
Fat	65 g	30% of kcalories
Saturated fat	20 g	10% of kcalories
Cholesterol	300 mg	Same regardless of kcalories
Carbohydrate (total)	300 g	60% of kcalories
Fiber	25 g	11.5 g per 1000 kcalories
Protein	50 g	10% of kcalories
Sodium	2400 mg	Same regardless of kcalories
Potassium	3500 mg	Same regardless of kcalories

Note: The DRV were established for adults and children over 4 years old. The values for energy-yielding nutrients are based on 2000 kcalories a day.
Source: Adapted from the first two of the *Dietary Reference Intakes Series*, National Academy Press. Copyright 1997 and 1998, by the National Academy of Sciences.
Courtesy of the National Academy Press, Washington, D.C.

Appendix 2

BMI Height/Weight Chart

Body Mass Index Table

	Normal							Overweight				Obese					
BMI	*19*	*20*	*21*	*22*	*23*	*24*	*25*	*26*	*27*	*28*	*29*	*30*	*31*	*32*	*33*	*34*	*35*
Height (inches)	Body Weight (pounds)																
58	91	96	100	105	110	115	119	124	129	134	138	143	148	153	158	162	167
59	94	99	104	109	114	119	124	128	133	138	143	148	153	158	163	168	173
60	97	102	107	112	118	123	128	133	138	143	148	153	158	163	168	174	179
61	100	106	111	116	122	127	132	137	143	148	153	158	164	169	174	180	185
62	104	109	115	120	126	131	136	142	147	153	158	164	169	175	180	186	191
63	107	113	118	124	130	135	141	146	152	158	163	169	175	180	186	191	197
64	110	116	122	128	134	140	145	151	157	163	169	174	180	186	192	197	204
65	114	120	126	132	138	144	150	156	162	168	174	180	186	192	198	204	210
66	118	124	130	136	142	148	155	161	167	173	179	186	192	198	204	210	216
67	121	127	134	140	146	153	159	166	172	178	185	191	198	204	211	217	223
68	125	131	138	144	151	158	164	171	177	184	190	197	203	210	216	223	230
69	128	135	142	149	155	162	169	176	182	189	196	203	209	216	223	230	236
70	132	139	146	153	160	167	174	181	188	195	202	209	216	222	229	236	243
71	136	143	150	157	165	172	179	186	193	200	208	215	222	229	236	243	250
72	140	147	154	162	169	177	184	191	199	206	213	221	228	235	242	250	258
73	144	151	159	166	174	182	189	197	204	212	219	227	235	242	250	257	265
74	148	155	163	171	179	186	194	202	210	218	225	233	241	249	256	264	272
75	152	160	168	176	184	192	200	208	216	224	232	240	248	256	264	272	279
76	156	164	172	180	189	197	205	213	221	230	238	246	254	263	271	279	287

Source: Adapted from *Clinical Guidelines on the Identification, Evaluation, and Treatment of Overweight and Obesity in Adults: The Evidence Report* and NHLBI, 2002.

				Extreme Obesity														
36	*37*	*38*	*39*	*40*	*41*	*42*	*43*	*44*	*45*	*46*	*47*	*48*	*49*	*50*	*51*	*52*	*53*	*54*
				Body Weight (pounds)														
172	177	181	186	191	196	201	205	210	215	220	224	229	234	239	244	248	253	258
178	183	188	193	198	203	208	212	217	222	227	232	237	242	247	252	257	262	267
184	189	194	199	204	209	215	220	225	230	235	240	245	250	255	261	266	271	276
190	195	201	206	211	217	222	227	232	238	243	248	254	259	264	269	275	280	285
196	202	207	213	218	224	229	235	240	246	251	256	262	267	273	278	284	289	295
203	208	214	220	225	231	237	242	248	254	259	265	270	278	282	287	293	299	304
209	215	221	227	232	238	244	250	256	262	267	273	279	285	291	296	302	308	314
216	222	228	234	240	246	252	258	264	270	276	282	288	294	300	306	312	318	324
223	229	235	241	247	253	260	266	272	278	284	291	297	303	309	315	322	328	334
230	236	242	249	255	261	268	274	280	287	293	299	306	312	319	325	331	338	344
236	243	249	256	262	269	276	282	289	295	302	308	315	322	328	335	341	348	354
243	250	257	263	270	277	284	291	297	304	311	318	324	331	338	345	351	358	365
250	257	264	271	278	285	292	299	306	313	320	327	334	341	348	355	362	369	376
257	265	272	279	286	293	301	308	315	322	329	338	343	351	358	365	372	379	386
265	272	279	287	294	302	309	316	324	331	338	346	353	361	368	375	383	390	397
272	280	288	295	302	310	318	325	333	340	348	355	363	371	378	386	393	401	408
280	287	295	303	311	319	326	334	342	350	358	365	373	381	389	396	404	412	420
287	295	303	311	319	327	335	343	351	359	367	375	383	391	399	407	415	423	431
295	304	312	320	328	336	344	353	361	369	377	385	394	402	410	418	426	435	443

Height & Weight Charts

Height & Weight Table For Women

Height (Feet/Inches)	Small Frame	Medium Frame	Large Frame
4′ 10″	102–111	109–121	118–131
4′ 11″	103–113	111–123	120–134
5′ 0″	104–115	113–126	122–137
5′ 1″	106–118	115–129	125–140
5′ 2″	108–121	118–132	128–143
5′ 3″	111–124	121–135	131–147
5′ 4″	114–127	124–138	134–151
5′ 5″	117–130	127–141	137–155
5′ 6″	120–133	130–144	140–159
5′ 7″	123–136	133–147	143–163
5′ 8″	126–139	136–150	146–167
5′ 9″	129–142	139–153	149–170
5′ 10″	132–145	142–156	152–173
5′ 11″	135–148	145–159	155–176
6′ 0″	138–151	148–162	158–179

Height & Weight Table For Men

Height (Feet/Inches)	Small Frame	Medium Frame	Large Frame
5′ 2″	128–134	131–141	138–150
5′ 3″	130–136	133–143	140–153
5′ 4″	132–138	135–145	142–156
5′ 5″	134–140	137–148	144–160
5′ 6″	136–142	139–151	146–164
5′ 7″	138–145	142–154	149–168
5′ 8″	140–148	145–157	152–172
5′ 9″	142–151	148–160	155–176
5′ 10″	144–154	151–163	158–180
5′ 11″	146–157	154–166	161–184
6′ 0″	149–160	157–170	164–188
6′ 1″	152–164	160–174	168–192
6′ 2″	155–168	164–178	172–197
6′ 3″	158–172	167–182	176–202
6′ 4″	162–176	171–187	181–207

Source: Adapted from *Clinical Guidelines on the Identification, Evaluation, and Treatment of Overweight and Obesity in Adults: The Evidence Report*, and NHLBI, 2002.

Appendix 3

Exchange Lists for Meal Planning

Everyone needs to eat nutritious foods. Good health depends on eating a variety of foods that contain the right amounts of carbohydrate, protein, fat, vitamins, minerals, fiber, and water. For adolescents and adults, a healthy daily meal plan should include at least 3 servings of vegetables; 2 servings of fruits; 6 servings of grains, beans, and starchy vegetables; 2 servings of low-fat or fat-free milk; about 6 oz of meat or meat substitutes; and *small* amounts of fat and sugar. The actual amounts will depend on the number of calories you need, which in turn depends on your size, age, and activity level. If you are an adult, eating the right number of calories can help you reach and stay at a reasonable weight. Children and adolescents must eat enough calories so they grow and develop normally.

EXCHANGE LISTS

Foods are listed with their serving sizes, which are usually measured after cooking. When you begin, measuring the size of each serving will help you learn to "eyeball" correct serving sizes.

The following chart shows the amount of nutrients in one serving from each list.

Groups/ Lists	Carbohydrate (grams)	Protein (grams)	Fat (grams)	Calories
Carbohydrate Group				
Starch	15	3	0–1	80
Fruit	15	—	—	60
Milk				
Fat-free	12	8	0–3	90
Reduced-fat	12	8	5	120
Whole	12	8	8	150
Sweets, dessert, and other carbohydrates	15	varies	varies	varies
Nonstarchy vegetables	5	2	—	25
Meat and Meat Substitutes Group				
Very lean	—	7	0–1	35
Lean	—	7	3	55
Medium-fat	—	7	5	75
High-fat	—	7	8	100
Fat Group	—	—	5	45

Starch List

Cereals, grains, pasta, breads, crackers, snacks, starchy vegetables, and cooked beans, peas, and lentils are starches. In general, one starch is:

- ½ cup of cooked cereal, grain, or starchy vegetable
- ⅓ cup of cooked rice or pasta
- 1 oz of a bread product, such as 1 slice of bread
- ¾ to 1 oz of most snack foods (some snack foods may also have added fat)

One starch exchange equals 15 grams carbohydrate, 3 grams protein, 0 to 1 gram fat, and 80 calories.

Bread

Bagel, 4 oz	¼ (1 oz)
Bread, reduced-calorie	2 slices (1½ oz)
Bread, white, whole-wheat, pumpernickel, rye	1 slice (1 oz)
Breadsticks, crisp, 4 inch × ½ inch.	4 (⅔ oz)
English muffin	½
Hot dog bun or hamburger bun	½ (1 oz)
Naan, 8 × 2 inches	¼
Pancake, 4 inches across, ¼ inch thick	1
Pita, 6 inches across	½
Roll, plain, small	1 (1 oz)
Raisin bread, unfrosted	1 slice (1 oz)
Tortilla, corn, 6 inches across	1
Tortilla, flour, 6 inches across	1
Tortilla, flour, 10 inches across	⅓
Waffle, 4 inches square or across, reduced-fat	1

Cereals and Grains

Bran cereals	½ cup
Bulgur	½ cup
Cereals, cooked	½ cup
Cereals, unsweetened, ready-to-eat	¾ cup
Cornmeal (dry)	3 Tbsp
Couscous	⅓ cup
Flour (dry)	3 Tbsp
Granola, low-fat	¼ cup
Grape-Nuts®	¼ cup
Grits	½ cup
Kasha	½ cup
Millet	⅓ cup
Muesli	¼ cup
Oats	½ cup
Pasta	⅓ cup
Puffed cereal	1½ cups
Rice, white or brown	⅓ cup
Shredded Wheat®	½ cup
Sugar-frosted cereal	½ cup
Wheat germ	3 Tbsp

Starchy Vegetables

Baked beans	⅓ cup
Corn	½ cup
Corn on cob, large	½ cob (5 oz)
Mixed vegetables with corn, peas, or pasta	1 cup
Peas, green	½ cup
Plantain	½ cup
Potato, boiled	½ cup or ½ medium (3 oz)
Potato, baked with skin	¼ large (3 oz)
Potato, mashed	½ cup
Squash, winter (acorn, butternut, pumpkin)	1 cup
Yam, sweet potato, plain	½ cup

Crackers and Snacks

Animal crackers	8
Graham cracker, 2 1/2 inches square	3
Matzoh	¾ oz
Melba toast	4 slices
Oyster crackers	24
Popcorn (popped, no fat added, or low-fat microwave)	3 cups
Pretzels	¾ oz
Rice cakes, 4 inches across	2
Saltine-type crackers	6
Snack chips, fat-free (tortilla, potato)	15–20 (¾ oz)
Whole-wheat crackers, no fat added	2–5 (¾ oz)

Beans, Peas, and Lentils (Count as 1 starch exchange, plus 1 very lean meat exchange)	
Beans and peas (garbanzo, pinto, kidney, white, split, black-eyed)	½ cup
Lima beans	⅔ cup
Lentils	½ cup
Miso*	3 Tbsp

* = 400 mg or more sodium per exchange.

Starchy Foods Prepared with Fat (Count as 1 starch exchange, plus 1 fat exchange)	
Biscuit, 2½ inches across	1
Chow mein noodles	½ cup
Corn bread, 2-inch cube	1 (2 oz)
Crackers, round butter-type	6
Croutons	1 cup
French-fried potatoes (oven-baked)	1 cup (2 oz)
Granola	¼ cup
Hummus	⅓ cup
Muffin, 5 oz	⅕ (1 oz)
Popcorn, microwaved	3 cups
Sandwich crackers, cheese or peanut butter filling	3
Snack chips (potato, tortilla)	9–13 (¾ oz)
Stuffing, bread (prepared)	⅓ cup
Taco shell, 6 inches across	2
Waffle, 4 inches square or across	1
Whole-wheat crackers, fat added	4–7 (1 oz)

Fruit List

Fresh, frozen, canned, and dried fruits and fruit juices are on this list. In general, one fruit exchange is:

- 1 small fresh fruit (4 oz)
- ½ cup of canned or fresh fruit or unsweetened fruit juice
- ¼ cup of dried fruit

One fruit exchange equals 15 grams carbohydrate and 60 calories. The weight includes skin, core, seeds, and rind.

Fruit	
Apple, unpeeled, small	1 (4 oz)
Applesauce, unsweetened	½ cup
Apples, dried	4 rings
Apricots, fresh	4 whole (5½ oz)
Apricots, dried	8 halves
Apricots, canned	½ cup

Banana, small	1 (4 oz)
Blackberries	¾ cup
Blueberries	¾ cup
Cantaloupe, small	⅓ melon (11 oz) or 1 cup cubes
Cherries, sweet, fresh	12 (3 oz)
Cherries, sweet, canned	½ cup
Dates	3
Figs, fresh	1½ large or 2 medium (3½ oz)
Figs, dried	1½
Fruit cocktail	½ cup
Grapefruit, large	½ (11 oz)
Grapefruit sections, canned	¾ cup
Grapes, small	17 (3 oz)
Honeydew melon	1 slice (10 oz) or 1 cup cubes
Kiwi	1 (3½ oz)
Mandarin oranges, canned	¾ cup
Mango, small	½ fruit (5½ oz) or ½ cup
Nectarine, small	1 (5 oz)
Orange, small	1 (6½ oz)
Papaya	½ fruit (8 oz) or 1 cup cubes
Peach, fresh, medium	1 (4 oz)
Peaches, canned	½ cup
Pear, fresh, large	½ (4 oz)
Pears, canned	½ cup
Pineapple, fresh	¾ cup
Pineapple, canned	½ cup
Plums, fresh, small	2 (5 oz)
Plums, canned	½ cup
Plums, dried (prunes)	3
Raisins	2 Tbsp
Raspberries	1 cup
Strawberries	1¼ cup whole berries
Tangerines, small	2 (8 oz)
Watermelon	1 slice (13½ oz) or 1¼ cup cubes

Fruit Juice, Unsweetened

Apple juice/cider	½ cup
Cranberry juice cocktail	⅓ cup
Cranberry juice cocktail, reduced-calorie	1 cup
Fruit juice blends, 100% juice	⅓ cup
Grape juice	⅓ cup
Grapefruit juice	½ cup
Orange juice	½ cup
Pineapple juice	½ cup
Prune juice	⅓ cup

Milk List

Different types of milk and milk products are on this list. Cheeses are on the Meat and Meat Substitutes list and cream and other dairy fats are on the Fat list. Based on the amount of fat they contain, milks are divided into fat-free/low-fat milk, reduced-fat milk, and whole milk. One choice of these includes:

	Carbohydrate (grams)	Protein (grams)	Fat (grams)	Calories
Fat-free/low-fat (½% or 1%)	12	8	0–3	90
Reduced-fat (2%)	12	8	5	120
Whole	12	8	8	150

One milk exchange equals 12 grams carbohydrate and 8 grams protein.

Fat-free and Low-fat Milk (0–3 grams fat per serving)	
Fat-free milk	1 cup
½% milk	1 cup
1% milk	1 cup
Buttermilk, low-fat or fat-free	1 cup
Evaporated fat-free milk	½ cup
Fat-free dry milk	⅓ cup dry
Soy milk, low-fat or fat-free	1 cup
Yogurt, fat-free, flavored, sweetened with nonnutritive sweetener and fructose	6 oz
Yogurt, plain, fat-free	6 oz

Reduced-fat Milk (5 grams fat per serving)	
2% milk	1 cup
Soy milk	1 cup
Sweet acidophilus milk	1 cup
Yogurt, plain, low-fat	6 oz

Whole Milk (8 grams fat per serving)	
Whole milk	1 cup
Evaporated whole milk	½ cup
Goat's milk	1 cup
Kefir	1 cup
Yogurt, plain (made from whole milk)	8 oz

Sweets, Desserts, and Other Carbohydrates List

One exchange equals 15 grams carbohydrate, 1 starch, 1 fruit, or 1 milk.

Food	Serving Size	Exchanges per Serving
Angel food cake, unfrosted	1/12th cake (about 2 oz)	2 carbohydrates
Brownie, small, unfrosted	2-inch square (about 1 oz)	1 carbohydrate, 1 fat
Cake, unfrosted	2-inch square (about 1 oz)	1 carbohydrate, 1 fat
Cake, frosted	2-inch square (about 2 oz)	2 carbohydrates, 1 fat
Cookie or sandwich cookie with cream filling	2 small (about 2/3 oz)	1 carbohydrate, 1 fat
Cookies, sugar-free	3 small or 1 large (3/4–1 oz)	1 carbohydrate, 1–2 fats
Cranberry sauce, jellied	1/4 cup	1½ carbohydrates
Cupcake, frosted	1 small (about 2 oz)	2 carbohydrates, 1 fat
Doughnut, plain cake	1 medium (1½ oz)	1½ carbohydrates, 2 fats
Doughnut, glazed	3¾ inches across (2 oz)	2 carbohydrates, 2 fats
Energy, sport, or breakfast bar	1 bar (1⅓ oz)	1½ carbohydrates, 0–1 fat
Energy, sport, or breakfast bar	1 bar (2 oz)	2 carbohydrates, 1 fat
Fruit cobbler	½ cup (3½ oz)	3 carbohydrates, 1 fat
Fruit juice bars, frozen, 100% juice	1 bar (3 oz)	1 carbohydrate
Fruit snacks, chewy (pureed fruit concentrate)	1 roll (¾ oz)	1 carbohydrate
Fruit spreads, 100% fruit	1½ Tbsp	1 carbohydrate
Gelatin, regular	½ cup	1 carbohydrate
Gingersnaps	3	1 carbohydrate
Granola or snack bar, regular or low-fat	1 bar (1 oz)	1½ carbohydrates
Honey	1 Tbsp	1 carbohydrate
Ice cream	½ cup	1 carbohydrate, 2 fats
Ice cream, light	½ cup	1 carbohydrate, 1 fat
Ice cream, low-fat	½ cup	1½ carbohydrates
Ice cream, fat-free, no sugar added	½ cup	1 carbohydrate
Jam or jelly, regular	1 Tbsp	1 carbohydrate
Milk, chocolate, whole	1 cup	2 carbohydrates, 1 fat
Pie, fruit, 2 crusts	⅙ of 8-inch commercially prepared pie	3 carbohydrates, 2 fats
Pie, pumpkin or custard	⅛ of 8-inch commercially prepared pie	2 carbohydrates, 2 fats
Pudding, regular (made with reduced-fat milk)	½ cup	2 carbohydrates
Pudding, sugar-free or sugar-free and fat-free (made with reduced-fat milk)	½ cup	1 carbohydrate
Reduced calorie meal replacement (shake)	1 can (10–11 oz)	1½ carbohydrates, 0–1 fat
Rice milk, low-fat or fat-free, plain	1 cup	1 carbohydrate
Rice milk, low-fat, flavored	1 cup	1½ carbohydrates
Salad dressing, fat-free*	¼ cup	1 carbohydrate
Sherbet, sorbet	½ cup	2 carbohydrates
Spaghetti or pasta sauce, canned*	½ cup	1 carbohydrate, 1 fat
Sports drinks	8 oz (about 1 cup)	1 carbohydrate
Sugar	1 Tbsp	1 carbohydrate
Sweet roll or Danish	1 (2½ oz)	2½ carbohydrates, 2 fats
Syrup, light	2 Tbsp	1 carbohydrate
Syrup, regular	1 Tbsp	1 carbohydrate
Syrup, regular	¼ cup	4 carbohydrates
Vanilla wafers	5	1 carbohydrate, 1 fat
Yogurt, frozen	½ cup	1 carbohydrate, 0–1 fat
Yogurt, frozen, fat-free	⅓ cup	1 carbohydrate
Yogurt, low-fat with fruit	1 cup	3 carbohydrates, 0–1 fat

* = 400 mg or more of sodium per exchange.

Nonstarchy Vegetable List

Vegetables that contain small amounts of carbohydrates and calories are on this list. In general, one vegetable exchange is:

- ½ cup of cooked vegetables or vegetable juice
- 1 cup of raw vegetables

Selection Tips

One vegetable exchange (½ cup cooked or 1 cup raw) equals 5 grams carbohydrate, 2 grams protein, 0 grams fat, and 25 calories.

Artichoke
Artichoke hearts
Asparagus
Beans (green, wax, Italian)
Bean sprouts
Beets
Broccoli
Brussels sprouts
Cabbage
Carrots
Cauliflower
Celery
Cucumber
Eggplant
Green onions or scallions
Greens (collard, kale, mustard, turnip)
Kohlrabi
Leeks
Mixed vegetables (without corn, peas, or pasta)
Mushrooms
Okra
Onions
Pea pods
Peppers (all varieties)
Radishes
Salad greens (endive, escarole, lettuce, romaine, spinach)
Sauerkraut*
Spinach
Summer squash
Tomato
Tomatoes, canned
Tomato sauce*
Tomato/vegetable juice*
Turnips
Water chestnuts
Watercress
Zucchini

---

* = 400 mg or more sodium per exchange.

Meat and Meat Substitutes List

Meat and meat substitutes that contain both protein and fat are on this list. In general, one meat exchange is:

- 1 oz of meat, fish, poultry, or cheese
- ½ cup of beans, peas, or lentils

Based on the amount of fat they contain, meats are divided into very lean, lean, medium-fat, and high-fat lists. One ounce (one exchange) of each of these includes:

	Carbohydrate (grams)	Protein (grams)	Fat (grams)	Calories
Very lean	0	7	0–1	35
Lean	0	7	3	55
Medium-fat	0	7	5	75
High-fat	0	7	8	100

Very Lean Meat and Substitutes List

One exchange equals 0 grams carbohydrate, 7 grams protein, 0–1 gram fat, and 35 calories.

One very lean meat exchange is equal to any one of the following items:

Poultry	
Chicken or turkey (white meat, no skin), Cornish hen (no skin)	1 oz
Fish	
Fresh or frozen cod, flounder, haddock, halibut, trout, lox (smoked salmon)*; tuna, fresh or canned in water	1 oz
Shellfish	
Clams, crab, lobster, scallops, shrimp, imitation shellfish	1 oz
Game	
Duck or pheasant (no skin), venison, buffalo, ostrich	1 oz
Cheese with 1 gram of fat or less per ounce	
Fat-free or low-fat cottage cheese	¼ cup
Fat-free cheese	1 oz
Other	
Processed sandwich meats with 1 gram fat or less per ounce, such as deli thin, shaved meats, chipped beef*, turkey ham	1 oz
Egg whites	2
Egg substitutes, plain	¼ cup
Hot dogs with 1 gram of fat or less per ounce*	1 oz
Kidney (high in cholesterol)	1 oz
Sausage with 1 gram of fat or less per ounce	1 oz

Count the following items as one very lean meat and one starch exchange.

Beans, peas, lentils (cooked)	½ cup

* = 400 mg or more sodium per exchange.

Lean Meat and Substitutes List

One exchange equals 0 grams carbohydrate, 7 grams protein, 3 grams fat, and 55 calories.	
One lean meat exchange is equal to any one of the following items:	
Beef	
USDA Select or Choice grades of lean beef trimmed of fat, such as round, sirloin, and flank steak; tenderloin; roast (rib, chuck, rump); steak (T-bone, porterhouse, cubed); ground round	1 oz
Pork	
Lean pork, such as fresh ham; canned, cured, or boiled ham; Canadian bacon*; tenderloin; center loin chop	1 oz
Lamb	
Roast, chop, or leg	1 oz
Veal	
Lean chop, roast	1 oz
Poultry	
Chicken, turkey (dark meat, no skin), chicken (white meat, with skin), domestic duck or goose (well-drained of fat, no skin)	1 oz
Fish	
Herring (uncreamed or smoked)	1 oz
Oysters	6 medium
Salmon (fresh or canned), catfish	1 oz
Sardines (canned)	2 medium
Tuna (canned in oil, drained)	1 oz
Game	
Goose (no skin), rabbit	1 oz
Cheese	
4.5%-fat cottage cheese	¼ cup
Grated Parmesan	2 Tbsp
Cheeses with 3 grams fat or less per ounce	1 oz
Other	
Hot dogs with 3 grams fat or less per ounce*	1½ oz
Processed sandwich meat with 3 grams of fat or less per ounce, such as turkey pastrami or kielbasa	1 oz
Liver, heart (high in cholesterol)	1 oz

Medium-fat Meat and Substitutes List

One exchange equals 0 grams carbohydrate, 7 grams protein, 5 grams fat, and 75 calories.	
One medium-fat meat exchange is equal to any one of the following items:	
Beef	
Most beef products fall into this category (ground beef, meatloaf, corned beef, short ribs, Prime grades of meat trimmed of fat, such as prime rib)	1 oz
Pork	

Top loin, chop, Boston butt, cutlet	1 oz
Lamb	
Rib roast, ground	1 oz
Veal	
Cutlet (ground or cubed, unbreaded)	1 oz
Poultry	
Chicken (dark meat, with skin), ground turkey or ground chicken, fried chicken (with skin)	1 oz
Fish	
Any fried fish product	1 oz
Cheese with 5 grams or less fat per ounce	
Feta	1 oz
Mozzarella	1 oz
Ricotta	¼ cup (2 oz)
Other	
Egg (high in cholesterol, limit to 3 per week)	1
Sausage with 5 grams of fat or less per ounce	1 oz
Tempeh	¼ cup
Tofu	4 oz or ½ cup

*= 400 mg or more sodium per exchange.

High-fat Meat and Substitutes List

One exchange equals 0 grams carbohydrate, 7 grams protein, 8 grams fat, and 100 calories.

Remember that these items are high in saturated fat, cholesterol, and calories and may raise blood cholesterol levels if eaten on a regular basis.

One high-fat meat exchange is equal to any one of the following items:

Pork	
Spareribs, ground pork, pork sausage	1 oz
Cheese	
All regular cheeses, such as American*, cheddar, Monterey Jack, Swiss	1 oz
Other	
Processed sandwich meats with 8 grams of fat or less per ounce, such as bologna, pimento loaf, salami	1 oz
Sausage, such as bratwurst, Italian, knockwurst, Polish, smoked	1 oz
Hot dog (turkey or chicken)*	1 (10/lb)
Bacon	3 slices (20 slices/lb)
Peanut butter (contains unsaturated fat)	1 Tbsp

Count the following items as 1 high-fat meat plus 1 fat exchange:

Hot dog (beef, pork, or combination)*	1 (10/lb)

*= 400 mg or more sodium per exchange.

Fat List

Fats are divided into three groups, based on the main type of fat they contain: monounsaturated, polyunsaturated, and saturated. In general, one fat exchange is:

- 1 teaspoon of regular margarine or vegetable oil
- 1 tablespoon of regular salad dressings

Monounsaturated Fats List

One fat exchange equals 5 grams fat and 45 calories.	
Avocado, medium	2 Tbsp (1 oz)
Oil (canola, olive, peanut)	1 tsp
Olives: ripe (black)	8 large
green, stuffed*	10 large
Nuts: almonds, cashews	6 nuts
mixed (50% peanuts)	6 nuts
peanuts	10 nuts
pecans	4 halves
Peanut butter, smooth or crunchy	½ Tbsp
Sesame seeds	1 Tbsp
Tahini or sesame paste	2 tsp

Polyunsaturated Fats List

One fat exchange equals 5 grams fat and 45 calories.	
Margarine: stick, tub, or squeeze	1 tsp
lower-fat spread (30% to 50% vegetable oil)	1 Tbsp
Mayonnaise: regular	1 tsp
reduced-fat	1 Tbsp
Nuts: walnuts, English	4 halves
Oil (corn, safflower, soybean)	1 tsp
Salad dressing: regular*	1 Tbsp
reduced-fat	2 Tbsp
Miracle Whip Salad Dressing®: regular	2 tsp
reduced-fat	1 Tbsp
Seeds: pumpkin, sunflower	1 Tbsp

*= 400 mg or more sodium per exchange.

Saturated Fats List

One fat exchange equals 5 grams fat and 45 calories.	
Bacon, cooked	1 slice (20 slices/lb)
Bacon, grease	1 tsp
Butter: stick	1 tsp
whipped	2 tsp
reduced-fat	1 Tbsp

Chitterlings, boiled	2 Tbsp (½ oz)
Coconut, sweetened, shredded	2 Tbsp
Coconut milk	1 Tbsp
Cream, half and half	2 Tbsp
Cream cheese: regular	1 Tbsp (½ oz)
reduced-fat	1½ Tbsp (¾ oz)
Fatback or salt pork	1 tsp
Shortening or lard	1 tsp
Sour cream: regular	2 Tbsp
reduced-fat	3 Tbsp

Free Foods List

A *free food* is any food or drink that contains fewer than 20 calories or 5 grams carbohydrate per serving. Foods with a serving size listed should be limited to 3 servings per day. Be sure to spread them out throughout the day. If you eat all 3 servings at one time, it could raise your blood glucose level. Foods listed without a serving size can be eaten whenever you like.

Fat-free or Reduced-fat Foods	
Cream cheese, fat-free	1 Tbsp (½ oz)
Creamers, nondairy, liquid	1 Tbsp
Creamers, nondairy, powdered	2 tsp
Mayonnaise, fat-free	1 Tbsp
Mayonnaise, reduced-fat	1 tsp
Margarine spread, fat-free	4 Tbsp
Margarine spread, reduced-fat	1 tsp
Miracle Whip®, fat-free	1 Tbsp
Miracle Whip®, reduced-fat	1 tsp
Nonstick cooking spray	
Salad dressing, fat-free or low-fat	1 Tbsp
Salad dressing, fat-free, Italian	2 Tbsp
Sour cream, fat-free, reduced-fat	1 Tbsp
Whipped topping, regular	1 Tbsp
Whipped topping, light or fat-free	2 Tbsp

Sugar-free Foods	
Candy, hard, sugar-free	1 candy
Gelatin dessert, sugar-free	
Gelatin, unflavored	
Gum, sugar-free	
Jam or jelly, light	2 tsp
Sugar substitutes[a]	
Syrup, sugar-free	2 Tbsp

[a]Sugar substitutes, alternatives, or replacements that are approved by the Food and Drug Administration (FDA) are safe to use. Common brand names include:
Equal® (aspartame)
Splenda® (sucralose)
Sprinkle Sweet® (saccharin)

Sweet One® (acesulfame K)
Sweet-10® (saccharin)
Sugar Twin® (saccharin)
Sweet 'N Low® (saccharin)

Drinks	
Bouillon, broth, consommé*	
Bouillon or broth, low-sodium	
Carbonated or mineral water	
Club soda	
Cocoa powder, unsweetened	1 Tbsp
Coffee	
Diet soft drinks, sugar-free	
Drink mixes, sugar-free	
Tea	
Tonic water, sugar-free	

Condiments	
Catsup	1 Tbsp
Horseradish	
Lemon juice	
Lime juice	
Mustard	
Pickle relish	1 Tbsp
Pickles, sweet (bread and butter)	2 slices
Pickles, sweet (gherkin)	½ oz
Pickles, dill*	½ large
Salsa	¼ cup
Soy sauce, regular or light*	1 Tbsp
Taco sauce	1 Tbsp
Vinegar	
Yogurt	2 Tbsp

Seasonings
Flavoring extracts
Garlic
Herbs, fresh or dried
Pimento
Spices
Tabasco® or hot pepper sauce
Wine, used in cooking
Worcestershire sauce
Be careful with seasonings that contain sodium or are salts, such as garlic or celery salt, and lemon pepper.

*= 400 mg or more of sodium per exchange.

Combination Foods List

Many foods are mixed together in various combinations. These combination foods do not fit into any one exchange list. Often it is hard to tell what is in a casserole dish or prepared food item. This is a list of exchanges for some typical combination foods. This list will help you fit these foods into your meal plan. Ask your dietitian for information about any other combination foods you would like to eat.

Food	Serving Size	Exchanges per Serving
Entrees		
Tuna noodle casserole, lasagna, spaghetti with meatballs, chili with beans, macaroni and cheese*	1 cup (8 oz)	2 carbohydrates, 2 medium-fat meats
Chow mein (without noodles or rice)*	2 cups (16 oz)	1 carbohydrate, 2 lean meats
Tuna or chicken salad	½ cup (3½ oz)	½ carbohydrate, 2 lean meats, 1 fat
Frozen entrees and meals		
Dinner-type meal*	generally 14–17 oz	3 carbohydrates, 3 medium-fat meats, 3 fats
Meatless burger, soy-based	3 oz	½ carbohydrate, 2 lean meats
Meatless burger, vegetable- and starch-based	3 oz	1 carbohydrate, 1 lean meat
Pizza, cheese, thin crust*	¼ of 12 inch (6 oz)	2 carbohydrates, 2 medium-fat meats
Pizza, meat topping, thin crust*	¼ of 12 inch (6 oz)	2 carbohydrates, 2 medium-fat meats, 1½ fats
Pot pie*	1 (7 oz)	2½ carbohydrates, 1 medium-fat meat, 3 fats
Entree or meal with less than 340 calories*	about 8–11 oz	2–3 carbohydrates, 1–2 lean meats
Soups		
Bean*	1 cup	1 carbohydrate, 1 very lean meat
Cream (made with water)*	1 cup (8 oz)	1 carbohydrate, 1 fat
Instant*	6 oz prepared	1 carbohydrate
Instant with beans/lentils*	8 oz prepared	2½ carbohydrates, 1 very lean meat
Split pea (made with water)*	½ cup (4 oz)	1 carbohydrate
Tomato (made with water)*	1 cup (8 oz)	1 carbohydrate
Vegetable beef, chicken noodle, or other broth-type*	1 cup (8 oz)	1 carbohydrate

*= 400 mg or more sodium per exchange.

Fast Foods[a]

Food	Serving Size	Exchanges per Serving
Burrito with beef*	1 (5–7 oz)	3 carbohydrates, 1 medium-fat meat, 1 fat
Chicken nuggets*	6	1 carbohydrate, 2 medium-fat meats, 1 fat
Chicken breast and wing, breaded and fried*	1 each	1 carbohydrate, 4 medium-fat meats, 2 fats
Chicken sandwich, grilled*	1	2 carbohydrates, 3 very lean meats
Chicken wings, hot*	6 (5 oz)	1 carbohydrate, 3 medium-fat meats, 4 fats
Fish sandwich/tartar sauce*	1	3 carbohydrates, 1 medium-fat meat, 3 fats
French fries*	1 medium serving (5 oz)	4 carbohydrates, 4 fats
Hamburger, regular	1	2 carbohydrates, 2 medium-fat meats
Hamburger, large*	1	2 carbohydrates, 3 medium-fat meats, 1 fat
Hot dog with bun*	1	1 carbohydrate, 1 high-fat meat, 1 fat
Individual pan pizza*	1	5 carbohydrates, 3 medium-fat meats, 3 fats
Pizza, cheese, thin crust*	¼ of medium (12 inch round) about 6 oz	2½ carbohydrates, 2 medium-fat meats, 1½ fats
Pizza, meat, thin crust*	¼ of medium (12 inch round) about 6 oz	2½ carbohydrates, 2 medium-fat meats, 2 fats
Soft-serve cone	1 small (5 oz)	2½ carbohydrates, 1 fat
Submarine sandwich (regular)*	1 sub (6 inch)	3½ carbohydrates, 2 medium-fat meats, 1 fat
Submarine sandwich*(less than 6 gm fat)	1 sub (6 inch)	3 carbohydrates, 2 very lean meats
Taco, hard or soft shell*	1 (3-3½ oz)	1 carbohydrate, 1 medium-fat meat, 1 fat

[a]= 400 mg or more of sodium per exchange. Ask at your fast-food restaurant for nutrition information about your favorite fast foods or check Web sites.

Index